SURGERY FOR HYPEROPIA

SURGERY FOR HYPEROPIA

Edited by

Neal A. Sher, MD, FACS

Clinical Professor of Ophthalmology, University of Minnesota Medical School
Attending Surgeon, Phillips Eye Institute
Minneapolis, Minn

SLACK
INCORPORATED
An innovative information, education, and management company
6900 Grove Road • Thorofare, NJ 08086

Library of Congress Cataloging-in-Publication Data

Surgery for hyperopia / [edited by] Neal A. Sher.
p. ; cm.
Includes bibliographical references and index.
ISBN 1-55642-651-8 (hardback)
1. Hyperopia--Surgery. 2. Lasers in ophthalmology.
[DNLM: 1. Hyperopia--surgery. 2. Ophthalmologic Surgical Procedures--methods. WW 300 S9603 2003] I. Sher, Neal A.
RE936 .S87 2003
617.7'55--dc22

2003016550

Printed by Imprelibros S.A.
Printed in Colombia

Published by: SLACK Incorporated
6900 Grove Road
Thorofare, NJ 08086 USA
Telephone: 856-848-1000
Fax: 856-853-5991
www.slackbooks.com

Last digit is print number: 10 9 8 7 6 5 4 3 2 1

Dedication

To my loving wife and children.
Your encouragement, support, and love make everything worthwhile.

TABLE OF CONTENTS

Acknowledgments

I am indebted to the encouragement, support, and friendship of Francis L'Esperance, Jr, MD. His vision and genius has made the use of lasers in ophthalmology an everyday occurrence, to the benefit of millions of patients facing blindness worldwide. L'Esperance, building on the prior work of Meyer-Schwickerath, Maiman, and Zweng, developed systems for photocoagulation of ophthalmic vascular disease in 1965. In the 1980s, not limiting his perspective to the retina, L'Esperance saw the potential of Srinivasan and Trokel's pioneering work with ultraviolet lasers and applied for a patent covering the various aspects of corneal sculpting. This led to the formation of Taunton Technologies, which later became VISX. I had the opportunity to participate in the early excimer clinical trials with the Taunton team and had the privilege of working with Dr. L'Esperance.

I wish to thank my friends and partners in my practice, Eye Care Associates in Minneapolis, including Irving Shapiro, MD, the founder and guiding light of the Phillips Eye Institute and a mentor to me in practice. Other colleagues in my practice, including Robert Warshawsky, MD; Marian Rubenfeld, MD, PhD; Trond Stockenstrom, MD; Daniel Durant, MD; Shobana Murali, MD; Jane West, MD; Ed Glur, OD; David Warshawsky, OD; and Holly O'Claire, OD, have been generous in their support to allow me to undertake this book.

I am also grateful to Richard Lindstrom, MD, a gifted surgeon, honest researcher, and generous teacher, for encouraging me to see the potential of refractive surgery and for his continued help and advice. His partner, David Hardten, MD, has also been generous with his insight and advice.

I wish to especially thank Shula Luck, who served as an editorial assistant for this project and has devoted her considerable intellect, perseverance, and organizational skills. I am indebted to Charlene Counsellor at SLACK Incorporated for the great job she has done as the overall editor. Autumn Arvidsen, Nancy Read, and Britta Erickson of Eye Care Associates have also provided much help. I am grateful to Amy McShane and Lauren Biddle Plummer and their colleagues at SLACK Incorporated for their skill and hard work in putting this book together as well as for their confidence in me.

About the Editor

A native of Long Beach, New York, Neal A. Sher, MD, FACS, received his BS and MD degrees with honors from Boston University by the age of 22.

After his pediatric internship at the University of Minnesota Hospitals, he entered the U.S. Public Health Service in 1972 and became a staff associate at the National Institute of Health (NIH). He spent the next 3 years at the NIH in Bethesda, Maryland performing tumor immunology and immunotherapy research and authoring a number of papers in that field. At that time, he became interested in ocular immunology and completed an ophthalmology residency at the University of Minnesota, followed by corneal and external disease fellowship training at Moorfield's Eye Hospital in London. Returning to Minneapolis, he went into private practice.

Dr. Sher is an attending surgeon at the Phillips Eye Institute where he was a founding member in 1984 and has served as chief of ophthalmology. Active in teaching other doctors and students, Dr. Sher has been on the adjunct faculty of the University of Minnesota Medical School since 1979 and currently holds the rank of clinical professor of ophthalmology.

Since 1988, Dr. Sher has devoted considerable time to studying and working in the field of refractive surgery. He holds several patents on related medical devices. He has authored or co-authored more than 75 scientific papers and book chapters, is a frequent lecturer, and is a reviewer for a number of scientific journals. In 1994, Dr. Sher was the first American to be awarded the prestigious Troutman Award by the International Society for Refractive Surgery for his work on the control of pain using diclofenac after PRK. He is the author of a textbook entitled *Surgery for Hyperopia and Presbyopia*, published in 1997 by Williams and Wilkins; this was the first book devoted to this topic. Dr. Sher authored a monograph on postoperative care after laser corneal surgery (PRK) published by the American Academy of Ophthalmology and edited an *Atlas of Refractive Surgery* for the AAO.

Dr. Sher has been the principal investigator or co-investigator for a number of ophthalmologic clinical trials, as well as a consultant for a number of ophthalmic-related companies (including VISX, Inc). He has served as a member of the Preferred Practice Patterns Panel of the American Academy of Ophthalmology for Refractive Errors and Refractive Surgery. Additionally, he is on the editorial board of *EyeWorld* and *Clinical Signs in Ophthalmology*.

Dr. Sher makes his home in Minneapolis with his wife and two adult daughters. He is an avid movie fan and enjoys photography and gardening.

Contributing Authors

Dimitri T. Azar, MD
Corneal and Refractive Surgery Service,
Massachusetts Eye and Ear Infirmary
Harvard Medical School
Boston, Mass

Robin F. Beran, MD, FACS
Columbus Ophthalmology Associates
Columbus, Ohio

William I. Bond, MD
Bond Eye Associates
Peoria, Ill

Mark A. Bullimore, MCOptom, PhD
The Ohio State University College of Optometry
Columbus, Ohio

Fabrizio I. Camesasca, MD
Vice-Chairman, Department of Ophthalmology
Istituto Clinico Humanitas
Milan, Italy

J. Stuart Cumming, MD, FACS, FRCOphth
C&C Vision
Aliso Viejo, Calif

Jonathan Davidorf, MD
Davidorf Eye Group
West Hills, Calif

David Deitz, Research Assistant
McDonald Eye Associates
Fayetteville, Ariz

Daniel S. Durrie, MD
Durrie Vision P.A.
Hunkeler Eye Institute
Overland Park, Kan

Bradley Fundingsland, BA
VISX, Inc.
Santa Clara, Calif

Adrian Glasser, PhD
Assistant Professor
College of Optometry
University of Houston
Houston, Tex

David R. Hardten, MD, FACS
Minnesota Eye Consultants
Clinical Associate Professor of Ophthalmology
University of Minnesota Medical School
St. Paul, Minn

Neelu Hira, OD
Minnesota Eye Consultants
University of Minnesota
St. Paul, Minn

W. Bruce Jackson, MD, FRCSC
Director General
University of Ottawa Eye Institute
The Ottawa Hospital
Professor and Chairman
Department of Ophthalmology
University of Ottawa
Ottawa, Canada

Peter G. Kansas, MD
Clinical Professor of Ophthalmology
Albany Medical College
Albany, NY

Herbert E. Kaufman, MD
Boyd Professor of Ophthalmology and
Pharmacology
Louisiana State University Health Science Center:
Ophthalmology
New Orleans, La

Stephen C. Kaufman, MD, PhD
Director of Cornea and Refractive Surgery
Henry Ford Health System: Ophthalmology
Detroit, Grosse Pointe, and Troy, Mich

Danish Khan, MB, BS
Massachusetts Eye and Ear Infirmary
Boston, Mass

Shula Luck, BA
Eye Care Associates
Minneapolis, Minn

Shareef Mahdavi, BA
Honors Psychology, University of Michigan
SM[2] Consulting
VISX, Inc.,
Humphrey Instruments
Pleasanton, Calif

Parag A. Majmudar, MD
Midwest Eye Physicians
Palos Heights, Ill

Magdi Mansour, MD, MSc
Michel Pop Clinics
Montreal, Canada

J. E. "Jay" McDonald II, MD
McDonald Eye Associates
Fayetteville, Ariz

Allyson Mertins, OD
McDonald Eye Associates
Fayetteville, Ariz

Laura T. Muller, MD
Pasco Eye Institute
New Port Richey, Fla

Donald O. Mutti, OD, PhD
The Ohio State University College of Optometry
Columbus, Ohio

Yves Payette, MSc
Research Assistant
Michel Pop Clinics
Montreal, Canada

Mihai Pop, MD
Medical Director
Michel Pop Clinics
Montreal, Canada

Louis E. Probst, MD
TLC Laser Eye Centers
Ann Arbor, Mich

Gayla Rowland, MD
University of South Florida College of Medicine
Tampa, Fla

James Salz, MD
Cedars Sinai Medical Center
Los Angeles, Calif

Amy Scally, OD
Massachusetts Eye and Ear Infirmary
Boston, Mass

Daljit Singh, MS, DSc
Daljit Singh Eye Hospital
Amritsar, India

Charles B. Slonim, MD, FACS
University of South Florida College of Medicine
Tampa, Fla

Jason Stahl, MD
Stahl Vision Center
Olathe, Kan

William Trattler, MD
Miami Baptist Hospital
Miami, Fla

Paolo Vinciguerra, MD
Chairman, Department of Ophthalmology
Istituto Clinico Humanitas
Milan, Italy

R. Bruce Wallace III, MD, FACS
Wallace Eye Surgery
Alexandria, La

Jeffrey J. Walline, OD, PhD
The Ohio State University College of Optometry
Columbus, Ohio

Kevin L. Waltz, OD, MD
Eye Surgeons of Indiana
Indianapolis, Ind

Trevor Woodhams, MD
Woodhams Eye Clinic
Atlanta, Ga

INTRODUCTION

One hundred years have passed since Dutch physician Leendert Jan Lans demonstrated that the cornea can be reshaped by incisions or thermal means. Despite recent remarkable advances in refractive surgery, there is still no general agreement on the best surgical procedure for either myopia or hyperopia. It has been 6 years since I edited the first text devoted to the surgery of hyperopia and presbyopia. The controversies over surface ablation or LASIK, thermokeratoplasty, and use of inlays or implants still persist.

Until recently, the surgical correction of hyperopia has lagged behind the surgery of myopia in terms of investigative efforts. In past years, the number of papers published on hyperopia has always been a fraction of the number of papers published on myopia. This is a result of a combination of physiology, demographics, and economics. It is easier to permanently flatten the cornea for myopia than to steepen it centrally for hyperopia. The preoperative uncorrected vision plays a significant role in the motivation to undergo refractive surgery. A 30-year-old with myopia is more likely to seek corrective surgery than a 30-year-old 3-diopter hyperopic individual.

The demographics of the population, especially in industrialized economies will see many millions of "baby boomers" entering their late 40s and 50s. The incidence of hyperopia in this population has been estimated to be 20%, increasing to almost 50% a decade later. The incidence of presbyopia is almost universal. This group will be a prime consumer of refractive surgery and will provide an impetus to develop safe and effective refractive surgical procedures to reduce visual handicaps.

Although it is impossible to completely separate presbyopia from hyperopia, this book will be devoted primarily to hyperopia. Dr. Glasser's excellent chapter will give the reader a concise summary of the latest theories of the physiology accommodation and the relevant anatomy. In addition, there have been several excellent texts published in the last year devoted to presbyopia and its surgical correction. Accordingly, areas such as scleral expansion and modification will not be covered. I have also omitted a chapter on spectacle correction of hyperopia as this has been covered in many excellent texts.

Due to proprietary considerations by the two companies involved in developing intrastromal ablation, a chapter could not be included on this fascinating area.

It is an honor to be able to edit this textbook consisting of the contributions of my colleagues, many of whom I consider friends, who shared their insights, perspectives, experiences—both good and bad—in an effort to advance this rapidly changing field for the benefit of our patients. I am indebted to them for the enormous amount of hard work and that went into the preparation of each chapter. For this text, there was an unusually brief preparation time from inception to publication in order to be timely in this changing field.

Neal A. Sher, MD, FACS
Clinical Professor of Ophthalmology, University of Minnesota Medical School
Attending Surgeon, Phillips Eye Institute
Minneapolis, Minn

Foreword

It is an honor and a great privilege to write a foreword to this magnificent book, *Surgery for Hyperopia*, edited by Neal A. Sher, MD, FACS. Dr. Sher, along with several other distinguished individuals, has been enormously instrumental in the creation of new procedures, the evaluation of existing concepts, and the academic and instructional propagation of the finest clinical techniques for the correction of hyperopia. His reputation as one of the world's outstanding refractive surgeons and a leading pioneer in excimer laser correction of refractive errors of the eye uniquely positions him to discuss the surgical correction of hyperopia.

In the first chapters of this textbook, Dr. Sher has wisely chosen to present background information concerning the etiology, epidemiology, physiology, and historical perspectives related to hyperopia. Subsequent chapters discuss the evaluation of the prospective patient and the use of contact lenses for the correction of hyperopia.

Following this description of the basic corrective avenues for hyperopia, more sophisticated techniques and approaches—chapters including the evaluation of the prospective refractive surgical patient—are documented in the subsequent section with special emphasis on the hyperopic patient.

The next section deals with the relationship of PRK, LASIK, LASEK, and hyperopic astigmatic correction. The possible complications and their management, the required surgical techniques for each of these entities, the results of the various surgical interventions, and the evaluation and interpretation of the ablation profile and wavefront analysis are all integral parts of this outstanding treatise.

Subsequent chapters describe the proper method of enhancement after overcorrected myopic refractive surgery following radial keratoplasty, LASIK, and PRK, and various pharmacologically induced corneal shaping techniques.

The final chapters discuss more recent surgical techniques for the correction of hyperopia and presbyopia. The use of the Holmium-YAG laser, conductive keratoplasty, corneal inlays, refractive lensectomy, phakic intraocular lens implantation, presbyopic lens exchange (PRELEX), and the use of accommodating IOLs all represent the very latest and most advanced clinical research techniques and applications that are directed toward the ultimate correction of hyperopia. No research or clinically established technical or surgical application for the correction of hyperopia and presbyopia has been omitted from this textbook.

This textbook, for which Dr. Sher should be congratulated, displays an exceptionally well-defined and brilliant view of the entire subject of hyperopia correction of the eye by all currently available surgical approaches. This volume brings together the finest clinical research scientists and ophthalmic intellects, and they have described their various surgical approaches and techniques to correct these refractive conditions. Each chapter is comprehensive in nature, exhaustive in scope, and representative of the most current thinking. Furthermore, the book has magnificent illustrations throughout the chapters. Combined with the information regarding the most recent statistics and surgical trends, they eloquently position this textbook as the foremost treatise of its kind. This fine work—in its comprehensive and outstanding compilation of information regarding the various forms of surgical treatment of hyperopia—is unparalleled in the world literature.

Francis A. L'Esperance, Jr, MD, FACS
Professor of Clinical Ophthalmology
Columbia University College of Physicians and Surgeons
New York, NY

Section One

Background

Chapter One

Hyperopia: Etiology and Epidemiology

Mark A. Bullimore, MCOptom, PhD; Jeffrey J. Walline, OD, PhD; and Donald O. Mutti, OD, PhD

Introduction

Hyperopia and presbyopia are unavoidably linked and confused in the minds of the lay public because they elucidate identical symptoms, namely difficulty with near vision. While the ramifications of these two conditions are very similar, the prevalence and etiology are dramatically different. Hyperopia affects a relatively small proportion of the young adult population, although the prevalence increases later in life. Conversely, presbyopia can be viewed in the same way as death and taxes; inevitable. Indeed, the literature suggests that few factors affect the onset of presbyopia, although a warmer climate is associated with earlier onset.[1] Hyperopia is caused by a mismatch in the refractive and axial components of the eye. On the other hand, presbyopia is a result of a failure of the accommodative mechanism, although, as can be seen in Chapter 2, the precise etiology remains the subject of some debate. This chapter focuses on the etiology and epidemiology of hyperopia.

Hyperopia occurs when the refracting optics of the eye are too weak relative to the length of the eye, with images of distant objects being brought to focus behind the retina (Figure 1-1). This occurs either when the cornea and/or lens power are too weak in an eye of normal size, or when the cornea and lens power are normal but the eye is too short. Recent biometric data from the Orinda Longitudinal Study of Myopia indicates that hyperopic children typically have a shorter axial length and a flatter, less powerful cornea compared to emmetropes.[2] Previous literature suggests that lens power is not correlated with hyperopia, but recent work suggests correlations of ~0.2, with hyperopes having steeper, more powerful lenses than other subjects.[2] In addition, the rate of axial growth is significantly slower in hyperopic children compared to emmetropes. This slower rate of growth results in a stable refractive error. Children more hyperopic than +2.00 D tend not to undergo significant changes in refractive error between the ages of 6 and 14 years.[3,4]

While there is a wealth of literature and energetic debate about the etiology of myopia,[5] hyperopia has been relatively ignored.[6] This imbalance in the scientific literature is likely due to a number of factors. First, myopia is progressive, whereas hyperopia is relatively stable from early childhood through early adulthood. Second, severe myopia has a number of unpleasant sequelae, such as retinal detachment, from which the hyperopic eye is relatively immune. Third, uncorrected distance visual acuity is relatively unaffected by low hype•opia and thus may go undetected. Conversely, even low myopia can reduce uncorrected distance visual acuity. Finally, myopia is

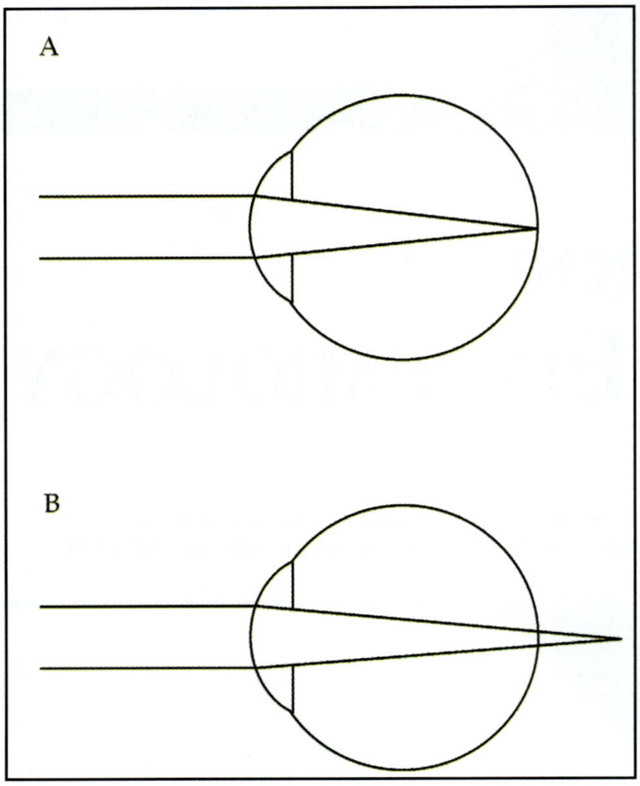

Figure 1-1. Schematic representations of A) the emmetropic eye and B) the hyperopic eye.

more prevalent, particularly among the more educated individuals[7-11] who might be inclined to study it and among higher income individuals[7,8,12] who are more likely to be able to afford the surgical correction of surgical refractive error.

Glasses, contact lenses, and refractive surgery are available to correct hyperopic refractive error. Glasses are typically the first treatment option provided to patients. Many hyperopic individuals may opt for refractive surgery or contact lenses because spectacle lenses may be heavy, they can magnify the eyes of the patient and the object being viewed, and they may distort the patient's peripheral vision. Contact lenses and refractive surgery can improve the cosmesis and comfort, as well as reduce the peripheral distortions and magnified image as viewed through glasses. Contact lenses for high hyperopia are thick, they allow less oxygen to reach the eye, and they may be more difficult to fit on the eye appropriately. Results of several studies with short-term follow-up have shown that refractive surgery for low to moderate hyperopia is safe and efficacious.[11,13,14] Thus far, refractive surgery in children has been limited to the correction of high anisometropia.[15-17]

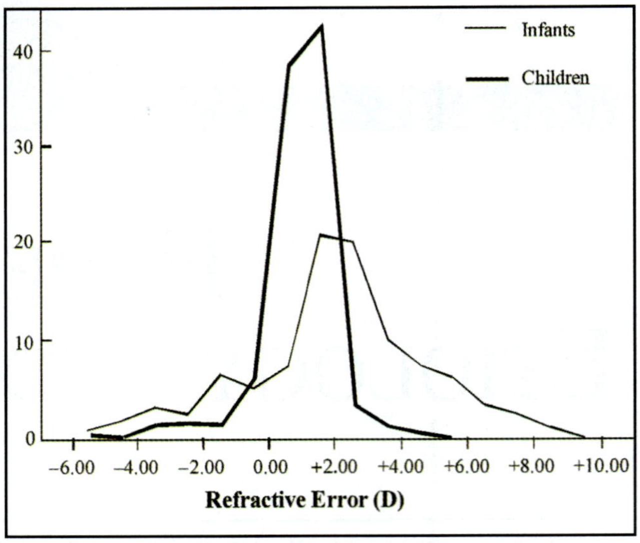

Figure 1-2. Distribution of refractive errors in newborn infants[56] and children.[2] Note that the distribution for children is narrower. Redrawn from Mutti and Zadnik.[2]

Hyperopia in Children

Most studies of infant refractive error conclude that newborns are moderately hyperopic and have a broad distribution of refractive errors. Between infancy and childhood the eye grows in such a way that the mean refractive error shifts toward emmetropia.[18-22] Concurrently, the distribution of refractive error narrows considerably (Figure 1-2). This process of emmetropization[23] results in a steady reduction in the prevalence of hyperopia and myopia in early childhood.

In contrast to myopia, which progresses steadily, hyperopia tends to persist throughout childhood. As mentioned above, most infants begin life with a moderate degree of hyperopia. Hyperopia could thus represent a failure of the emmetropization mechanism or an initial level of hyperopia so extreme that emmetropization could not overcome it. Recent longitudinal evidence suggests that the former is true. In a study of 93 infants with at least +4.00 D of hyperopia at age 9 months, the average change by age 3.5 years was a decrease in hyperopia, but only by –0.50 to –0.75 D.[24] In a study of 65 infants examined during the first 6 months of life and again between ages 9 and 16 years, 18 of 20 children with some degree of hyperopia in infancy were nonmyopic in childhood.[25]

It is then perhaps curious that Hirsch[26] found a prevalence of hyperopia around 25% in 13- to 14-year-olds. There are also some reports that hyperopia increases between the ages of 3 and 7 years[11,27-29] but it is very likely that these data arise from sam-

Table 1-1

The Prevalence of Hyperopia in Children

Author(s)	*N*	*Criterion*	*Method*	*Age (years)*	*Prevalence*
Kempf et al[27]		>+1.00 D	Cycloplegic retinoscopy	6 to 8	35.4%
				9 to 11	25.2%
				≥12	15.2%
Blum et al[30]	>1,000	≥+1.50 D	Non-cycloplegic retinoscopy	5 to 15	6%
Hirsch[26]	261	>+1.00 D	Non-cycloplegic retinoscopy	13 to 14	26.4%
Laatikainen and Erkkila[31]	162	≥+2.00 D	Cycloplegic retinoscopy	7 to 8	19.1%
	218			9 to 10	6.9%
	222			11 to 12	11.7%
	220			14 to 15	3.6%
Dandona et al[32]	804	>+0.50 D	Cycloplegic retinoscopy	6 to 9	65.8%
	1006		Cycloplegic retinoscopy	10 to 15	51.0%
Zadnik et al[4]	512	>+1.00 D	Cycloplegic auto-refraction	6 to 14	6.4%

pling artifacts. Table 1-1 shows a number of estimates of the prevalence of hyperopia in children.[4,26,27, 30-32] As might be expected, prevalence varies with the criterion level of hyperopia. The prevalence of hyperopia >+1.00 D from Kempf et al is considerably higher than the prevalence of 7.6% for hyperopia >+2.00 D in the sample as a whole from the same study.[27] This is similar to a recent prevalence of 6.5% for the same level of hyperopia (>+2.00 D) found in a sample of children 6 to 14 years of age.[4] Some of the published studies of hyperopia in children can, of course, be criticized because of the measurement technique used (eg, near retinoscopy), the lack of the use of cycloplegia, or both.

Slow ocular growth may be both the reason for the appearance of hyperopia as well as why it does not disappear with time. Recent longitudinal data from the Berkeley Infant Biometry Study show that increasing axial length is the major factor reducing infant hyperopia during emmetropization. The crystalline lens and the cornea decrease in power in tandem with axial growth, but not in a 1:1 relationship in terms of diopters of refractive error. Without axial growth, these losses of lenticular and corneal power would actually increase the hyperopic refractive error of infants. Axial growth typically exceeds these power losses, resulting in a net decrease in hyperopia. Failure to emmetropize in infancy is essentially a failure of sufficient axial growth. In spite of this and other recent studies, much is still to be learned about the developing eye, particularly with respect to hyperopia.

The Correction of Hyperopia in Children

While the majority of young hyperopic patients do not require spectacles, contact lenses, or refractive surgery in order to see clearly and comfortably, individuals with higher amounts of hyperopia may benefit from some type of refractive error correction. The refractive correction may help to alleviate visual complaints such as blur or double vision, or it may decrease the frequency or severity of asthenopic complaints such as headaches or eyestrain. Optical correction for hyperopia may be worn full time, or it may be worn only while the person is performing near work activities.

Due to the interactions of hyperopic refractive error, accommodation, and convergence, the level of hyperopia that requires correction and the method used to determine the refractive error correction to prescribe vary greatly.[33,34] One survey found that two-thirds of optometrists would prescribe hyperopic correction for a 2-year-old child without any other signs at +3.00 to +4.00 D of hyperopia, but two-thirds of ophthalmologists would not prescribe correction for the same child until the child had +5.00 to +6.00 D of hyperopia.[33] A separate survey of 334 American Association for Pediatric Ophthalmology & Strabismus members found that 50% would prescribe for a hyperopic child younger than 2 years "in routine clinical practice" at +4.00 D or less, but one-fourth would not prescribe until at least +5.50 D.[34] The amount of refractive error correction to prescribe for an individual with hyperopia is also controversial. One survey found that 16.3% of eye care practitioners would prescribe one-half the amount of hyperopia found under cycloplegia, 23.6% would prescribe two-thirds the cycloplegic amount, and 11.8% would prescribe three-fourths of the full cycloplegic amount.[33] Two-fifths of the practitioners prescribe for hyperopia in a manner other than deciding the proportion of cycloplegic hyperopia to correct optically.

The Effect of Correction of the Development of Amblyopia and Emmetropia

Controversy exists not only for when and how to prescribe for hyperopia—relatively little is also known about the effects of optical correction on the development of amblyopia, the onset of accommodative esotropia, the emmetropization process in young children, and/or academic performance. Outcomes regarding each of these areas may influence whether or not refractive error correction is prescribed for a hyperopic individual.

Accommodative esotropia is a convergent strabismus that can be partially or completely corrected with refractive error correction. Controversy exists as to whether or not prophylactic correction of hyperopia decreases the risk of accommodative esotropia onset.[35,36] A randomized clinical trial of 124 subjects with +3.50 D or more in one or more meridians showed that subjects without refractive error correction were 13 times more likely to be strabismic and 6 times more likely to have reduced visual acuity (presumably due to amblyopia) than subjects who received refractive error correction at 6 months of age.[36] A separate study of 285 children with +4.00 D or more hyperopia in any meridian did not find a significant difference between the groups with and without refractive error correction in the proportion of subjects who had strabismus or visual acuity worse than 20/40.[35] While the results of the two clinical trials are contradictory, they show that spectacle correction does not increase the incidence of esotropia or amblyopia. As long as optical correction for hyperopia does not affect normal development of the eye, it should be considered even before the onset of symptoms.

The role of spectacle correction in emmetropization has been postulated, especially since it was shown that the development of primate eyes may be partially regulated by visual feedback.[37,38] Two studies looked at the effect of spectacle correction on emmetropization of hyperopic children.[39,40] Atkinson et al recruited infants with between +3.50 and +6.00 D of hyperopia in at least one meridian.[40] Subjects were randomly assigned to receive partial hyperopic correction or no correction at 9 months of age. Cycloplegic retinoscopy was performed at approximately 9 months, 18 months, and 36 months. Although the hyperopic refractive error reduced significantly more in the untreated group than the treated group over the first 9 months, the overall reduction of hyperopia was not significantly different between the two groups after 3 years.[40] A separate study reported that spectacles interfered with the emmetropization process.[39] The refractive error of subjects with spectacles changed less than the refractive error of subjects without spectacles. The contradictory findings of the two studies illustrate the fact that there is much more to learn about the regulation of eye growth and the process of emmetropization.

There is also much to learn about the effects of optical correction for hyperopia on reading skills and academic standing. Several studies have found a higher prevalence of hyperopia among learning disabled children,[41] children in low and medium ability classes,[42] and poor reading groups.[43] Hyperopes also had lower mean scores on a written test of intelligence.[42] A meta-analysis also showed that hyperopia was associated with below average reading skills.[44] While the results of these studies illustrate a relationship between hyperopia and poorer reading skills or intelligence, no study has shown that optical correction reduces the deficit.

Little is known about the risks and benefits of optical correction for hyperopia because results of studies vary or because there are few well-designed studies that explore this topic. Refractive error correction should be the primary treatment for patients with symptoms, but the role of prophylactic correction for hyperopia should be further examined to better assess the risk versus benefit ratio for young children.

Hyperopia in Adulthood

Refractive error is relatively stable in adulthood. Slataper showed an increase in average myopia up

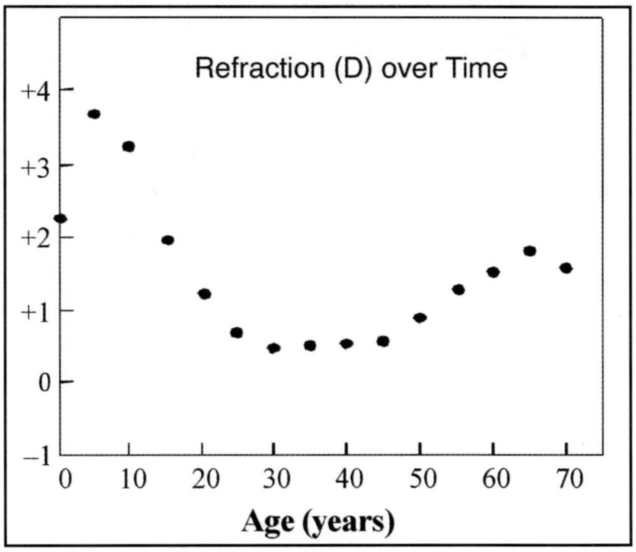

Figure 1-3. Average refractive error as a function of age (after Slataper[29]).

to age 20 years but little mean change between 20 and 50 years in a large clinical sample of over 30 thousand eyes examined by cycloplegic refractions (Figure 1-3).[29] This is consistent with the notion that eye growth and the progression of myopia are largely complete by adulthood. More recently, Midelfart et al[45] found that the prevalence of hyperopia of at least +0.50 D in 20- to 25-year-olds (13%) was similar to that in 40- to 45-year-olds (17.4%).

Although little change in refraction occurs in patients in their 30s and 40s, a marked increase in hyperopia occurs in patients 50 years and over. Wang et al. reported the prevalence of refractive errors in 4926 adults over 43 years of age (Table 1-2) in the Beaver Dam Eyes Study.[8] They found that hyperopia is much more common at age 65 to 74 years (67%) than it is at age 43 to 54 years (22%). This finding has been replicated by others authors in a range of studies of different racial groups.[7,9,11,12,46-51] The data are summarized in Table 1-2. Most studies show a three-fold increase in the prevalence of hyperopia, regardless of the criteria used. The increase may be less marked in some Asian populations but the data are remarkably consistent in white populations. As would be expected, the mean refractive error shifts in a hyperopic direction. In the cross-sectional Baltimore Eye Survey, Katz et al[9] found that the mean refractive error was –0.74 D in 40- to 49-year-old white patients compared to +0.86 D in 60- to 69-year-old white patients.

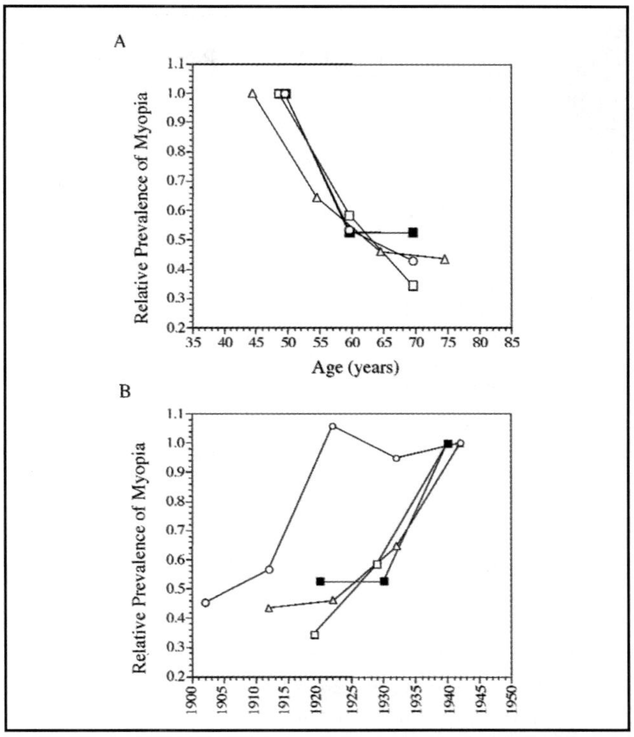

Figure 1-4. Prevalences of myopia scaled relative to a reference group and plotted as a function of age. (A) Data are plotted as a percentage of the prevalence for ages 44.5 to 49.5 years (set at 1.0). (B) Data are plotted as a percentage of the prevalence for those born from 1940 through 1942 (set at 1.0). Data from the Baltimore Eye Survey are plotted as the average for the four groups. (o): NHANES data from Table 1 in Mutti and Zadnik[52]; (□): Beaver Dam Eye Study[8]; (Δ): Baltimore EyeSurvey[9]; and (■): Framingham Offspring EyeStudy.[57] (Reprinted with permission from Mutti D, Zadnick K. Age-related decreases in the prevalence of myopia: longitudinal change or cohort effect? *Invest Ophthalmol Vis Sci*. 2000;41:1022-1030.)

The Age-Related Hyperopic Shift: Cohort Effect or a True Age-Related Change?

The decline in the prevalence of myopia and the increase in the prevalence of hyperopia with age that is demonstrated in cross-sectional studies may represent an increase in the prevalence of myopia in younger generations, possibly through increased exposure to near work, or an intrinsic age-related decline in myopia prevalence. Mutti and Zadnik[52] analyzed data from 4 published studies to determine which of these two alternatives better explains the data. They found that the pattern of change in the prevalence of myopia as a function of age was consistent across all studies when data were scaled relative to the prevalence of myopia at age-range midpoints from 44.5 to 49.5 years (Figure 1-4). The pattern of change was not consistent as a function of

Table 1-2

The Prevalence of Hyperopia in Older Adults

Note the dramatic increase in prevalence in the older age group.

Author(s)	*Race/Ethnicity*	*Criterion*	*40 to 49 year olds*		*60 to 69 year olds*	
			N	*Prevalence*	*N*	*Prevalence*
Wang et al[8]	Predominantly White	> +0.50 D	1468[a]	22.1%	1089[b]	67.2%
Katz et al[9]	Black	> +0.50 D	613	16.0%	568	51.4%
	White		531	15.6%	852	57.3%
Katz et al[9]	Black	> +2.00 D	613	4.9%	568	15.3%
	White		531	6.0%	852	27.8%
Attebo et al[10]	Predominantly white	> +0.50 D	465[c]	26.9%	1093[b]	68.0%
Dandona et al[11]	Indian	> +0.50 D	382	18.8%	145	29.7%
Wu et al[50]	Black	> +0.50 D	1235	28.8%	936	58.9%
Wong et al[7]	Chinese	> +0.50 D	275	12.1%	307	42.0%
Saw et al[12]	Indonesian	> +1.00 D	184	10.9%	174[d]	29.3%

a 43- to 54-year-olds
b 65- to 74-year-olds
c 49- to 54-year-olds
d 50 years and above

year of birth. They concluded that the decline in the prevalence of myopia, and presumably the increase in the prevalence of hyperopia, in older adults between the early 1970s and the late 1980s can be better explained by age than by year of birth. The prevalence of myopia appears to decrease because of an intrinsic age-related decrease in the amount of an individual's myopia rather than because of a cohort effect of increasing prevalence over time. Bengtsson and Grodum[46] reached similar conclusions to Mutti and Zadnik although they believed that there was a myopic shift of –0.25 D from one generation to the next. Longitudinal data from the Beaver Dam Eye Study suggests both a cohort effect of increasing prevalence over time and an age-related hyperopic shift.[49] By comparing people of the same age across examinations, those born in more recent years had more myopia and less hyperopia than those born in earlier years.

Etiology of Age-Related Hyperopic Shift

The underlying cause of this hyperopic shift is still unknown. It is well known that the crystalline lens both thickens and steepens during this time,[53] but this implies that eyes should become more myopic with age, leading to a phenomenon often referred to as "the lens paradox." Grosvenor has suggested that the length of the eye actually shrinks with age in order to prevent this myopia.[54] Recent studies propose that the gradient refractive index structure of the lens changes so that the net equivalent index of the lens decreases, and so does its equivalent power.[55] In summary, the lens radii of curvature may steepen, but this refractive index change causes a net shift toward hyperopia.

Risk Factors for Hyperopia

Little has been published on risk factors for hyperopia. A number of the studies of adults listed in Table 1-2 found significant associations. For example, hyperopia has been shown to be associated with less education[7-11] and lower incomes.[7,8,12] Hyperopia is also less prevalent in professionals and office workers than in production workers and laborers.[7]

Summary

Many infants are born with significant hyperopia, but due to the emmetropization process this dissipates in early childhood. The ophthalmic community does not correct low to moderate hyperopia in young children and the impact of correction on the emmetropization process is equivocal.

Hyperopia remains constant in older children and young adults. Above the age of 50, there is pronounced hyperopic shift. This shift has a number of ramifications for refractive surgery. First, in studies of emerging or existing procedures, it may be difficult to distinguish between true regression of the procedure and the physiological age-related hyperopic shift. Second, it is very likely that emmetropes, who prior to refractive surgery were myopes, will develop functionally significant hyperopia in their 50s and 60s and thus be prime candidates for the surgical correction of hyperopia. We are reminded of the Dr. Seuss book *The Sneetches* in which Sylvester McMonkey McBean develops a successful and lucrative practice sequentially adding and removing stars from the bellies of the Sneetches. The refractive surgery practice of the near future could resemble this scenario with 30- and 40-year-olds having their myopia treated and 50- and 60-year-olds having surgery for hyperopia.

References

1. Miranda MN. The environmental factor in the onset of presbyopia. In: Stark LW, Obrecht G, eds. *Presbyopia*. New York: Fairchild Publications; 1987:19-27.
2. Mutti DO, Zadnik K. Refractive error. In: Zadnik K, ed. *The Ocular Examination: Measurements and Findings*. Philadelphia: WB Saunders;1997.
3. Jones LA, Mitchell GL, Zadnik K, et al. Growth of ocular components as a function of refractive error groups. *Invest Ophthalmol Vis Sci*. 2002;43:abstract nr 2025.
4. Zadnik K, Mitchell GL, Jones LA, Mutti DO. Ocular component development as a function of refractive error. *Optom Vis Sci*. 2001;78(Suppl):237.
5. Mutti DO, Zadnik K, Adams AJ. Myopia. The nature versus nurture debate goes on. *Invest Ophthalmol Vis Sci*. May 1996;37(6):952-957.
6. Grosvenor T. The neglected hyperope. *Am J Optom Arch Am Acad Optom*. May 1971;48(5):376-382.
7. Wong TY, Foster PJ, Hee J, et al. Prevalence and risk factors for refractive errors in adult Chinese in Singapore. *Invest Ophthalmol Vis Sci*. Aug 2000;41(9):2486-2494.
8. Wang Q, Klein BE, Klein R, Moss SE. Refractive status in the Beaver Dam Eye Study. *Invest Ophthalmol Vis Sci*. 1994;35(13):4344-4347.
9. Katz J, Tielsch JM, Sommer A. Prevalence and risk factors for refractive errors in an adult inner city population. *Invest Ophthalmol Vis Sci*. 1997;38(2):334-340.
10. Attebo K, Ivers RQ, Mitchell P. Refractive errors in an older population: The Blue Mountains Eye Study. *Ophthalmology*. Jun 1999;106(6):1066-1072.
11. Dandona R, Dandona L, Naduvilath TJ, Srinivas M, McCarty CA, Rao GN. Refractive errors in an urban population in Southern India: the Andhra Pradesh Eye Disease Study. *Invest Ophthalmol Vis Sci*. Nov 1999;40(12):2810-2818.
12. Saw SM, Gazzard G, Koh D, et al. Prevalence rates of refractive errors in Sumatra, Indonesia. *Invest Ophthalmol Vis Sci*. Oct 2002;43(10):3174-3180.
13. Lian J, Ye W, Zhou D, Wang K. Laser in situ keratomileusis for correction of hyperopia and hyperopic astigmatism with the Technolas 117C. *J Refract Surg*. Jul-Aug 2002;18(4):435-438.
14. Salz JJ, Stevens CA. LASIK correction of spherical hyperopia, hyperopic astigmatism, and mixed astigmatism with the LADARVision excimer laser system. *Ophthalmology*. Sep 2002;109(9):1647-1656; discussion 1657-1648.
15. Nassaralla BR, Nassaralla JJ, Jr. Laser in situ keratomileusis in children 8 to 15 years old. *J Refract Surg*. Sep-Oct 2001;17(5):519-524.
16. Primack JD, Azar NF, Azar DT. Pediatric refractive surgery. *Int Ophthalmol Clin*. Fall 2001;41(4):19-34.
17. Nucci P, Drack AV. Refractive surgery for unilateral high myopia in children. *J AAPOS*. Dec 2001;5(6):348-351.
18. Mohindra I, Held R. Refraction in humans from birth to five years. *Doc Ophthalmol Proc Series*. 1981;28:19-27.
19. Wood IC, Hodi S, Morgan L. Longitudinal change of refractive error in infants during the first year of life. *Eye*. 1995;9 (Pt 5):551-557.
20. Saunders KJ, Woodhouse JM, Westall CA. Emmetropization in human infancy: Rate of change is related to initial refractive error. *Vision Res*. May 1995;35(9):1325-1328.
21. Ehrlich DL, Atkinson J, Braddick O, Bobier W, Durden K. Reduction of infant myopia: a longitudinal cycloplegic study. *Vision Res*. May 1995;35(9):1313-1324.
22. Mayer DL, Hansen RM, Moore BD, Kim S, Fulton AB. Cycloplegic refractions in healthy children aged 1 through 48 months. *Arch Ophthalmol*. Nov 2001;119(11):1625-1628.
23. van Alphen GWHM. On emmetropia and ametropia. *Ophthalmologica Suppl*. 1961;142:1-92.
24. Atkinson J. Infant vision screening: prediction and prevention of strabismus and amblyopia from refractive screening in the Cambridge Photorefraction Program. In: Simons K, National Research Council (US) Committee on Vision, eds. *Early visual development, normal and abnormal*. New York: Oxford University Press;1993.
25. Gwiazda J, Thorn F, Bauer J, Held R. Emmetropization and the progression of manifest refraction in children followed from infancy to puberty. *Clin Vis Sci*. 1993;8:337-344.
26. Hirsch MJ. Predictability of refraction at age 14 on the basis of testing at age 6-interim report from the Ojai Longitudinal Study of Refraction. *Am J Optom Arch Am Acad Optom*. Dec 1964;41:567-573.
27. Kempf GA, Collins SD, Jarman BL. *Refractive errors in the eyes of children as determined by retinoscopic examination with a cycloplegic*. Washington, DC: USPHS; 1928.

28. Brown EVL. Net average yearly changes in refraction of atropinized eyes from birth to beyond middle life. *Arch Ophthalmol.* 1938;13:719-734.

29. Slataper M. Age norms of refraction and vision. *Arch Ophthalmol.* 1950;43:466-481.

30. Blum HL, Peters HB, Bettman JW. *Vision screening for elementary schools; The Orinda study*. Berkeley: University of California Press; 1959.

31. Laatikainen L, Erkkila H. Refractive errors and other ocular findings in school children. *Acta Ophthalmol (Copenh).* 1980;58(1):129-136.

32. Dandona R, Dandona L, Srinivas M, Giridhar P, McCarty CA, Rao GN. Population-based assessment of refractive error in India: the Andhra Pradesh eye disease study. *Clin Experiment Ophthalmol.* Apr 2002;30(2):84-93.

33. Lyons SA, Carlson NB, Moore BD, et al. The Hyperopic Infants Study: a survey of clinical prescribing philosophies. *Optom Vis Sci.* 1999;76(Suppl):140.

34. Miller JM, Harvey EM. Spectacle prescribing recommendations of AAPOS members. *J Pediatr Ophthalmol Strabismus.* Jan-Feb 1998;35(1):51-52.

35. Ingram RM, Arnold PE, Dally S, Lucas J. Results of a randomised trial of treating abnormal hypermetropia from the age of 6 months. *Br J Ophthalmol.* Mar 1990;74(3):158-159.

36. Atkinson J, Braddick O, Robier B, et al. Two infant vision screening programmes: prediction and prevention of strabismus and amblyopia from photo- and videorefractive screening. *Eye.* 1996;10 (Pt 2):189-198.

37. Wildsoet CF. Active emmetropization—evidence for its existence and ramifications for clinical practice. *Ophthalmic Physiol Opt.* Jul 1997;17(4):279-290.

38. Hung LF, Crawford ML, Smith EL. Spectacle lenses alter eye growth and the refractive status of young monkeys. *Nat Med.* Aug 1995;1(8):761-765.

39. Ingram RM, Gill LE, Lambert TW. Effect of spectacles on changes of spherical hypermetropia in infants who did, and did not, have strabismus. *Br J Ophthalmol.* Mar 2000;84(3):324-326.

40. Atkinson J, Anker S, Bobier W, et al. Normal emmetropization in infants with spectacle correction for hyperopia. *Invest Ophthalmol Vis Sci.* Nov 2000;41(12):3726-3731.

41. Rosner J. Comparison of visual characteristics in children with and without learning difficulties. *Am J Optom Physiol Opt.* Jul 1987;64(7):531-533.

42. Grosvenor T. Refractive state, intelligence test scores, and academic ability. *Am J Optom Arch Am Acad Optom.* May 1970;47(5):355-361.

43. Grisham JD, Simons HD. Refractive error and the reading process: a literature analysis. *J Am Optom Assoc.* Jan 1986;57(1):44-55.

44. Simons HD, Gassler PA. Vision anomalies and reading skill: A meta-analysis of the literature. *Am J Optom Physiol Opt.* Nov 1988;65(11):893-904.

45. Midelfart A, Kinge B, Midelfart S, Lydersen S. Prevalence of refractive errors in young and middle-aged adults in Norway. *Acta Ophthalmol Scand.* Oct 2002;80(5):501-505.

46. Bengtsson B, Grodum K. Refractive changes in the elderly. *Acta Ophthalmol Scand.* Feb 1999;77(1):37-39.

47. Haegerstrom-Portnoy G, Schneck ME, Brabyn JA, Lott LA. Development of refractive errors into old age. *Optom Vis Sci.* Oct 2002;79(10):643-649.

48. Lee KE, Klein BE, Klein R. Changes in refractive error over a 5-year interval in the Beaver Dam Eye Study. *Invest Ophthalmol Vis Sci.* Jul 1999;40(8):1645-1649.

49. Lee KE, Klein BE, Klein R, Wong TY. Changes in refraction over 10 years in an adult population: the Beaver Dam Eye study. *Invest Ophthalmol Vis Sci.* Aug 2002;43(8):2566-2571.

50. Wu SY, Nemesure B, Leske MC. Refractive errors in a black adult population: The Barbados Eye Study. *Invest Ophthalmol Vis Sci.* Sep 1999;40(10):2179-2184.

51. Gudmundsdottir E, Jonasson F, Jonsson V, Stefansson E, Sasaki H, Sasaki K. "With the rule" astigmatism is not the rule in the elderly. Reykjavik Eye Study: a population based study of refraction and visual acuity in citizens of Reykjavik 50 years and older. Iceland-Japan co-working study groups. *Acta Ophthalmol Scand.* Dec 2000;78(6):642-646.

52. Mutti DO, Zadnik K. Age-related decreases in the prevalence of myopia: longitudinal change or cohort effect? *Invest Ophthalmol Vis Sci.* Jul 2000;41(8):2103-2107.

53. Brown N. The change in lens curvature with age. *Exp Eye Res.* Aug 1974;19(2):175-183.

54. Grosvenor T. Reduction in axial length with age: an emmetropizing mechanism for the adult eye? *Am J Optom Physiol Opt.* Sep 1987;64(9):657-663.

55. Hemenger RP, Garner LF, Ooi CS. Change with age of the refractive index gradient of the human ocular lens. *Invest Ophthalmol Vis Sci.* Mar 1995;36(3):703-707.

56. Cook RC, Glasscock RE. Refractive and ocular findings in the newborn. *Am J Ophthalmol.* 1951;34:1407-1413.

57. Familial aggregation and prevalence of myopia in the Framingham Offspring Eye Study. The Framingham Offspring Eye Study Group. *Arch Ophthalmol.* Mar 1996;114(3):326-332.

Chapter Two

Physiology of Accommodation and Presbyopia

Adrian Glasser, PhD

Lens, Ciliary Body, and Mechanisms of Accommodation

The Helmholtz Accommodative Mechanism

Accommodation is defined as a dioptric change in optical power of the eye.[1]

Accommodation occurs due to an increase in the optical power of the lens due to an increase in curvature of the anterior and posterior lens surfaces. The increase in surface curvatures occurs as a consequence of the lens undergoing a change from the relatively flattened unaccommodated form to a more spherical, accommodated form. In order for the lens surface curvatures to increase with accommodation, the lens axial thickness increases and lens cross-sectional diameter decreases. At rest, in the unaccommodated state, tension on the zonular fibers at the lens equatorial region holds the lens in the relatively flattened and unaccommodated form. With an accommodative effort, the ciliary muscle contracts and the apex of the ciliary body moves forward and toward the axis of the eye. Resting tension on the zonular fibers spanning the circumlental space between the ciliary processes and the lens equator is relaxed. The release in tension allows the elasticity of the lens capsule surrounding the lens to mold the lens substance into the more spherical accommodated state.

With accommodation, the vertex of the anterior lens surface moves forward and toward the cornea resulting in a decrease in anterior chamber depth. The vertex of the posterior lens surface moves backward toward the retina, resulting in an increase in anterior segment length (the sum of anterior chamber depth and lens thickness) and a decrease in vitreous chamber depth. The accommodative increase in optical power of the eye is due to the combined optical effects of the increase in lens surface curvatures and lens thickness, and the decrease in anterior chamber depth and vitreous chamber depth.

This is essentially the accommodative mechanism originally proposed by Helmholtz[2] (Figures 2-1A and B). Although Helmholtz described the most comprehensive mechanism of accommodation consistent with the established facts of the time, he did not fully appreciate or accurately describe all the accommodative changes that are now known to occur. Helmholtz[2,3] provided no explanation as to how it is that the lens assumes the more accommodative form when the zonular tension at the lens equator is released and he believed that the posterior lens surface was stationary during accommodation. Significant further knowledge of the accommodative mechanisms became available from studies following the work of Helmholtz. For example, due to the work of Fincham, it is now generally recognized that

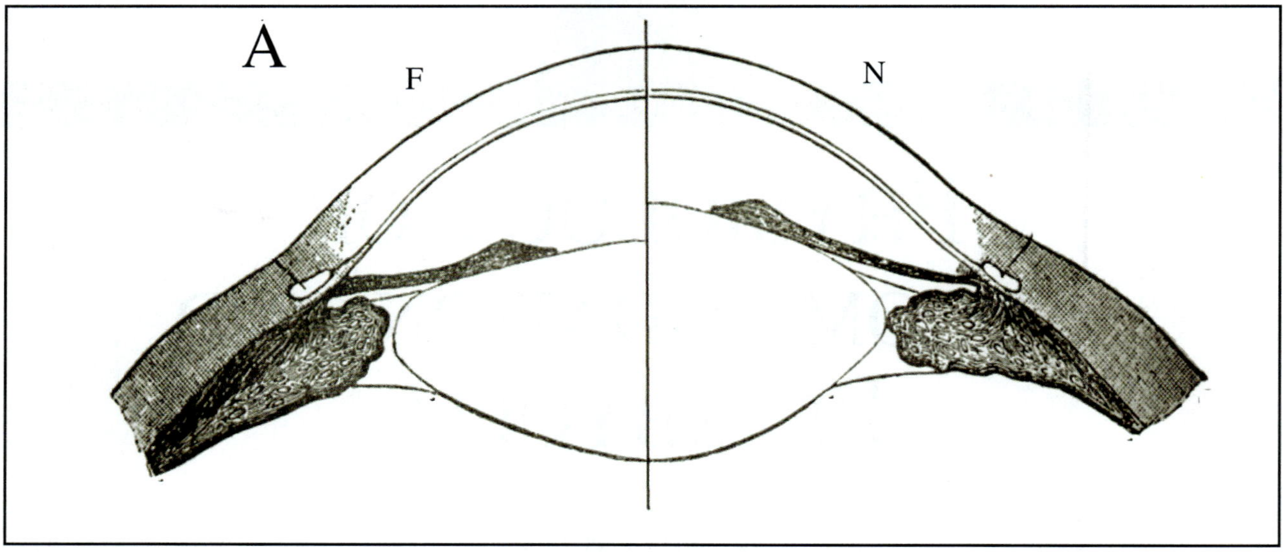

Figure 2-1A. The accommodative mechanism as depicted by Helmholtz. On the left the eye is focused for far (F) and on the right for near (N). In the unaccommodated state, tension on the zonular fibers at the lens equatorial region holds the lens in a relatively flattened form. With accommodation, the apex of the ciliary body moves forward and toward the axis of the eye to release the resting zonular tension, allowing the lens to undergo an increase in axial thickness and an increase in surface curvatures.[3] (Reproduced from the Helmholtz Treatise on Physiological Optics, 1909.)

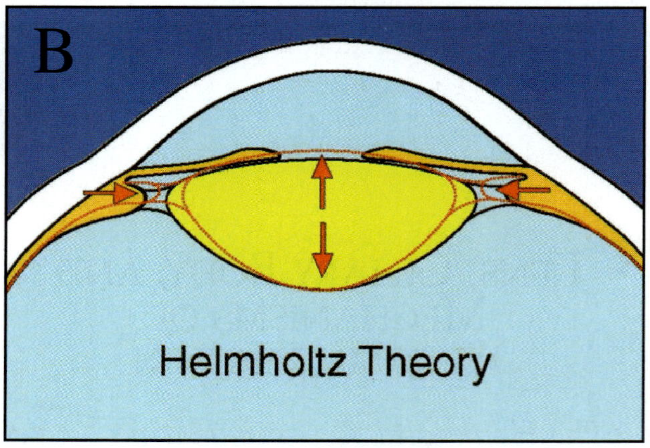

Figure 2-1B. A depiction of the Helmholtz accommodative mechanism shows the accommodative movements of the ciliary muscle and the lens. The accommodated lens (red dashed lines) show that with accommodation, lens diameter decreases, lens thickness increases, and the lens surface curvatures increase. This diagram depicts no movement of the posterior lens surface, as Helmholtz believed occurred, but it is now widely recognized that the posterior lens surface moves toward the retina with accommodation (down in this diagram).

the lens capsule plays an important role in accommodating the lens.[4] In addition, anatomical studies with scanning electron microscopy have provided significant additional information on the arrangements of the zonular fibers and how they contribute to the accommodative mechanism.[5,6] A-scan ultrasound[7] and partial coherence interferometry[8] have documented forward movement of the anterior lens surface and backward movement of the posterior lens surface with accommodation.

Schachar's Mechanism of Accommodation

Schachar[9-11] has proposed that accommodation occurs in a manner quite different from that originally proposed by Helmholtz. This is essentially the mechanism originally proposed by Tscherning.[12] Schachar's explanation of how this theory of accommodation works requires significant modification in terms of what is known about the anatomy of the accommodative structures. Schachar describes that the zonular fibers at the lens equator are composed of 3 distinct subgroups comprising the anterior, equatorial and posterior zonular fibers.[10] Schachar believes that these 3 groups insert into discreet locations into the ciliary body with the anterior and posterior zonular fibers coursing through the valleys between the ciliary processes to insert more posteriorly in the ciliary body and the equatorial zonular fibers inserting to the anterior face of the ciliary muscle beneath the iris.[10] In fact no such anatomical arrangement of zonular fibers exists. Scanning electron microscope (SEM) images of the zonular fibers at the lens equator may give the appearance of three distinct subgroups (Figure 2-2A).[13] However, the harsh chemical processing required to prepare the tissues for histology or SEM results in cohesion of the individual fibers resulting in "clumping" of

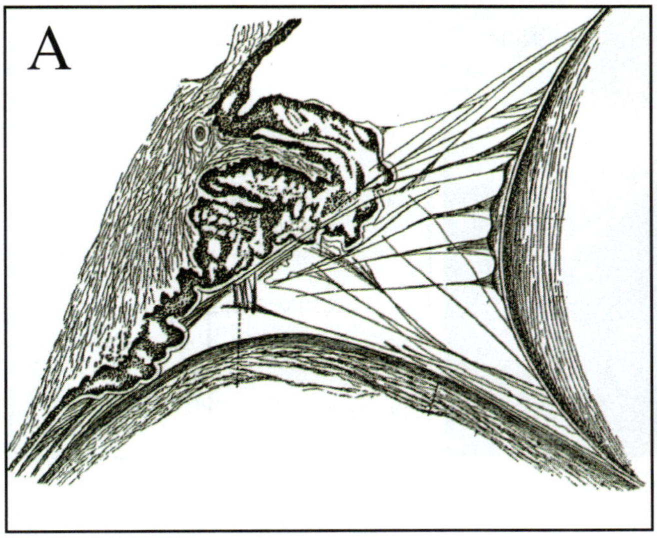

Figure 2-2A. Diagram of a histological section of the accommodative apparatus. The diagram shows the ciliary muscle within the ciliary body, the zonular fibers spanning from the ciliary processes to the equatorial region of the lens to insert in the lens capsule surrounding the lens. The zonular fibers originate all along the pars plicata region of the ciliary body and there is extensive crossing of the zonular fiber bundles. The diagrammatic representation shows some adhesion and clumping of zonular fibers characteristic of tissues chemically processed for histology.[3] (Reproduced from Helmholtz Treatise on Physiological Optics, 1909.)

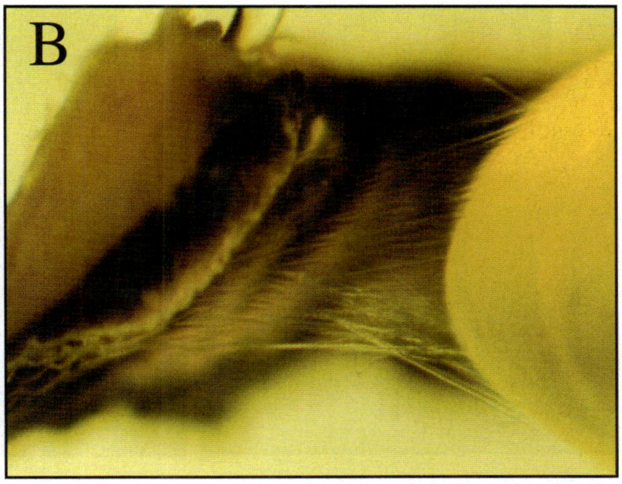

Figure 2-2B. Photograph of a partially dissected, unfixed human eye (age 43 years). The ciliary body is cut through to show (from left to right) the ciliary muscle, the pars plicata region of the ciliary processes, and the zonular fibers extending from the ciliary body to the lens equatorial region.[14] (Reproduced from *Vision Research,* 38[2], Glasser A, Campbell MCW, Presbyopia and the optical changes in the human crystalline lens with age, 209-229, Copyright 1998, with permission from Elsevier.)

fibers and the artifactual appearance of distinct subgroups.[14] When the zonular fibers at the lens equator are observed in fresh anatomical preparations, there is a continuum of zonular insertion all around the lens equator and no discreet anterior, posterior, or equatorial insertions (Figure 2-2B).[14] The fresh, unfixed specimens show that zonular fibers spanning the circumlental space originate along the base of the pars plicata region of the ciliary body and distinct crossing of zonular fibers can also be observed. There are no zonular fibers that insert into the anterior face of the ciliary muscle as required by Schachar.[10]

Schachar suggests that with an accommodative effort, the anterior face of the ciliary muscle moves posteriorly toward the sclera to selectively increase the tension on what he describes as the equatorial zonular fibers, and that the anterior and posterior zonular tension is released during accommodation.[11] The anatomical basis for this description of how the ciliary muscle selectively increases equatorial zonular tension while releasing the anterior and posterior zonular tension comes from Schachar's analysis of the shape of two previously published rhesus monkey ciliary muscle histological sections, one atropinized and the other treated with pilocarpine. No physiological evidence exists to support this theory of ciliary muscle contraction. In fact, extensive evidence shows that the entire bulk of the ciliary body moves forward and toward the axis of the eye with accommodation (Figures 2-3A through C).[15-19]

Schachar believes that equatorial zonular tension is increased and anterior and posterior zonular tension is released during accommodation, to move the lens equator toward the sclera resulting in an accommodative increase in lens equatorial diameter.[20] Schachar believes this results in a flattening of the peripheral lens surfaces and an increase in the central lens surface curvatures. Experiments aimed at exploring the accommodative mechanism in iridectomized monkey eyes found no evidence for the accommodative mechanism described by Schachar. Accommodation was induced by electrical stimulation of the Edinger-Westphal nucleus of the brain as well as using topical pharmacological stimulation of accommodation.[18] Extensive testing showed that the lens equator moves away from the sclera and lens cross-sectional diameter decreases with accommodation (Figures 2-3D through F). The entire lens diameter can be observed when a Goldmann lens is placed on the cornea. There is a concentric decrease in lens diameter with accommodation (Figure 2-4). The lens is seen to sag down under the influence of gravity with accommodation, irrespective of the ori-

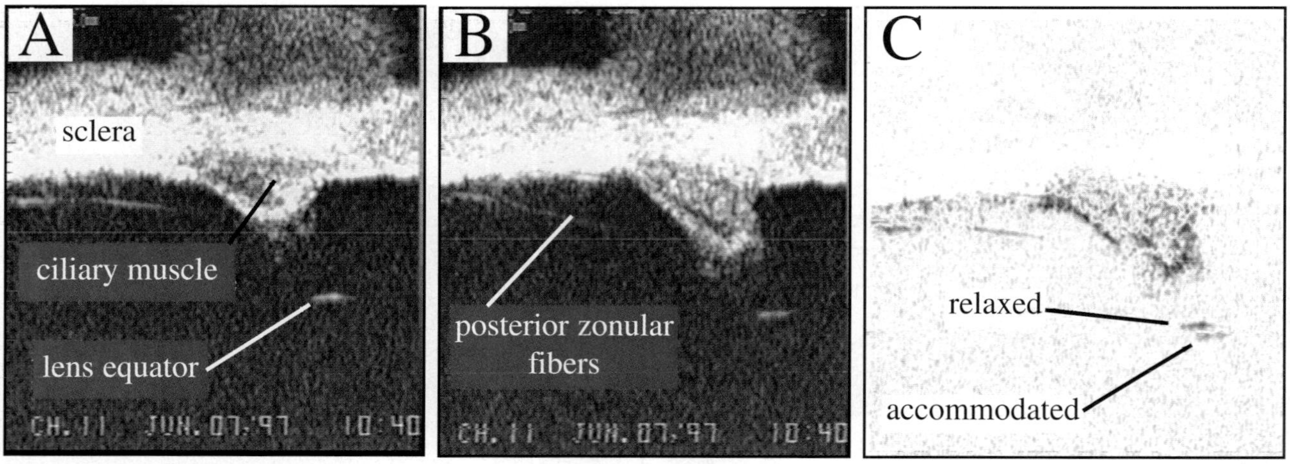

Figures 2-3A, B, & C. Ultrasound biomicroscopy of the temporal ciliary region of a young, iridectomized cynomolgus monkey eye accommodating 10 D. For orientation, the cornea extends off to the right of the image. A) The sclera, the ciliary region and the lens equator (visible as a short bright horizontal line at lower right) as viewer in the unaccommodated eye. B) With accommodation, the apex of the ciliary body moves forward and toward the axis of the eye. The lens equator moves away from the sclera of the eye. The posterior zonular fiber bundle that extends from the anterior aspect of the ciliary processes to the posterior attachment of the ciliary muscle is stretched during accommodation. C) The subtracted image pair shows the accommodative movements as darkened parts of the image. There is about 250 µm of movement of the lens equator away from the sclera with 10 D of accommodation.

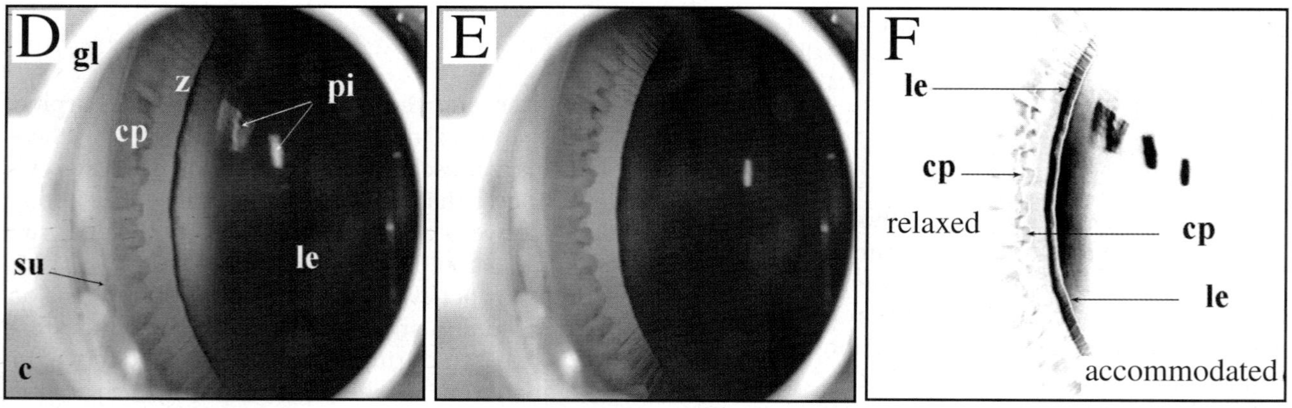

Figures 2-3D, E, & F. Swan-Jakob gonioscopy of the ciliary body and lens equator of an iridectomized rhesus monkey eye. D) The eye is in the unaccommodated state. The ciliary processes, circumlental space with zonular fibers evident and the lens equator can clearly be observed. E) With accommodation, the ciliary processes and lens equator move away from the sclera in accordance with the Helmholtz accommodative mechanism. F) The subtracted image pair shows that accommodative movements of the lens and ciliary processes are both in the same direction and away from the sclera in accordance with the Helmholtz accommodative mechanism. Although eye movements cannot be completely eliminated (as with any living system), the extent of the eye movements that occur are negligible and cannot account for the accommodative movements observed. (gl: gonioscopy lens; cp: ciliary processes; z: zonular fibers; pi: Purkinje images reflected off the lens; su: 9-0 nylon suture tied at the limbus of the eye to provide a landmark against which to monitor the extent of eye movements that occur with accommodation; le: lens equator; c: conjunctiva).[18] (Reproduced from *Ophthalmology,* 106[5], Glasser A, Kaufman PL. The mechanism of accommodation in primates, 863-872, Copyright 1999, with permission from Elsevier.)

entation of the head, thus demonstrating that zonular tension is reduced with accommodation. Pharmacological stimulation of accommodation produces results that are qualitatively and quantitatively similar. While electrical stimulation causes systematic convergence eye movements, the eye movements that occur with pharmacological stimulation are random and nonsystematic. The accommodative movements of the ciliary body, ciliary processes, and lens equator cannot be explained by eye movements, but rather reflect the actual accommodative changes that are occurring. Experiments on living human eyes also show a decrease in lens cross-sectional diameter with accommodation. Infrared retroillumination of the eye of a young subject with ocular albinism allowed the entire lens equatorial circum-

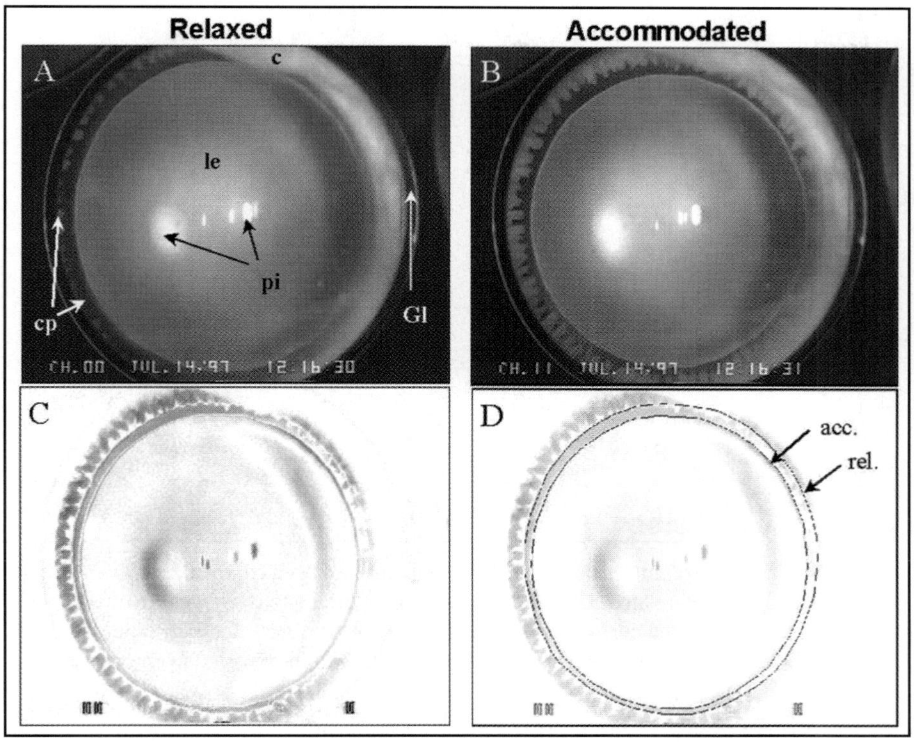

Figure 2-4. Goldmann lens imaging of an iridectomized rhesus monkey eye accommodating about 10 D. A) The eye is in the unaccommodated state. Because the corneal power is effectively neutralized by the Goldmann lens, the entire lens diameter can be observed. (cp: ciliary processes; le: lens; pi: Purkinje images; c: conjunctiva; Gl: Goldmann gonioscopy lens). B) The eye in the accommodated state. C) The subtracted image pair. D) The subtracted image pairs with the graphic overlay superimposed to show the concentric accommodative decrease in the diameter of the lens.[18] (Reproduced from *Ophthalmology,* 106[5], Glasser A, Kaufman PL. The mechanism of accommodation in primates, 863-872, Copyright 1999, with permission from Elsevier.)

ference to be observed.[21] In accordance with the monkey results, an accommodative effort resulted in a concentric decrease in cross sectional lens diameter and a movement of the lens equator away from the sclera. These experiments provide no support for the Schachar theory and overwhelming support for the accommodative mechanism originally described by Helmholtz.

Presbyopia

Presbyopia is the gradual age related loss of accommodative ability. In humans, the progressive loss of accommodation begins early in life and culminates in a complete loss of accommodative ability of the lens by about age 55 years. Classically presbyopia is attributed to sclerosis or "hardening" of the crystalline lens. There is substantial evidence for multiple age-related changes in human and monkey eyes, all of which potentially contribute to the progressive age related loss of accommodation. The age changes in the eye can broadly be grouped in two categories; those that affect the accommodative apparatus other than the lens (extralenticular factors) and those that affect the lens (lenticular factors).

Extralenticular Factors

The human and monkey ciliary muscle undergoes age-related anatomical changes as observed with electron microscopy.[15,22-24] These changes include increasing amounts of connective tissue in the aging rhesus monkey ciliary muscle.[23] In addition, anatomical studies show that there is a reduced accommodative configurational change of the aging rhesus monkey ciliary muscle to pilocarpine stimulation.[15] This is not due to a reduced force of contraction of the rhesus monkey ciliary muscle[25] or due to a loss of cholinergic receptors within the ciliary muscle,[26] but is due to a loss of elasticity of the posterior attachment of the ciliary muscle.[16] Anatomical evidence for this exists[24] and histological studies show that when this posterior attachment is severed, the aging ciliary muscle is able to undergo accommodative configurational changes in response to pilocarpine stimulation.[16]

The atropinized unaccommodated human ciliary muscle undergoes an age-related change in configuration as observed in histological sections of human eye-bank eyes. The old unaccommodated human ciliary muscle looks more like a young, accommodated ciliary muscle, with the internal apex of the ciliary body adopting a more centripetally oriented configuration with increasing age (Figure 2-5).[17] This might suggest that unaccommodated zonular tension is reduced with increasing age as the ciliary muscle adopts a more inwardly oriented configuration, but this does not occur.

Although the accommodative movements of the rhesus monkey ciliary muscle are reduced with increasing age and the human ciliary muscle undergoes age-related configurational changes, the human ciliary muscle/body is still capable of undergoing

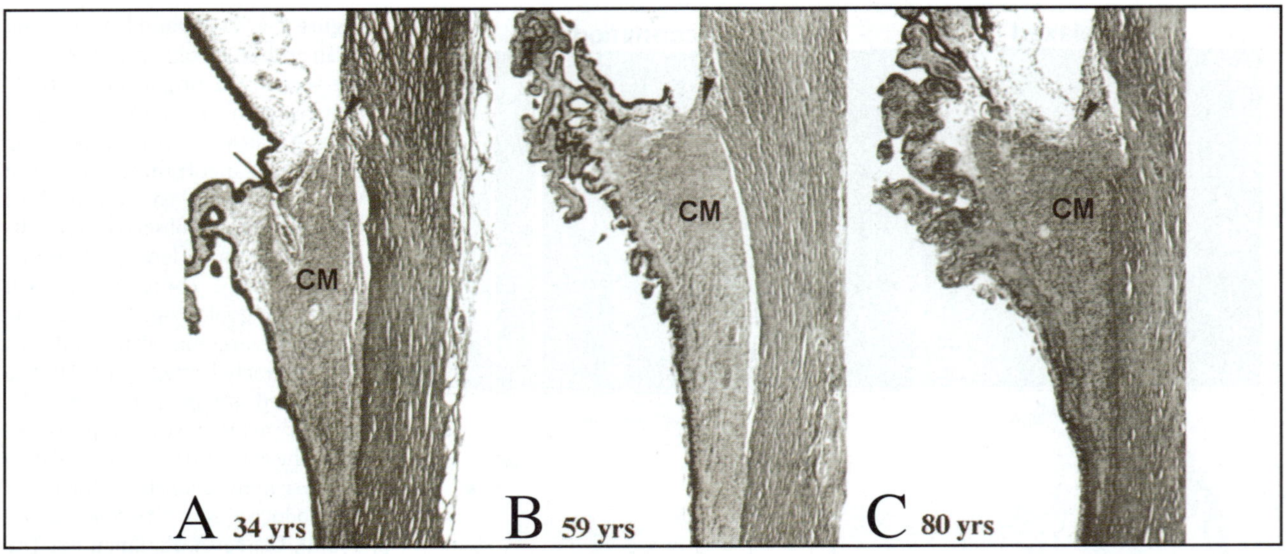

Figure 2-5. Histological sections of the ciliary muscle from atropinized donor eyes. The unaccommodated ciliary muscle from a A) 34-year-old, B) 59-year-old, and C) 80-year-old donor show an age-related configurational change. With increasing age, the unaccommodated ciliary muscle looks like it takes on a more accommodated configuration.[17] (Reproduced from *Mech Age Dev,* 62[2], Tamm S, Tamm E, Rohen JW. Age-related changes of the human ciliary muscle, 209-221, Copyright 1992, with permission from Elsevier.)

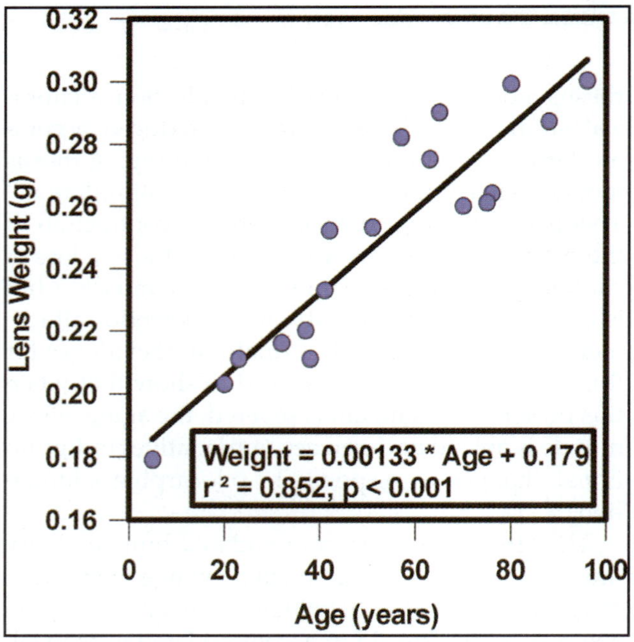

Figure 2-6. The human crystalline lens undergoes an linear age-related increase in mass, from 5 to 96 years of age. The graph show the wet weight of fresh, unfixed lenses extracted from donor eyes.[30] (Reproduced from *Vision Research,* 39[11], Glasser A, Campbell MCW. Biometric, optical, and physical changes in the isolated human crystalline lens with age in relation to presbyopia, 1991-2015, Copyright 1999, with permission from Elsevier.)

changes in configuration with an accommodative effort in the eyes of presbyopes. Magnetic resonance imaging (MRI) of the eyes of human subjects 22 to 83 years of age showed that there is still an accommodative movement of the ciliary body in the eyes of presbyopes, even when there is no discernable accommodative change in the lens.[27] Similarly, ultrasound biomicroscopy shows accommodative movements of the ciliary muscle/body in the eyes of presbyopes.[19]

Lenticular Factors

Numerous studies have documented age-related changes in the lens. For example, SEM studies show that there is an anterior shift of the zonular fibers on the anterior lens surface with increasing age.[28] This study also shows that the distance from the zonular insertion on the anterior lens surface to the ciliary body is unchanged with age. Thus there is no indication that the unaccommodated resting zonular tension is reduced with the inward shift of the ciliary muscle. The crystalline lens continues to grow through out life adding more lens fiber cells, but never losing cells.[29] This results in a lens of increasing size and mass (Figure 2-6).[29,30] The unaccommodated lens undergoes an increase in axial thickness as can readily be measured in the unaccommodated eye with A-scan ultrasonography.[31-33] The lens also undergoes an increase in anterior and posterior surface curvatures as determined from Scheimpflug imaging.[33-35] Thus, based on the external profile, older lenses tend to look more like accommodated young lenses. However, it is well established that accommodative changes in the lens are due to a change in thickness of the nucleus while the cortical thickness is unchanged with accommodation.[36,37] As age increases, there is a constancy of the unaccommodated lens nuclear thickness and so it is clear that the aging lens is not simply becoming more accommodated with increasing age.[38]

Schachar's Theory of Presbyopia

Schachar believes that presbyopia occurs due to continued growth of the crystalline lens and a resulting increase in lens equatorial diameter.[39] Schachar cites a book chapter by Rafferty,[40] rather than an original study, as the sole source for his evidence of a growth related increase in lens diameter.[9,20,39,41,42,43] In this chapter, Rafferty refers to data from an original study by Smith[44] who measured the diameters of 91 human lenses extracted from human donor eyes aged 20 to 90. Rafferty states that Smith's data show an age-related increase in diameter of the extracted lenses. The data do indeed show this trend. However, Smith[44] was aware that the increase in diameter of the isolated lenses does not reflect an age-related growth of the lens, but rather an increase in diameter of lenses that occurs because the lenses are extracted. Smith recognized that when the zonular fibers at the lens equator are cut and the lens is extracted from the eye, young lenses tend to take on an accommodated form whereas the older, more presbyopic and harder lenses undergo no change in shape with extraction. Smith recognized that his measurements are of young lenses in an accommodated form and older lenses in an unaccommodated form. Helmholtz,[3] Fincham,[4] and other subsequent investigations of human lenses[14,30] also recognized this drawback of attempting to make such inferences from extracted lenses. There is in fact no evidence to support the notion that the lens diameter grows with increasing age. Only one study exists that has measured lens diameter as a function of age in vivo in living human eyes. MRI measurements in the unaccommodated eyes of subjects aged 22 to 83 found no age-related increase in lens diameter.[27] The study also measured lens diameter as a function of age as the subjects accommodated to an 8 D stimulus. The accommodated lens diameters as a function of age reported from the in vivo MRI measurements agree well with Smith's lens diameter data from extracted lenses, thus confirming that the extracted lens measurements reflect the diameter of the lens in the maximally accommodated state.

Age Changes in the Lens and Capsule

The lens assumes an accommodated form due to the molding forces of the elastic capsule on the lens substance. Presbyopia is classically attributed to "sclerosis" or hardening of the lens. However, age-related changes in the elasticity of either the lens or the capsule could contribute to presbyopia. Anterior capsular thickness increases up to about age 70 and then decreases thereafter and undergoes a decrease in Young's modulus of elasticity.[45,46] In general, the anterior capsule gets thicker, is less extensible and more brittle with increasing age.[46] The mechanical strength of the posterior lens capsule decreases with age.[47]

The human lens undergoes an age-dependent increase in resistance to changes in shape due to high-speed rotational forces and a more than three-fold increase in Young's modulus of elasticity.[48] Fisher calculated that the decrease in elastic modulus of the capsule and the increase in the elastic modulus of the lens can fully account for the loss of accommodation by age 60.[49] Mechanical stretching experiments show that the human lens loses the ability to undergo accommodative optical changes with increasing age (Figure 2-7). These experiments rely on the fact that when zonular tension is released in the young lens, the capsule molds the lens into a maximally accommodated form. Mechanical stretching of the lens of partially dissected human eyes through the intact ciliary body and zonule results in a decrease in optical power as the lens is stretched into an unaccommodated form.[14,50] However, lenses over the age of about 55 years show no change in optical power with the same extent of stretching.[14] These results suggest that loss of accommodative capacity of the lens is an important factor in the progression of presbyopia.

The young lens, when extracted from the eye, is maximally accommodated due to the capsule molding the lens into the accommodative form.[3,4,30,44] If the capsule is removed from a young 5-year-old human or a young monkey lens, the decapsulated lens substance assumes a relatively unaccommodated form (Figure 2-8).[4,30] This provides evidence that the capsule is responsible for molding the lens into an accommodated state and that the inherent shape of the decapsulated lens substance is more unaccommodated. However, when the capsule is removed from a 23-year-old human lens, the change in lens shape on removing the capsule is less than that of the 5-year-old lens. When the capsule is removed from an 84-year-old human lens, there is no change in shape of the decapsulated lens. The changes in shape of the young lens and the absence of a change in the old lens are matched by a change or an absence of a change in focal length of the lens with decapsulation. The focal length of young lenses increase after removal of the capsule but there is no systematic change in focal length of lenses over 55 years of age after removal of the capsule.[30]

Human lenses show an exponential increase in hardness with an over four-fold increase in resistance to mechanical compression over the human life span (Figure 2-9).[30] This increase in hardness begins early in life and extends well beyond that age at which accommodation is lost in presbyopes.

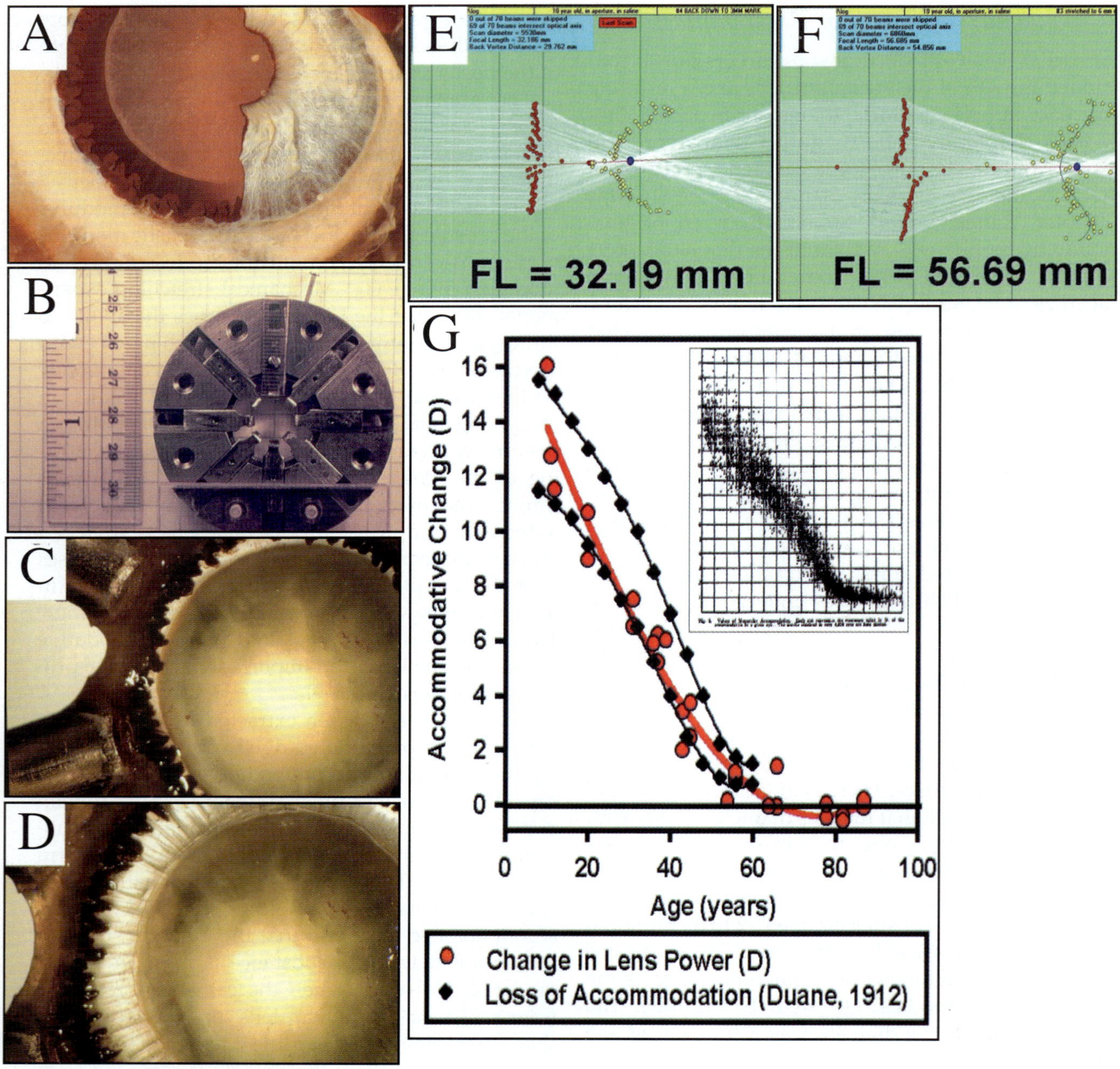

Figure 2-7. Mechanical stretching experiments to measure the age related loss of accommodative ability of the human crystalline lens from donor eyes. A) The eyes were partially dissected to remove the anterior sclera and the iris. The anterior segment of partially dissected, unfixed eyes, comprised of the ciliary body and the lens, still naturally suspended by the intact zonular fibers, was separated from the globe. B) The anterior segment tissue was glued to eight arms of a mechanical stretching apparatus. Tension on the zonular fibers, and hence the lens, could be mechanically released (C) to allow the lens to accommodate or mechanically stretched (D) to unaccommodated the lens. This experiment relies on the capsule providing the accommodative molding force to the lens. Lens focal length was measured with a scanning-laser ray-tracing technique as a function of the stretch applied to the tissues. E) The unstretched (accommodated) focal length of a 10-year-old human lens is 32.19 mm and this increases (F) to 56.69 mm in the maximally stretched (unaccommodated) state. G) The change in optical power in 27 human lenses ranging in age from 10 to 86 years (red symbols) shows that the human lens gradually and completely loses the ability to undergo accommodative changes in optical power. This data is plotted together with the maximum and minimum accommodative amplitudes of 1500 human subjects (black symbols) as measured by Duane[58] using a subjective push-up test. Duane's graph of accommodative amplitude (y-axis) as a function of age (x-axis) is shown inset.[14] (Reproduced from *Vision Research,* 38[2], Glasser A, Campbell MCW. Presbyopia and the optical changes in the human crystalline lens with age, 209-229, Copyright 1998, with permission from Elsevier.)

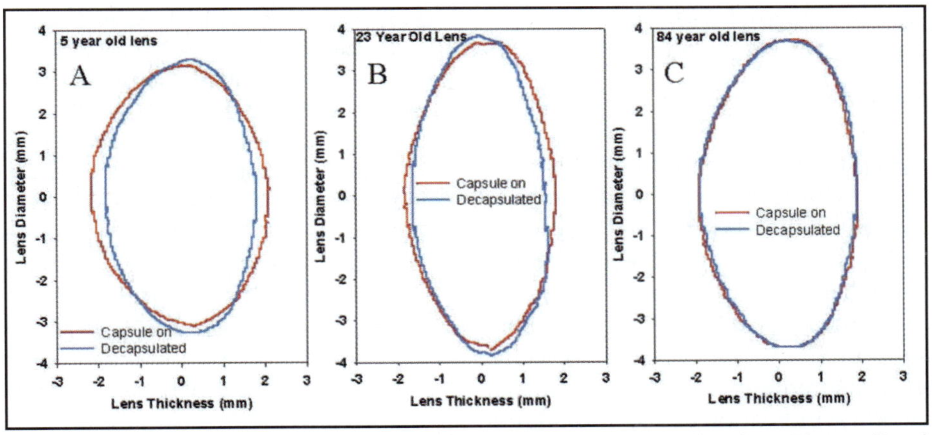

Figure 2-8. The effect of the lens capsule on the aging human crystalline lens. The profile of crystalline lenses extracted from A) 5-year-old, B) 23-year-old and C) 84-year-old donor eyes by cutting the zonular fibers with the capsule still intact (red outlines). The capsules were then removed from each lens and the profile of the decapsulated lens (blue profiles) was traced. There is considerable change in form of the 5-year-old lens from an accommodated form to an unaccommodated form with removal of the capsule (A). This change in form of the lens substance is reduced in the 23-year-old lens (B) and completely absent in the 84-year-old lens (C).[59] (Reproduced from *International Ophthalmology Clinics,* Glasser A, Croft MA, Kaufman PL. Aging of the human crystalline lens and presbyopia, 1-15, Copyright 2001, with permission from Lippincott Williams & Wilkins.)

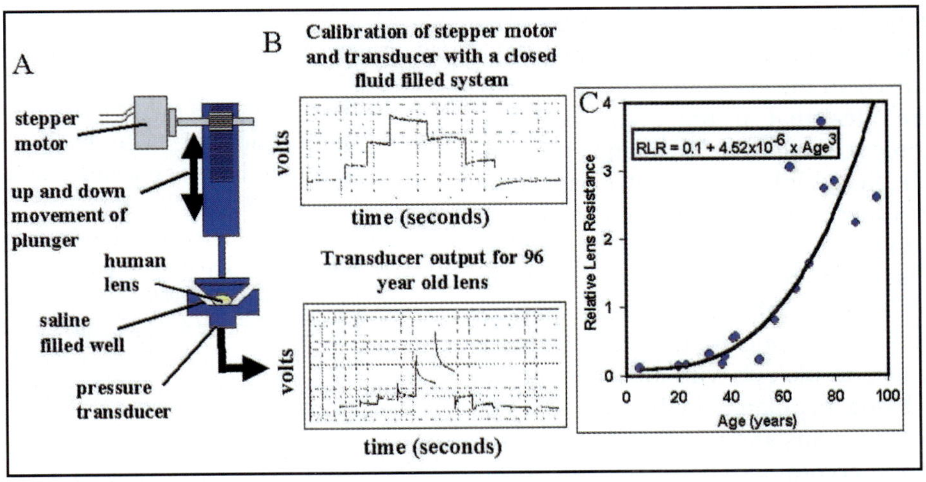

Figure 2-9. Measurements of the relative resistance of the human lens to mechanical compression tests. A) Unfixed human lenses extracted from human donor eyes were placed on a pressure transducer beneath a plunger attached to a stepper motor. For each lens tested, the plunger was first stepped down on the lens and then stepped up off the lens in six successive steps. B) The response from the transducer was recorded as a change in the output voltage. To characterize the performance of the measurement system it was first calibrated with a closed, fluid filled system (upper trace). The complete raw output signal from a 96-year-old human lens (lower trace) is shown. C) Graph of the maximum responses recorded from 19 human lenses aged 5 to 96 years. Human lenses show an over four-fold increase in resistance to mechanical compression over the human life span.[30] (Reproduced from *Vision Research,* 39[11], Glasser A, Campbell MCW. Biometric, optical, and physical changes in the isolated human crystalline lens in relation to presbyopia, 1991-2015, Copyright 1999, with permission from Elsevier.)

In summary, the lens from the eye of a presbyope does not undergo accommodative changes to mechanical stretching, is not altered in shape or optical power on removal of the capsule, and is roughly 3 times harder than the young human lens. This shows that the presbyopic lens is incapable of undergoing capsule-induced accommodative changes. This provides strong support for lenticular hardening as an important factor in the progression of presbyopia.

Restoration of Accommodation in Presbyopes

Overwhelming evidence in favor of the Helmholtz accommodative mechanism and evidence showing that the human crystalline lens gradually loses the ability to undergo accommodative changes suggest that accommodation cannot be restored by scleral expansion procedures. Expanding the scleral diameter overlying the ciliary muscle cannot restore the accommodative capacity to the presbyopic human lens. This is supported by the fact that objective accommodation measurements in scleral expansion band patients show no indication of accommodation restoration[51] and also from subjective evaluations of accommodative performance after scleral expansion procedures which show either no benefit, transient benefit, or limited benefits in only half of the patients.[52-54] The overwhelming body of experimental evidence suggests that if accommodation is to be restored in human presbyopes, the accommodative capacity of the crystalline lens must be restored or the presbyopic lens must be replaced with a lens capable of undergoing accommodative changes. The presence of some accommodative movements of the ciliary body/muscle in the eyes of presbyopes lends credence to the idea that if the accommodative capacity is restored to the lens, or an artificial accommodative lens is placed into the capsular bag, some accommodative function may be restored to presbyopes. Refilling the human lens capsular bag with a soft polymer restores the accommodative ability to even presbyopic lenses.[55] Intraocular lenses that are designed to allow the optic to translate forward along the optic axis in the eye with an accommodative effort are being evaluated in human cataract patients.[56,57] Forward translation of the lens is not a normal part of the accommodative response of the natural crystalline lens, but such movement could potentially provide limited accommodation within the constraints of how much forward movement such lenses can achieve.

REFERENCES

1. Keeney AH, Hagman RE, Fratello CJ. *Dictionary of Ophthalmic Optics*. Newton, MA: Butterworth-Heinemann; 1995.
2. Helmholtz von HH. Ueber die Accommodation des Auges. *Archiv für Ophthalmologie*. 1855;1(2),1-74.
3. Helmholtz von HH. Mechanism of accommodation. In: JPC Southall, ed. *Helmholtz's Treatise on Physiological Optics*. New York: Dover; 1909:143-173.
4. Fincham EF. The mechanism of accommodation. *British Journal of Ophthalmology, Monograph VIII*. 1937;7-80.
5. Rohen JW, Rentsch FJ. Architecture and function of the human zonula ciliaris. Morphological principles for a new theory of accommodation. *Albrecht Von Graefes Arch Klin Exp Ophthalmol*. 1969;178(1):1-19.
6. Rohen JW. Scanning electron microscopic studies of the zonular apparatus in human and monkey eyes. *Invest Ophthalm Vis Sci*. 1979;18(2):133-144.
7. Beauchamp R, Mitchell B. Ultrasound measures of vitreous chamber depth during ocular accommodation. *Am J Optom Physiol Opt*. 1985;62(8):523-532.
8. Drexler W, Baumgartner A, Findl O, Hitzenberger CK, Fercher AF. Biometric investigation of changes in the anterior eye segment during accommodation. *Vision Res*. 1997; 37(19):2789-2800.
9. Schachar RA, Black TD, Kash RL, Cudmore DP, Schanzlin DJ. The mechanism of accommodation and presbyopia in the primate. *Annals of Ophthalmology*. 1995;27(2):58-67.
10. Schachar RA. Zonular function: a new hypothesis with clinical implications. *Arch Ophthalmol*. 1994;26:36-38.
11. Schachar RA, Anderson D. The mechanism of ciliary muscle function. *Annals of Ophthalmology*. 1995;27(3):126-132.
12. Tscherning M. Accommodation. In Tscherning M, ed. *Physiological Optics*. 4th ed. Philadelphia: Keystone Publishing; 1924:192-228.
13. Farnsworth PN, Burke P. Three-dimensional architecture of the suspensory apparatus of the lens of the rhesus monkey. *Exp Eye Res*. 1977;25:563-576.
14. Glasser A, Campbell MCW. Presbyopia and the optical changes in the human crystalline lens with age. *Vision Res*. 1998;38(2):209-229.
15. Lütjen-Drecoll E, Tamm E, Kaufman PL. Age-related loss of morphologic responses to pilocarpine in rhesus monkey ciliary muscle. *Arch Ophthalmol*. 1988;106(11):1591-1598.
16. Tamm E, Croft MA, Jungkunz W, Lütjen-Drecoll E, Kaufman PL. Age-related loss of ciliary muscle mobility in the rhesus: role of the choroid. *Arch Ophthalmol*. 1992;110:871-876.
17. Tamm S, Tamm E, Rohen JW. Age-related changes of the human ciliary muscle. A quantitative morphometric study. *Mech Ageing Dev*. 1992;62(2):209-221.
18. Glasser A, Kaufman PL. The mechanism of accommodation in primates. *Ophthalmologe*. 1999;106(5):863-872.
19. Bacskulin A, Gast R, Bergmann U, Guthoff R. Ultrasound biomicroscopy imaging of accommodative configuration changes in the presbyopic ciliary body. *Ophthalmologe*. 1996;93(2):199-203.
20. Schachar RA, Tello C, Cudmore DP, Liebmann JM, Black TD, Ritch R. In vivo increase of the human lens equatorial diameter during accommodation. *Am J Physiol*. 1996; 271(3.2):R670-R676.
21. Wilson RS. Does the lens diameter increase or decrease during accommodation? Human accommodation studies: a new technique using infrared retro-illumination video photography and pixel unit measurements. *Trans Am Ophthalmol Soc*. 1997;95:261-267.
22. Rohen JW, Lütjen-Drecoll E. Age changes in the morphology of the anterior segment of the eye. *Atti Fond. G Ronchi*. 1985;Sept-Dec:635-645.

23. Lütjen-Drecoll E, Tamm E, Kaufman PL. Age changes in rhesus monkey ciliary muscle: light and electron microscopy. *Exp Eye Res*. 1988;47(6):885-899.
24. Tamm E, Lütjen-Drecoll E, Jungkunz W, Rohen JW. Posterior attachment of ciliary muscle in young, accommodating old, presbyopic monkeys. *Invest Ophthalmol Vis Sci*. 1991;32(5):1678-1692.
25. Poyer JF, Kaufman PL, Flugel C. Age does not affect contractile responses of the isolated rhesus monkey ciliary muscle to muscarinic agonists. *Curr Eye Res*. 1993;12(5):413-422.
26. Gabelt BT, Kaufman PL, Polansky JR. Ciliary muscle muscarinic binding sites, choline acetyltransferase, and acetylcholinesterase in aging rhesus monkeys. *Invest Ophthalmol Vis Sci*. 1990;31(11):2431-2436.
27. Strenk SA, Semmlow JL, Strenk LM, Munoz P, Gronlund-Jacob J, DeMarco KJ. Age-related changes in human ciliary muscle and lens: a magnetic resonance imaging study. *Invest Ophthalmol Vis Sci*. 1999;40(6):1162-1169.
28. Farnsworth PN, Shyne SE. Anterior zonular shifts with age. *Exp Eye Res*. 1979;28:291-297.
29. Scammon R, Hesdorffer M. Growth in mass and volume of the human lens in postnatal life. *Arch Ophthalmol*. 1937;17:104-112.
30. Glasser A, Campbell MCW. Biometric, optical and physical changes in the isolated human crystalline lens with age in relation to presbyopia. *Vision Res*. 1999;39(11):1991-2015.
31. Sorsby A, Leary GA, Richards M, Chaston J. Ultrasonographic measurements of the components of ocular refraction in life. *Vision Res*. 1963;3:499-505.
32. Weekers R, Delmarcelle Y, Luyckx-Bacus J. Biometrics of the crystalline lens. In Bellows J, ed. *Cataract and Abnormalities of the Lens*. New York: Grune & Stratton, Inc; 1975:134-147.
33. Koretz JF, Kaufman PL, Neider MW, Goeckner PA. Accommodation and presbyopia in the human eye—aging of the anterior segment. *Vision Res*. 1989;29(12):1685-1692.
34. Brown N. The change in lens curvature with age. *Exp Eye Res*. 1974;19:175-183.
35. Dubbelman M, Van Der Heijde GL. The shape of the aging human lens: curvature, equivalent refractive index and the lens paradox. *Vision Res*. 2001;41(14):1867-1877.
36. Brown N. The change in shape and internal form of the lens of the eye on accommodation. *Exp Eye Res*. 1973;15:441-459.
37. Koretz JF, Cook CA, Kaufman PL. Accommodation and presbyopia in the human eye. Changes in the anterior segment and crystalline lens with focus. *Invest Ophthalmol Vis Sci*. 1997;38(3):569-578.
38. Koretz JF, Cook CA, Kuszak JR. The zones of discontinuity in the human lens: development and distribution with age. *Vision Res*. 1994;34(22):2955-2962.
39. Schachar RA. Cause and treatment of presbyopia with a method for increasing the amplitude of accommodation. *Annals of Ophthalmology*. 1992;24(12):445-452.
40. Rafferty NS. Lens morphology. In Maisel H, ed. *The Ocular Lens Structure, Function, and Pathology*. New York: Marcel Dekker, Inc; 1985:1-60.
41. Schachar RA. Pathophysiology of accommodation and presbyopia: understanding the clinical implications. *Journal of the Florida Medical Association*. 1994;81(4): 268-271.
42. Schachar RA. Is Helmholtz's theory of accommodation correct? *Annals of Ophthalmology*. 1999;31(1):10-17.
43. Schachar RA. Theoretical basis for the scleral expansion band procedure for surgical reversal of presbyopia (SRP). *Annals of Ophthalmology*. 2000;32(4):271-278.
44. Smith P. Diseases of the crystalline lens and capsule: On the growth of the crystalline lens. *Transactions of the Ophthalmological Society of the United Kingdom*. 1883;3:79-102.
45. Fisher RF. Elastic constants of the human lens capsule. *J Physiol*. 1969;201:1-19.
46. Krag S, Olsen T, Andreassen TT. Biomechanical characteristics of the human anterior lens capsule in relation to age. *Invest Ophthalmol Vis Sci*. 1997;38(2):357-363.
47. Krag S, Andreassen TT. Mechanical Properties of the human posterior lens capsule. *Invest Ophthalmol Vis Sci*. 2003;44(2):691-696.
48. Fisher RF. The elastic constants of the human lens. *J Physiol*. 1971;212:147-180.
49. Fisher RF. Presbyopia and the changes with age in the human crystalline lens. *J Physiol*. 1973;228:765-779.
50. Fisher RF. The force of contraction of the human ciliary muscle during accommodation. *J Physiol*. 1977;270:51-74.
51. Mathews S. Scleral expansion surgery does not restore accommodation in human presbyopia. *Ophthalmology*. 1999;106(5):873-877.
52. Malecaze FJ, Gazagne CS, Tarroux MC, Gorrand JM. Scleral expansion bands for presbyopia. *Ophthalmology*. 2001;108(12):2165-2171.
53. Hamilton DR, Davidorf JM, Maloney RK. Anterior ciliary sclerotomy for treatment of presbyopia: a prospective controlled study. *Ophthalmology*. 2002;109(November):1970-1977.
54. Qazi MA, Pepose JS, Shuster JJ. Implantation of scleral expansion band segments for the treatment of presbyopia. *Am J Ophthalmol*. 2002;134(Dec):808-815.
55. Koopmans SA, Terwee T, Barkhof J, Haitjema HJ, Kooijman AC. Polymer refilling of presbyopic human lenses in vitro restores the ability to undergo accommodative changes. *Invest Ophthalmol Vis Sci*. 2003;44(1):250-257.
56. Cumming JS, Slade SG, Chayet A. Clinical evaluation of the model AT-45 silicone accommodating intraocular lens: results of feasibility and the initial phase of a Food and Drug Administration clinical trial. *Ophthalmology*. 2001; 108(11):2005-2009.
57. Küchle M, Nguyen NX, Langenbucher A, et al. Implantation of a new accommodative posterior chamber intraocular lens. *J Refract Surg*. 2002;18(May-Jun):208-216.
58. Duane A. Normal values of the accommodation at all ages. *JAMA*. 1912;Sept:1010-1013.
59. Glasser A, Croft MA, Kaufman PL. Aging of the human crystalline lens and presbyopia. *Int Ophthalmol Clin*. 2001;41(2):1-15.

Chapter Three

Surgery for Hyperopia: Historical Perspectives

Bradley Fundingsland, BA; William I. Bond, MD; and Neal A. Sher, MD, FACS

Introduction

At various stages, the surgical correction of myopia through radial keratotomy (RK), photoreactive keratotomy (PRK), and laser-assisted in-situ keratomileusis (LASIK) has gained overwhelming support in the literature and among the ophthalmic community as a whole. In contrast, hyperopic refractive error has yet to find a broadly accepted means of definitive surgical correction.

Myopes are typically confronted with their refractive error very early in life. They have had to wear correction from childhood and therefore, very often make peace with spectacles or contact lenses at an early age.

Not so for the hyperope. Manifest hyperopia usually begins in the patient's mid-to-late 30s as what will seem to be an early presbyopia. Soon, a drop in the uncorrected distance vision and further worsening of close vision occur. Because the far point of the hyperopic eye degrades both near and far vision, the patient becomes completely dependent on glasses, usually bifocals, for the rest of his or her life. This represents a profoundly unwelcome change to a person whose vision has been apparently normal up to that point in life.

This substantial group of hyperopic patients has historically been anxious to have this problem resolved without being forced into glasses or contact lenses. Not everyone in the age group is eager to embrace contact lenses. The demand of this large hyperopic group for an alternative to glasses or contacts has led ophthalmic surgeons to a variety of options. Casebeer called hyperopia (when accompanied by astigmatism) "the most uncomfortable refractive error".[1]

Surgical techniques for hyperopia have been attempted with fluctuating frequency over this and the previous century. A partial list includes the reshaping of the cornea through incisions, burns, laser ablations, lamellar cuts, the addition of corneal tissue, and the replacement of the posterior lens.[2] This chapter will briefly review the historical development of some of these procedures.

Hexagonal Keratotomy

Definition

Hexagonal keratotomy (HK) is a surgical technique where 6 incisions, usually non-connecting and approximately 90% deep, are placed in a hexagonal pattern around a clear optical zone of 5- to 6-mm diameter. The incisions may be accompanied by non-connecting transverse relaxing incisions placed peripheral to the hexagonal incisions. The incision

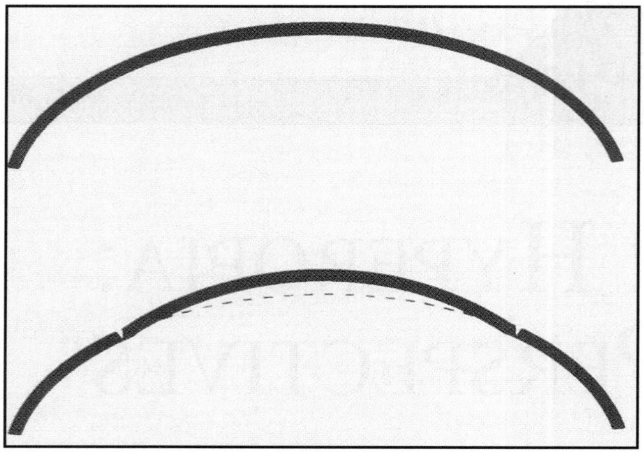

Figure 3-1. Schematic of HK. (Reproduced from *Ophthalmology Clinics of North America*, 5[4], Casebeer JC, Phillips SG. HK: an historical review an assessment of 46 cases, 727-744, Copyright 1992, with permission from Elsevier.)

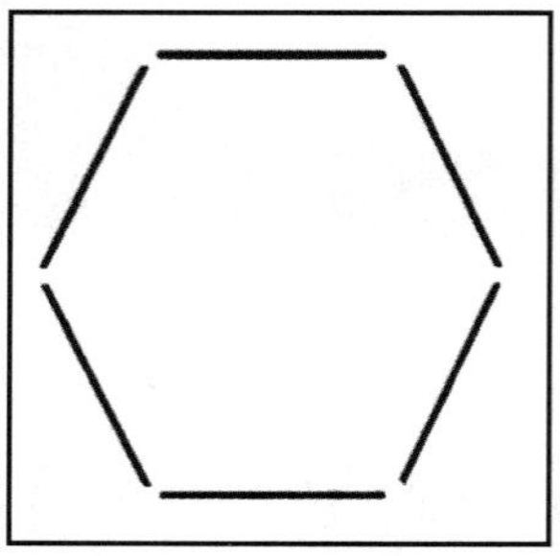

Figure 3-2A. A hexagonal pattern is thought to be the most practical approach—technically feasible yet a good approximation of a circle.

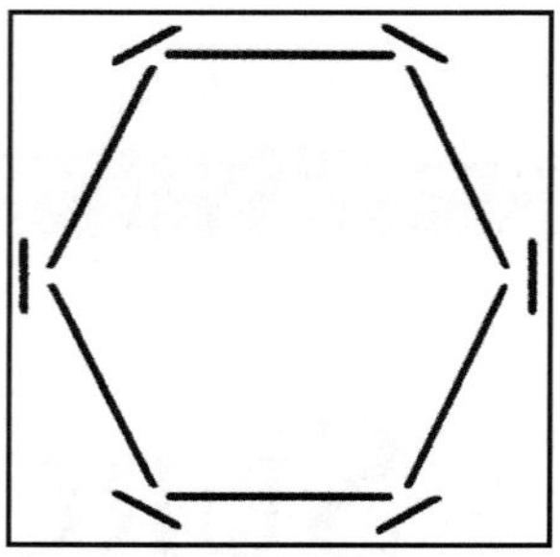

Figure 3-2B. Mendez HK as modified by R. Jensen, MD. Two or more pairs of transverse keratotomies are oriented to produce an outline of a regular polygon, centered around the pupil, and placed on an optical zone of 6.0 mm or less.

pattern causes weakening of the paracentral cornea and a compensatory steepening of the central cornea (Figure 3-1).[3]

The Early Evolution of HK

Refractive surgical techniques designed to decrease hyperopia include traditional (lathe) keratomileusis, automated lamellar keratoplasty, epikeratoplasty (epikeratophakia), thermokeratoplasty, transverse keratotomy, PRK, and LASIK.[4]

With incisional technique, the central corneal steepening necessary to reduce hyperopia requires incisions aligned in a circumferential pattern around the visual axis. In theory, any symmetrical geometric figure could be used, because they all describe a circle when the tangents of the inside of the sides are connected. A hexagonal pattern is thought to be the most practical approach—technically feasible, yet a good approximation of a circle (Figure 3-2A).[5]

Partial-thickness corneal trephination using a diameter of 7.0 mm in cadaver eyes caused central corneal flattening.[6] However, partial-thickness paracentral trephination was shown to cause central corneal steepening. Unpredictable wound healing and resultant astigmatism precluded trephination from being a useful technique.[7]

Paired transverse incisions made perpendicular to the steepest meridian will reduce corneal astigmatism.[8,9] If 2 or more pairs of transverse keratotomies are oriented to produce an outline of a regular polygon, centered around the pupil, and placed on an optical zone of 6.0 mm or less, central corneal steepening rather than flattening occurs (Figure 3-2B). The central corneal steepening requires incisions to be continuous or nearly so. Six-sided regular polygonal (hexagonal) keratotomy achieves central corneal steepening.[10-13]

In 1952, Akiyama, working with innovations developed by Sato in the 1940's, first described the ability of posterior hexagonal incisions to correct hyperopia in rabbits. In 1979, Yamashita experimented with an anterior corneal incisional technique in rabbits for creating peripheral flattening and consequent central steepening. He reported his results in 1986.[14] Yamashita and Gaster, in 1983, reported on trials of what they termed hexagonal keratotomy in rabbits, finding the hex to be more effective than trephination in rabbits that had undergone RK.[15] Gills did additional work relating to the trephination technique.[16]

Later Evolution of HK

Mendez first presented discussion of HK in humans in 1985. He also first presented clinical data from humans in 1986.[17]

Mendez reported on 46 eyes undergoing HK beginning in 1983. A regular hexagonal pattern was used with optical zones of 5.0, 5.5, and 6.0 mm outside diameter and with the incisions intersecting at the apices. Average reductions of 3.5, 2.5, and 1.5 D of hyperopia were achieved. These seem to have been the first contemporary reports of HK for the correction of hyperopia in humans, although Sato had described a similar procedure in Japan in the 1940s.[18]

In 1988 Mendez reported a larger series,[18] presenting data from 102 eyes of 53 patients. Incisions were created at 87% depth of the thinnest pachymetry

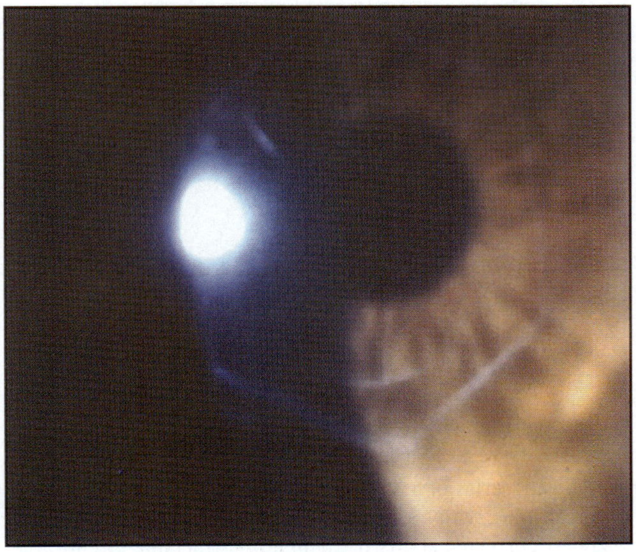

Figure 3-3. Clinical photo of Mendez HK with intersecting incision.

reading of the chosen optical zone. Mendez used his prior nomogram. All incisions were connected at the apices.

He found slightly less correction per optical zone than with his earlier series. An average of 1.50 ± 0.75 D was achieved with the 6.0mm central zone, 2.0 ± 0.75 D with a 5.5 mm zone, and 3.0 ± 0.75 D with a 5.0 mm zone. Astigmatism up to 1.5 D was treated by making a transverse incision 0.5 mm inside the hexagon.

Overcorrections (7.8%) and induced astigmatism (20%) were reported. Mendez believed that irregularity in the outline of the hexagon, non-uniform incision depth, and excessive depth were responsible for these complications.

Postoperative corneal thickness also increased approximately 50 µm, which Mendez ascribed to retraction of the central corneal collagen, thought to produce the central corneal steepening.[19]

In 1988, Neumann and McCarty reported results from HK in rabbits dating from 1985 that were very similar to those of Yamashita and Gaster.[15] They also performed HK on 1 eye of a patient blinded by optic atrophy, achieving a 3.1 D reduction in hyperopia with an optical zone 5.0 mm.

Neumann and McCarty then performed HK on sighted eyes. A total of 15 eyes of 11 patients underwent HK. The surgery was performed in the manner originally described by Mendez. The mean preop equivalent sphere was 3.21 D and the average reduction in hyperopia was 2.16 D. This correlated with an average keratometric increase of +2.22 D. Clear zone diameters of 5.0, 5.5, and 6.0 mm were employed. Follow-up was 9.5 months, and 93% of eyes had an improvement in uncorrected visual acuity.[20]

The Mendez technique was shown to definitely reduce hyperopia. However, the technique tended to isolate the central cornea with a considerable tendency to poor wound healing, persistent healing defects, and scarring, along with a good deal of unpredictability.[21] Figure 3-3 shows an example of a patient with Mendez HK. Some patients were left with high astigmatism, often irregular, and a loss of best-correctable visual acuity. Several patients required suturing for wound gapes. There was also, as was true in RK, an increased tendency toward ruptured globe.[21-24]

To try to correct these problems, Jensen introduced an altered technique where the incisions did not intersect. The Jensen modification increased relative safety but somewhat reduced the amount of hyperopic correction.[25] Jensen reported a series of 483 eyes operated between 1987 and 1990.[26] He reported a mean decrease in hyperopia, but presented little data on complications. Hollis in 1994 reported a series of 900 eyes done in this manner over a 7-year period. He noted "good results" with induced astigmatism "often" and a 10% undercorrection rate, as well as some scarring and a 1% irregular astigmatism rate reducing vision to the "20/30 to 20/50 range at best."

Mendez also modified the technique by using 6 non-intersecting incisions with an extension of one at each apex. This was intended to increase the effectiveness of the procedure. Casebeer reported that in his experience with the modified Mendez and Jensen technique, relatively small differences in the size of the uncut apices (which were referred to as "pillars") led to significant amounts of astigmatism. The modification suggested by Casebeer was to make the pillar as small as technically feasible (about 50 to 100 µm) and to make a transverse incision of 2.5 to 3.0 mm in length about 250 µm outside each apex. He termed this technique a "T-hex." It was widely taught to refractive surgeons in the United States as well as internationally. Gilbert, Friedlander, and Grant[27] independently arrived at a similar HK-with-transverse-incision technique with work on cadaver eyes.

In 1991, Casebeer reported a series of 46 eyes in 24 patients with the T-hex technique with good results. At that time, he advocated treating the astigmatism first with astigmatic keratotomy (AK), then treating residual hyperopia with the hexagonal component at least 6 weeks later. Another 1995 modification of

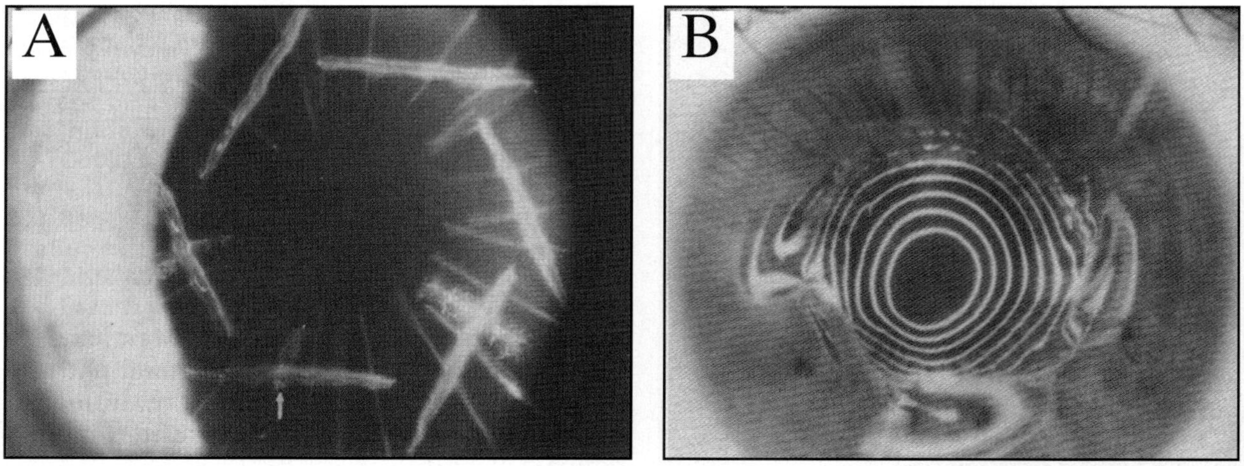

Figure 3-4A and B. A slit lamp photo and photokeratograph from the Basuk series of a 35-year-old woman who had previously undergone radial keratotomy with 24 incisions and had HK for presbyopic symptoms. The patient had scars 80 to 90% of the corneal thickness and were irregularly spaced. The patient had best corrected acuity of 20/40 and intractable foreign body sensation and symptoms of visual distortion. She was fitted with a rigid gas permeable contact lens but was intolerant because of pain.[21] (Reproduced from *Am J Ophthalmol,* 117, Basuk WL, Zisman M, Waring GO, et al. Complications of hexagonal keratotomy, 37-49, Copyright 1994, with permission from Elsevier.)

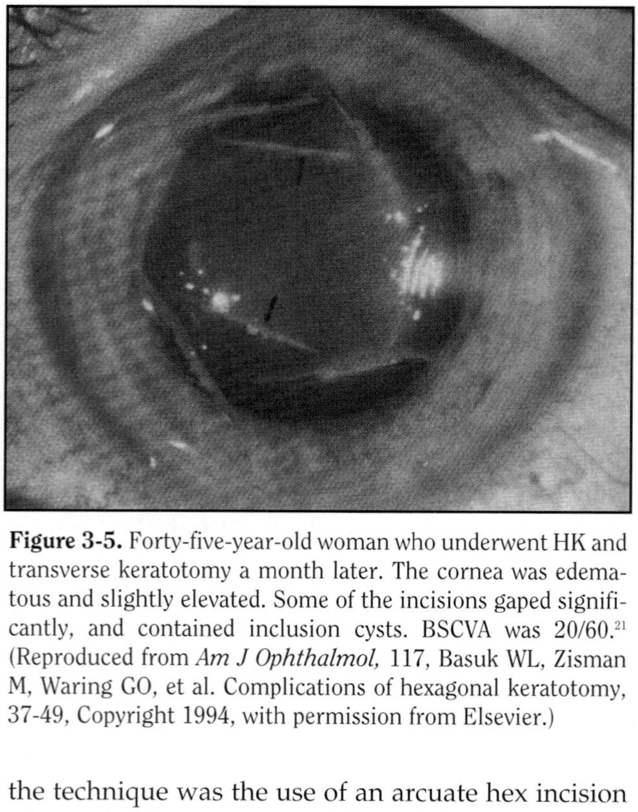

Figure 3-5. Forty-five-year-old woman who underwent HK and transverse keratotomy a month later. The cornea was edematous and slightly elevated. Some of the incisions gaped significantly, and contained inclusion cysts. BSCVA was 20/60.[21] (Reproduced from *Am J Ophthalmol,* 117, Basuk WL, Zisman M, Waring GO, et al. Complications of hexagonal keratotomy, 37-49, Copyright 1994, with permission from Elsevier.)

the technique was the use of an arcuate hex incision where the hexagon was followed by two arcuate incisions 6 to 8 months postoperatively.[1] This was thought to be a good way to treat the induced astigmatism that was shown to be frequent after hex by virtually every author.

Complications of HK

Results of HK for consecutive hyperopia following RK were almost uniformly dismal. Casebeer reported that the 3 patients of this type that he operated experienced "remarkable difficulties." He ascribed this to too many intersecting incisions. All 3 had wound gapes, migration of epithelium into wounds, persistent epithelial defects, and induction of large amounts of regular and irregular astigmatism. The experience of Grady was similar.[11]

Basuk et al[21] reported a series of complications after HK in 15 selected eyes of 10 patients. These complications included glare, photophobia, polyopia, visual fluctuation, overcorrection, irregular astigmatism, corneal edema, corneal perforation, bacterial keratitis, and endophthalmitis. Wound healing abnormalities were common in these selected eyes. Eight of the 15 eyes lost best spectacle-corrected visual acuity (BSCVA) of 2 or more Snellen lines. Three of these selected eyes underwent penetrating keratoplasty (PKP) (Figures 3-4A and B). Figure 3-5 shows another case from the same series, a 45-year-old woman who underwent HK and transverse keratotomy a month later. The cornea was edematous and slightly elevated. Some of the incisions gaped significantly, and contained inclusion cysts. BSCVA was 20/60. In Figure 3-6 we see another example of the severe scarring that can occur after hexagonal incisions cross radial incisions.

Nordan and Maxwell in 1992[28] strongly advocated the abolition of HK due to the complications of

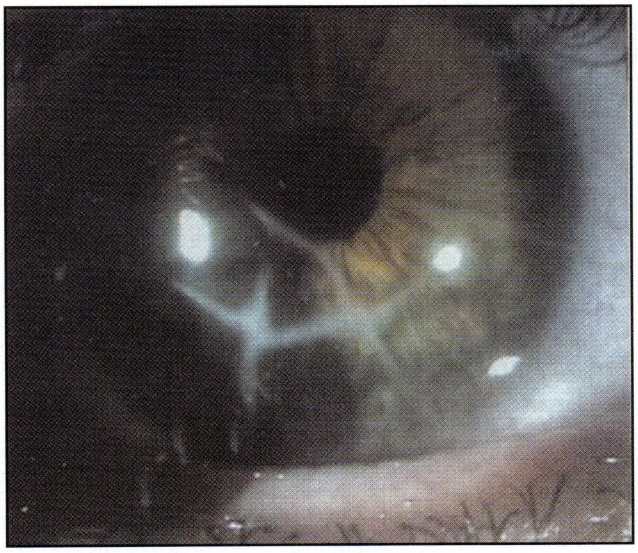

Figure 3-6. Another example of the severe scarring which can occur after hexagonal incisions cross radial incisions.[21] (Reproduced from *Am J Ophthalmol,* 117, Basuk WL, Zisman M, Waring GO, et al. Complications of hexagonal keratotomy, 37-49, Copyright 1994, with permission from Elsevier.)

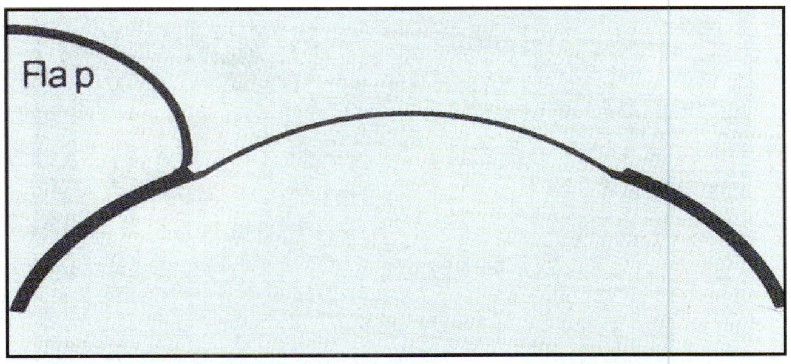

Figure 3-7. Schematic of ALK and "controlled ectasia."

irregular astigmatism with consequent loss of BSCVA, which they said occurred in almost every case. Their statement was disputed by many surgeons.[29,30]

Conclusion

The central problems of HK were (1) the induction of regular and irregular astigmatism with loss of BSCVA, and (2) its unpredictability, often ascribed to surgeon-dependent factors. Almost every series of HK results reported a fairly large number of eyes with extremely variable outcomes. Some eyes would show no effect at all; others a startling effect. Even when carefully performed, there was an unacceptable loss of BSCVA and induced amount of irregular astigmatism.

Werblin in 1997[31] said his experience with HK was "limited but positive," reporting a series of 18 consecutive eyes during 1993. (The author's own experience [WB] with a larger number of eyes was also "limited but positive.") I will close with Dr. Werblin's observation; despite his "positive experience," he said, "because of the highly variable results noted in the literature and several reports of significant complications, I no longer perform or recommend HK."[31]

Automated Lamellar Keratoplasty

Dr. Jose Barraquer in Bogota, Colombia, originated keratomileusis as a surgical treatment for refractive error. Keratomileusis with a cryolathe was problematic because of the inconsistent speed of passage of the keratome across the cornea.[32,33]

Dr. Luis Antonio Ruiz worked with Dr. Barraquer for many years. Ruiz addressed the keratome problem (as well as many others) by automating the instrument. The mechanized keratome was integrated into a machine to perform automated lamellar keratoplasty (ALK). One component, the adjustable suction ring, was meant to lock onto the sclera surrounding the cornea. The second component, the keratome itself, was motorized and external gears were added. The keratome head had tongues that were placed in a groove set on top of the suction ring. The gears then powered the keratome across the cornea on a gear track, also on top of the suction ring.

The automated machine eliminated the cryolathe and its technical problems. It also minimized handling of the tissue and freezing of the keratocytes.[34] Ruiz made the observation that one deep lamellar pass could treat hyperopia.[35] He discovered this when refractive change resulted even after aborted keratomileusis cases where the cryolathe did not work.

Procedure

Ruiz developed a nomogram, later modified by Casebeer and others, for the use of an ALK machine to treat hyperopia. The stroma was excised based on these nomograms, which related pachymetry to depth of cut. The desired depth was between 60% and 80% of the total depth. If the incision was less than 60%, the effect was minimal. If the depth was over 80%, ectasia was regarded as more likely.[36]

The action mechanism of hyperopic ALK was a "controlled ectasia" (Figure 3-7).[37,38]

Loss of the cap was one early problem with the procedure. The incidence was quite high, in the range of 5% to 10% of eyes done. Casebeer dealt with this problem by adding a stopper to the keratome. It

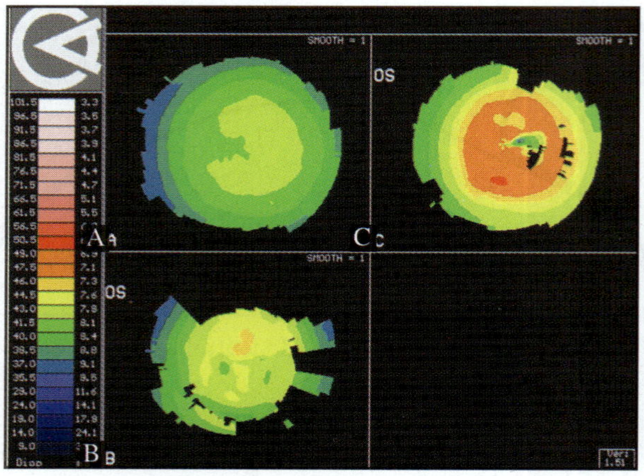

Figure 3-8. Topography following ALK for hyperopia. The preoperative (A), 2-week (B), and 3-week postoperative map (C) is shown.[37]

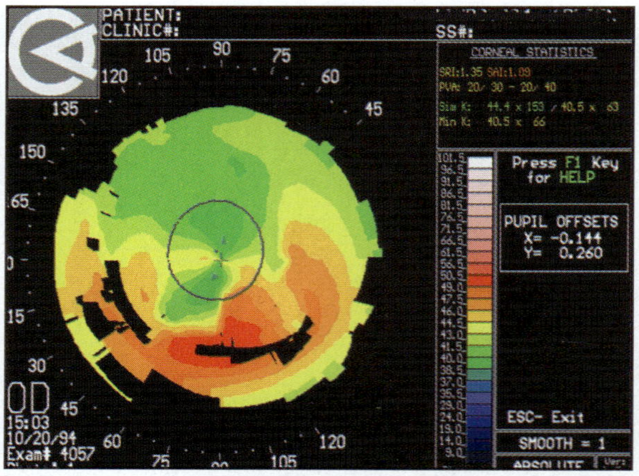

Figure 3-9. Topography of a patient who underwent hyperopic ALK postprogressive hyperopia after RK. Severe ectasia is present. (Courtesy of David Hardten, MD.)

automatically stopped the machine after its pass across the central cornea, creating a hinged flap rather than a free cap.

Hollis reported a series of 700 cases of hyperopic ALK[38] with some early undercorrections with the Ruiz nomogram, which he modified. This included a sub-group of 90 patients who had undergone previous Mendez HK with undercorrection. He also reported a series of 65 patients who had hyperopic ALK for hyperopia induced by RK overcorrection. No complication data was given. He reported a "success rate of 90%." Many people had the ability to see both near and far one day postop. This was attributed to an aspheric effect. Near vision was unfortunately lost over the next few months as the presumed aspheric shape regressed.

Kezirian and Gremillion reported a retrospective study of 85 eyes in 49 patients done in 1993.[37] Early cases were done with the Ruiz nomogram, which tended to produce 1 D to 1.5 D of residual hyperopia and adjustments were made to subsequent procedures. There was no tendency for myopic progression (which would have indicated unstable ectasia) in the 8 months of the study. Forty percent of the eyes underwent simultaneous AK for astigmatism.

The procedure was quite effective and the results were quite stable over the study period. The most significant complication was a reduction in BSCVA of 1 to 3 lines in 11 of 85 eyes; this was transient in 6 eyes. Figure 3-8 shows a topography following ALK for hyperopia. The preoperative (A), 2-week (B), and 3-week postoperative map (C) is shown.

Manche et al in 1996[39] reported a series of 24 eyes of 17 patients done in 1993 to 1994. The same early undercorrection was noted with the Ruiz nomogram and the usual modifications were made. The procedure was found to be effective and safe. There were no vision-threatening complications. There was no evidence of progressive myopia in 6 months. No eye lost two or more lines of BSCVA at 3 or 6 months postoperatively.

Complications of Hyperopic ALK

The Ruiz nomogram, although it produced undercorrections, had very little scatter.[40] Modifications generally used the same nomogram but manipulated the intended outcome (in other words, use what the nomogram said to do for +3 D to correct +2 D in the patient, with other modifications for higher corrections).

The results were often inconsistent and very unpredictable in any given case. A fair number of patients would show little if any effect. Enhancements were problematic.[41] The deep lamellar cut tended to be invisible at the slit lamp. It was difficult to know what to do if a case needed further correction.

Furthermore, it was easy to produce severe complications, particularly if the machine was set up at all incorrectly. A surgeon could easily remove an entire anterior segment by mistake not only by forgetting to include a removable metal block above the blade, but by not having the metal block pushed all the way in.[42] Late ectasia, feared by early authors, proved to be an unfortunate fact in some cases, particularly if the procedure was done after an overcorrected RK.

Figure 3-9 shows a patient who underwent hyperopic ALK post progressive hyperopia after RK. Severe ectasia is present.

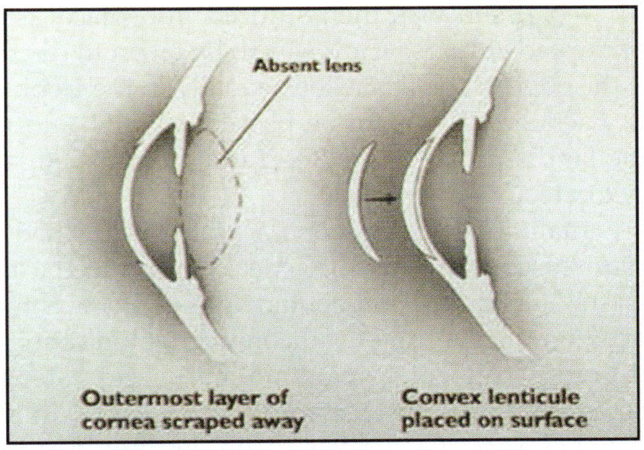

Figure 3-10A. Schematic of epikeratophakia in aphakia shows the outermost layer of the cornea scraped away so a convex lenticule can be placed on the surface.

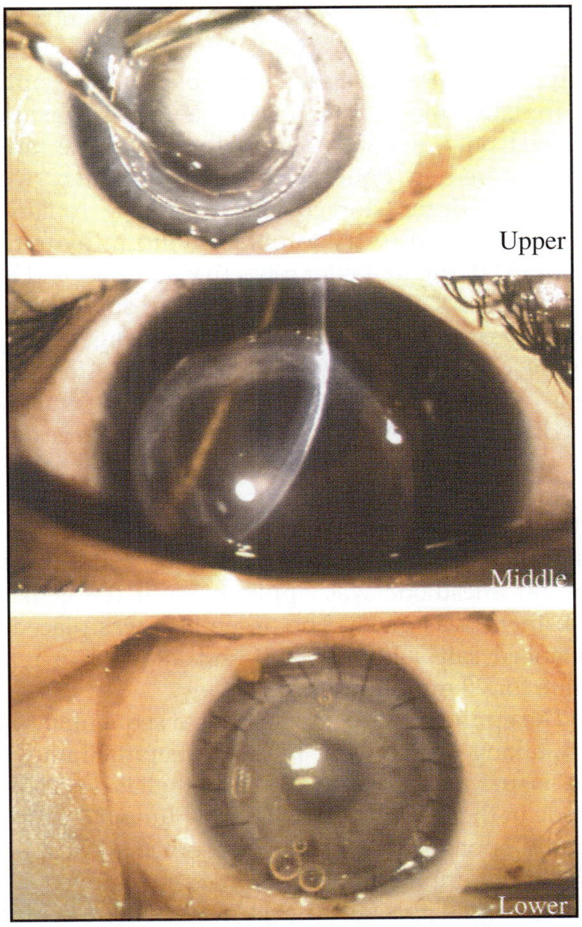

Figure 3-10B. Clinical photo of epikeratophakia button being placed into lamellar pocket and sutured into place.

EPIKERATOPHAKIA

Dr. HE Kaufman introduced epikeratophakia (EK) in 1979 as an alterative to then-current modes of aphakic correction[43] following a suggestion to Dr. Kaufman by Dr. TP Werblin, then an LSU corneal fellow. The shaped refractive lenticule in classical keratomileusis was placed into a dissected pocket in the central stroma (Figures 3-10A and B [upper, middle, lower]). Werblin's suggestion was that a properly shaped lenticule could just as effectively and far more simply be fastened to the front of the cornea after epithelial removal (the author was in the room at the time the suggestion was made and enthusiastically received).

EK was hailed as an answer to pediatric aphakia[44-47] keratoconus[48-50] myopia[51,52] and hyperopia[53] (initially from aphakia) in adults. "Tissue lenses" from donor corneal tissue that were screened by eye banks as unusable for transplants were lathed, commercially prepared, and could then be ordered in desired diameters and presumed dioptric powers. Bed sizes in the recipient could also be varied with a different-sized tissue lens for better approximation to the desired curvature or correction.

The surgical technique of EK continually evolved.[54] Originally, the powers of the tissue lenses were designated as one of 3 types: low, medium, or high. The first tissue lenses for aphakia were either 7.5 or 8.0 mm in diameter. They were sutured onto a bed of identical size, made by trephining a circular groove 0.2 mm deep after removing epithelium. A keratectomy of 0.5 mm width, which was cut from the inner wall of the keratectomy site, was later added. This was done to create a broader area of contact between the tissue lens and the host stroma in the hope that host keratocytes could more easily populate the tissue lens.[55]

The lathing process destroyed the viable keratocytes in the tissue lens (made from donor stroma). Early work with tissue lenses in primates showed that the tissue lens had achieved a normal density of keratocytes 7 weeks postoperatively. Other studies showed differing densities of host keratocytes in the tissue lens, ranging from a relative paucity to normal levels.[57-59]

Making a consistent keratectomy was technically difficult. An irregularly cut keratectomy significantly increased the chance of severe postoperative irregular astigmatism. Keratectomies wider than 0.5 mm also led to severe undercorrection in the EK done for myopia. A modified Hessburg-Barron vacuum trephine was developed with two concentric blades 0.5 mm apart and a stop to prevent entry into the anterior chamber. The keratectomy was finally eliminated for adult aphakia and phakic hyperopia.[60]

Initially, the lathing of tissue lenses was performed only at LSU.[61] Originally, the tissue lenses were stored in liquid nitrogen. Later, they were freeze-dried for storage and shipping. A cornea press was used to try to obtain uniform hydration prior to lathing for better refractive accuracy and less astigmatism.[62] Techniques were also developed to compensate for thermally induced changes caused by the cryolathe.[63] In 1983, the technology for tissue lens manufacture was transferred to American Medical Optics (AMO) commercial laboratories.[64]

Surgical Technique

The technique originally described in 1988 is described here. The visual axis was marked after topical anesthetic was applied. Local (or general) anesthetic was given. The tissue lens was placed in balanced salt solution (BSS) and allowed to rehydrate for 20 minutes preoperatively.

The epithelium was removed in a sequential fashion, taking care to leave the central epithelium with the visual axis mark. A small epithelial defect was made in the midperiphery using a blunted cellulose-tipped sponge soaked in unpreserved 4% cocaine. The mid-peripheral epithelium was removed in a circle around the visual axis mark with a spatula. The debris was swept centrally and removed. A keratotomy was made with a 7.0 Hessurg-Barron single blade trephine. The cutting blade was rotated until flushed with the inner suction ring and then retracted counter-clockwise 3 quarter turns. The trephine was subsequently placed on the eye centered on the visual axis mark and advanced 5.5 quarter turns, advancing the blade into the stroma 2.5 quarter turns or about 0.2 mm.

The depth of the keratectomy was inspected with a cellulose-tipped sponge. If uneven, it was recommended to try to compensate with a superblade or diamond knife. The remaining central epithelial island was then removed. Filtered BSS and a pediatric suction tube hooked to low suction were used to clear the corneal surface and conjunctive fornices.

For hyperopia, the diameter of the tissue lens was 8.5 mm placed into the keratotomy diameter of 7.0 mm. A lamellar dissection was then made at the base of the outer lip of the keratotomy using a Suarez spreader (see 3-10A and B). This was designed to create a horizontal dissection 1 mm wide peripheral to the keratectomy. Both sides of the tissue lens were then cleaned with the filtered BSS and suction. The hydrated tissue was then sutured into place using interrupted sutures. Care was to be taken to distribute the edge of the tissue lens equally in the trephine cut. Each suture was to be passed radially into the lamellar dissection and exited 1 mm from the edge of the keratectomy.

A qualitative keratoscope was then attached to the microscope and used to check for induced astigmatism. A bandage soft contact lens (CTL) was then placed on the eye, and a subconjunctival injection of antibiotic (typically Gentamycin) and steroid (Methylprednisolone acetate 80 mg) given in the inferior fornix. Cycloplegic and antibiotic drops were applied topically. A pressure patch was placed over the closed eyelids.

The patient was usually discharged from the hospital the same day. The eye was examined every 24 to 48 hours until epithelial healing was reasonably complete, usually 4 to 7 days. Temporary tarsorrhaphy was done when the epithelium failed to heal in 10 days or so.

Sutures were left in place for 3 to 4 weeks, with loose or vascularized sutures removed earlier. Pronounced cylinder was modified by early removal of stitches in the steep axis (for this reason, earliest possible refraction was recommended). Figure 3-11 shows one of the author's (NAS) patients after an epikeratophakia (in this case, for keratoconus) demonstrating the tissue onlay and dual interface.

Ehrlich and Nordan, in 1989, presented a refinement of the epikeratophakia concept.[65] No recipient keratectomy was performed, and a reverse 50-degree bevel was lathed onto the periphery of the tissue lens for easier tucking into the keratotomy pocket. This was thought to give more direct stromal apposition between recipient and tissue lens on both sides of the wing, promoting better and faster healing and quicker repopulation of the donor by keratocytes.[66] Fresh donor tissue was also used, (frozen for lenticule preparation but never freeze dried for storage.) A microkeratome was used to prepare the tissue lenses before freezing and lathing. Fresh donor tissue was used for epikeratophakia in another earlier series of 13 patients, who all "achieved 20/50 or better acuity."[67]

Results

The early studies of epikeratophakia were done on aphakia in children and adults.[68,69] Age was found to influence visual recovery, with patients older than 70 less likely to be correctable to within one line of preop spectacle correction and more likely to lose 3 or more lines of best-correctable vision. Recovery of

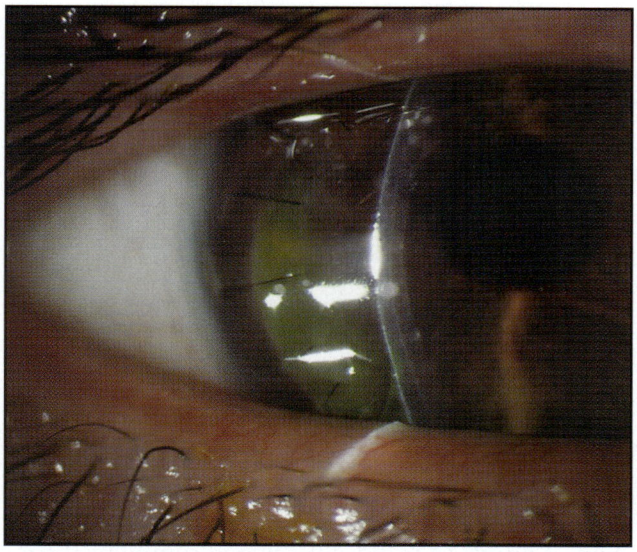

Figure 3-11. One of the author's (NAS) patients after an epikeratophakia (in this case, for keratoconus) demonstrating the tissue onlay and dual interface.

vision tended to progress slowly with time, usually as a result of slow clearing of graft haze and irregular astigmatism. The major improvement in vision occurred between 4 and 12 months postop yet even at 12 months irregular astigmatism was often pronounced.

In 1987, results of the first 519 procedures for aphakia in adults, as part of the nationwide study, were reported.[69] Average follow-up from date of surgery was 189 days and average time from suture removal was 114 days. Visual outcome was significantly affected by the length of time after suture removal. Of the 519 operations, 22 resulted in removal of the tissue lens, due to failure to epithelialize or refractive error. Eight patients received second tissue lenses. One anterior chamber was entered requiring secondary surgery, one pre-existing corneal edema persisting after tissue lens removal and necessitating penetrating keratoplasty, and one case each of hypopyon, uveitis, suture abscess, and infection within ulceration of the tissue lens. The most common problem was failure to re-epithelialize. This was attributed to advancing age, dry eye, and blepharitis, with noncompliance to treatment regimens for these problems leading to scarring or melting of the tissue lens. There was also a wide scatter of intended versus achieved correction.

Conclusions

Epikeratophakia was a technically demanding technique that even if perfectly done yielded very approximate results. This was marginally acceptable for huge refractive errors like aphakia in adults, or in areas where there was no good alternative at the time, like aphakia in children. Results were very approximate even in the most meticulously done studies. Recovery was slow and labor-intensive. Significant and vision-threatening complications were not rare.

The procedure was also not truly reversible and repeatable, as its earlier proponents had said it might be. Best-corrected acuities tended to be lost in significant percentages of the patients, whether due to irregular astigmatism additional corneal thickness (often nearly double now, and with two Bowman's membranes) compromised corneal endothelium, or other causes.

The problematic results as well as the complexity and expense of epikeratophakia led to its abandonment by the profession.

Intrastromal Procedures

Thermokeratoplasty

Thermokeratoplasty involves making a series of deep burns in radially oriented spots throughout the cornea (Figures 3-12A and B). These burns shrink the cornea periphery, increasing the central corneal curvature.

In 1898, Lans[70] first demonstrated the ability of superficial corneal burns to shrink tissue and change the refractive power of the cornea. Subsequently, this procedure was not further investigated until the late 1970s when it was used to treat keratoconus.[71-75]

In 1981, Fyodorov applied this concept to the correction of hyperopia in the form of radial burns and termed the procedure thermokeratoplasty.[76] With this procedure, a heat probe was used to perform 16 radial burns at a temperature of 600°C at 90% of corneal depth. These radial burns caused shrinkage and subsequent flattening in the periphery while steepening the central portion of the cornea.

Neumann's prospective evaluation of Fyodorov's 117 thermokeratoplasty eyes found that the technique reduced hyperopia from a mean of +5.27 D preoperatively to a mean of +1.84 D 12 months postoperatively with minimal regression. Other studies[77-79] have found similar amounts of undercorrection with this technique while experiencing greater amounts of regression. Speculation asserts that regression was due to burn-induced scars, even 1 year after the surgery caused by the high temperature of the heat probe.

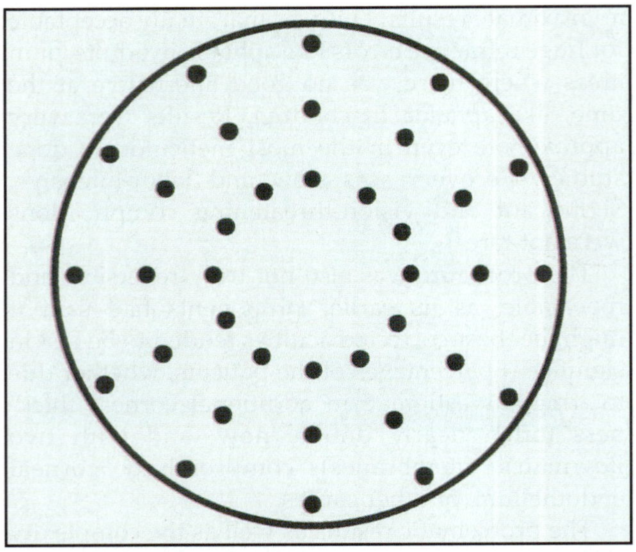

Figure 3-12A. Schematic of thermokeratoplasty demonstrating pattern of series radially oriented spots throughout the mid peripheral cornea.

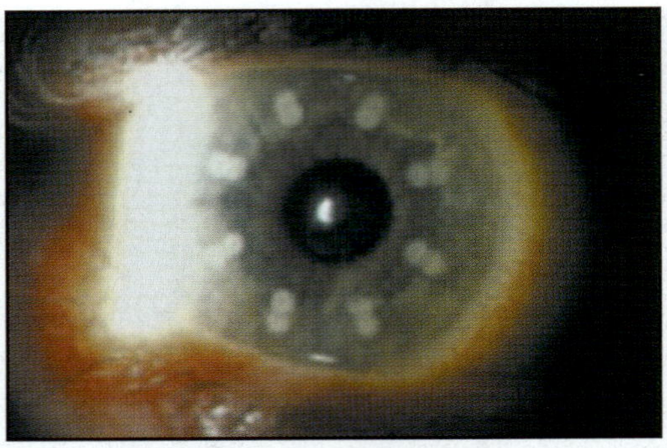

Figure 3-12B. Postoperative appearance 1 month after Holmium laser LTK using the Hyperion system (photo courtesy of Douglas Koch MD).

In 1990 Seiler reported a new technique using a Holmium-YAG laser instead of a heat probe, which would increase the predictability of thermokeratoplasty. In laser thermokeratoplasty (LTK), as this technique is called, infrared Holmium-YAG laser light is delivered to the cornea in a series of spots placed in a circular pattern. The diameter of these spots is a least 5.0 mm and tightens the corneal periphery, creating a central steepening. Seiler's initial data found hyperopic corrections up to 5.0 D with stability over the initial four months postoperatively. Subsequent studies[80-82] illustrate similar stability.

This technology was commercially developed by Sunrise Technologies (Fremont, Calif) and was approved by the FDA in 2000. However, indications on the labeling reading "for the temporary reduction of hyperopia..." were a condition of FDA approval, and the ophthalmic devices panel made very clear that patients should be fully informed their correction may not be permanent. The panel also recommended that labeling include outcome and satisfaction data stratified by age, data on night driving and glare, the number of patients who still need to wear glasses or contact lenses postoperatively, and a disclaimer that data on retreatment are insufficient. The FDA-submitted study included data revealing a 1.5-D regression at the 2-year mark, with models predicting near full regression at 3 to 5 years. Due to data from this study and others,[83] indicating regression of effect, LTK did not achieve commercial success and Sunrise Technologies went out of business in 2002. This topic is discussed further in Chapter 16 by Dr. Kansas, Dr. Sher, and Ms. Luck.

Conductive Keratoplasty

Conductive keratoplasty (CK), developed by Antonio Mendez, MD, uses a needle-like probe to deliver radio-frequency energy to the corneal collagen in a ring of individually placed spots to steepen the cornea. The Refractec Company (Irvine, Calif), has developed this technology for commercial use. Treatment spots can be placed at the 6-, 7-, or 8-mm optical zone and can range from 8 to 32 spots. The number and placement of the spots may vary, but the energy per spot is constant (Figure 3-13).

On April 11, 2002, the US Food and Drug Administration approved conductive keratoplasty for hyperopic patients with refractions of +0.75 to +3.25 D and no more than 0.75 D of astigmatism. Because of mild regression and a lack of long-term results on submission, the treatment was labeled as "temporary." Data from the FDA clinical trial submission on 335 eyes at 1-year follow-up, with an average of 0.47 D of regression from 3 to 12 months postoperatively, and 56% of eyes at 20/20 or better at 1 year postoperatively.[84] For more details, see Chapter 17 by Dr. Davidorf and Dr. Durrie.

Other potential future applications of CK, in addition to treating hyperopia, may eventually include astigmatism, under corrected hyperopic laser in-situ keratomileusis and photorefractive keratectomy, overcorrected myopic LASIK and PRK, post-cataract astigmatism, closing gaping radial keratotomy incisions, decreasing post-transplant astigmatism, and keratoconus.

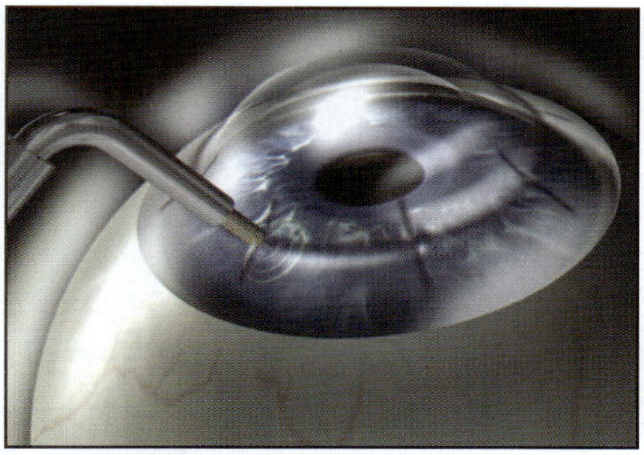

Figure 3-13. Conductive keratoplasty showing a Refractec machine and probe.

Diode Thermal Keratoplasty

Diode laser thermal keratoplasty (DTK) involves individual coagulation spots that are placed peripherally around the optic center with the contact handpiece of a continuous-wave (CW) diode laser. Applied energy is modulated based on preoperative corneal thickness measurements; therefore, spots reportedly penetrate at a more predictable corneal depth. Collagen within the spots shrinks, tightening the ring of spots like a belt, which pushes up the central cornea. This technology is being commercially developed by ProLaser Medical Systems (Germany).

The technology was developed at the University Eye Hospital in Tübingen, Germany. After DTK received the CE Mark in Europe in 1998, it was commercially available in Europe in 2000, and US clinical trials are planned.

Corneal Inlays

In reviews of this subject, Choyce[85] and Lane and Lindstrom[86] discussed their early work with fenestrated intracorneal lenses made of polysulfone. They reviewed the early work in this field, which dates back to 1949. At that time, Barraquer originated the idea of placing intracorneal lenses made of flint glass (6 mm in diameter) and tested these lenses in rabbits and cats. Despite modifications and the use of other materials such acrylic, there was a loss of transparency with vascularization and extrusion of lenses.[87] Knowles suggested that the degeneration of the stroma and epithelium anterior to the intracorneal lenses was caused by interference with diffusion of metabolites and the selective desiccation of the corneal epithelium anterior to the lens. Epithelial integrity may be maintained by nutrients from the aqueous.[88] This led to the fenestration of polysulfone intracorneal lenses, which led to better metabolic diffusion but a significant number of nebular opacities. A more recent approach includes the use of high water-content hydrogels.[89] These lenses allow diffusion of metabolites and are well tolerated.

The newest development of this technology involves a microporous hydrogel lens centered over the pupil under a lamellar flap. This technology is being commercially developed under the name PermaVision intracorneal lens by Anamed (Lake Forest, Calif).

The lens, designed to treat hyperopia from +1.00 D to +6.00 D, is 5 mm in diameter and the edge is beveled to less than 10 µm. Thicknesses range from 25 to 60 µm, determining the degree of correction. Its water content is similar to the cornea, approximately 78%.

The lens has received the CE mark in Europe, where Anamed hopes to launch the product and start FDA clinical trials soon. Although the PermaVision lens appears suitable for monovision applications, Anamed plans to develop a multifocal lens. Investigators also are studying lens versions for myopia.

Dr. Stephen Kaufman and Dr. Herbert Kaufman will be expanding on this innovation in Chapter 18.

Another derivation of this type of technology involves a photoablative inlay (PAI) that is placed under a lamellar flap. This inlay is then ablated with the use of an excimer laser, based on the patient's refraction. This technology was developed by Dr. Gholam A. Peyman, and is being commercially developed by Stromax Technologies (Pittsboro, NC).

Lenticular Implants

Clear Lens Extraction

Intraocular lens (IOL) correction of hyperopia has also joined with cataract technology to produce a surgical technique termed clear lens extraction for hyperopia. This procedure entails removing the normally functioning, non-cataractous lens with phacoemulsification through a scleral tunnel. An IOL of the appropriate power is then inserted and placed in the capsular bag. This procedure was first reported for myopia by Fukala in 1889[90] and applied to hyperopia by Lyle and Jin in 1994.[91] This and subsequent studies[92,93] provide encouraging possibilities for correcting high degrees of hyperopia with the safety and precision of cataract technology.

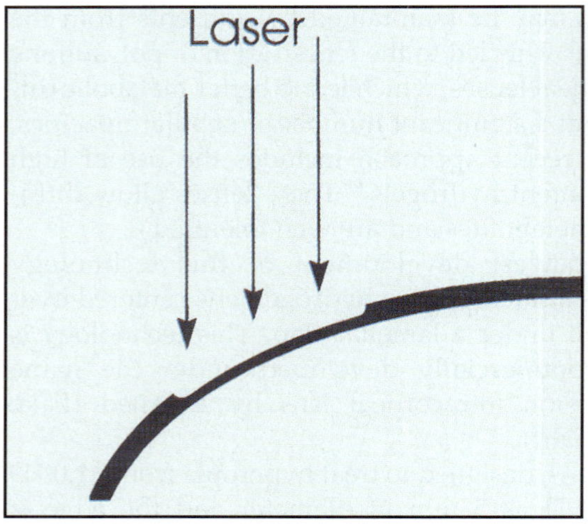

Figure 3-14. Hyperopic laser correction with peripheral tissue ablation.

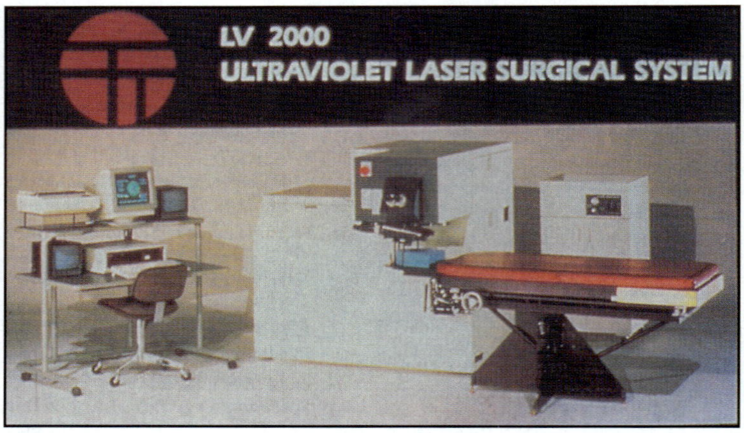

Figure 3-15. Early prototype excimer laser, Taunton Technologies, LV 2000 introduced in 1989.

Phakic Intraocular Lenses

Phakic lenses have been in development for well over a decade, while a single design has yet to achieve widespread acceptance.

Currently, several lenses are being commercially developed. The Staar Surgical (Monrovia, Calif) Implantable Contact Lens is lathe-manufactured from a proprietary porcine collagen/HEMA known as Collamer. The lens is foldable, enabling insertion through a small incision (3 mm), and is placed in the posterior chamber. Data reported from the Phase III clinical trial reveal that postoperatively, 40% of eyes had an uncorrected visual acuity of 20/20 or better.[94]

Ophtec (Boca Raton, Fla) is developing the Artisan lens, which are made of Perspex CQ-UV and PMMA materials, with uniquely designed haptics that hook into the iris. European data demonstrates reasonable safety and predictability for various levels of hyperopia.[95,96]

IOLTech (France) is developing the Vivarte/GBR, which is a foldable phakic anterior chamber lens. This lens is made of hydrophilic acrylic with PMMA haptic and soft foot plates for three-point fixation. Bausch & Lomb's (Rochester, NY) NuVita phakic lens (placed in front of the iris) an angle-supported anterior-chamber rigid PMMA. Medennium (Irvine, Calif), with Ciba Vision, is also developing a phakic lens called the phakic refractive lens (PRL).

Excimer Laser Surgery

The most common procedure for correcting hyperopia is with the use of the excimer laser. The initial application of this technology was hyperopic photorefractive keratectomy, termed H-PRK. Francis L'Esperance first proposed the principle of hyperopic correction with the laser in 1983.[97,98] In excimer laser surgery, a 193-nm argon fluoride (ArF) excimer laser beam is used to ablate superficial tissue and create a central corneal steepening, resulting in a more hyperopic eye (Figure 3-14). Similar work was done with the early prototypes of the VISX laser. The Taunton LV 2000 excimer laser, pictured in Figure 3-15, an early prototype excimer laser, had a rotating series of apertures with an expanding central area, which shielded the center of the cornea and allowed for a peripheral ablation (Figure 3-16). Sher et al in 1991[99] described a technique using the Taunton (Monroe, CT) LV 2000 excimer laser in which a peripheral steepening using the laser is performed after the central cornea is treated to remove scars. This technique, called a "unity cut," reduced the amount of hyperopic shift seen after the central cornea is treated. A similar technique can be performed with the Summit excimer laser by using a masking agent such as methylcellulose in the central cornea.

The mechanism for ablating the peripheral tissue varies with laser manufacturers. Techniques for creating a peripheral ablation range use a variety of techniques from wide area ablations with central

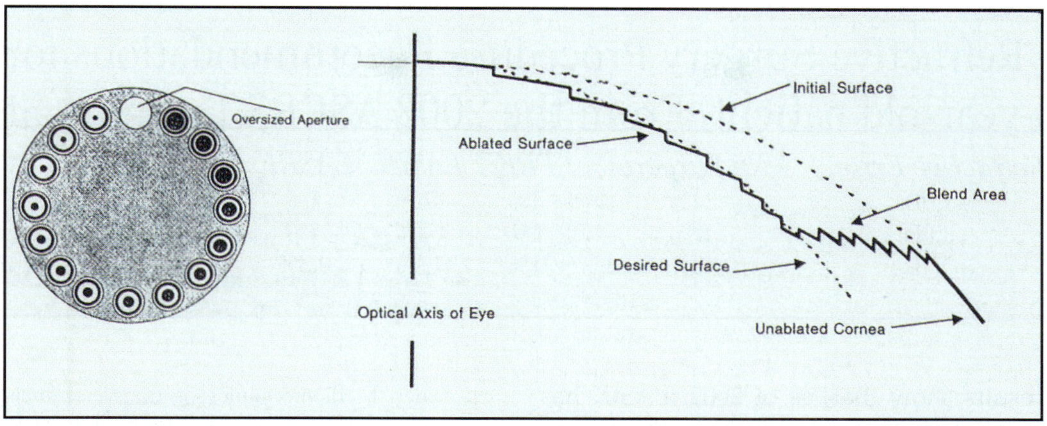

Figure 3-16. Schematic of hyperopic correction wheel in Taunton Technologies LV 2000. Series of apertures with expanding central masked area steepened peripheral cornea.

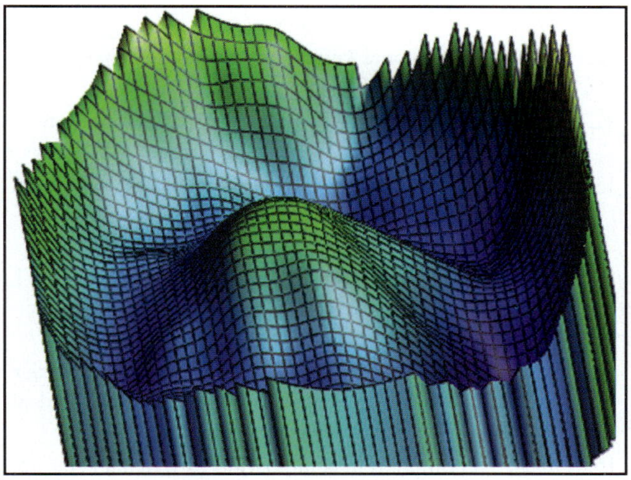

Figure 3-17. A 3-dimensional profile of a wavefront ablation shape that is intended to correct hyperopia and presbyopia refractive errors. (VISX Inc, Santa Clara, Calif.)

corneal sparing to scanning slit, flying spot, blocking agents, and masks.

Clinical investigations of PRK with hyperopia were initiated in 1991 by Dausch, Klein and Anschutz and reported in 1993.[100] This report corrected 15 low hyperopic eyes (+2.00 to +7.50 D) to +0.53 D and 8 highly hyperopic eyes (+11.00 to +16.00 D) to +2.50 D. Regression between 1 and 9 months was +0.70 D for the low group and +3.0 D for the high group. Anschutz[101] acquired similar data in unpublished reports of 81 hyperopic eyes.

Regression of effect, undercorrection and a higher complication rate presents the greatest problem to the effectiveness of hyperopic PRK. Deep ablations created in the periphery of highly hyperopic patients induce epithelial hyperplasia and other healing patterns that reduce predictability. Postoperative haze is also more of a problem with hyperopic PRK than with myopic PRK.

LASIK has also been advocated for hyperopia and is the most widely practiced procedure to address hyperopia today.[102]

Results for hyperopic LASIK[103-106] are very similar to those for hyperopic PRK but refractive stability occurs sooner with less regression, and there is less discomfort and follow-up.[107] LASIK may solve the problems of epithelial hyperplasia and is believed to control some of the healing problems associated with hyperopic PRK. It is for these reasons that hyperopic LASIK is the current preferred procedure. A review of the literature by Nagy[108] led to the conclusion that the refractive results, efficacy, and predictability depend more on the type of excimer laser beam delivery system than on the refractive procedure used (PRK or LASIK).

The next step in the development of hyperopic LASIK is the use of wavefront driven ablations. Results of these ablations will be reported on in Chapter 10 by Dr. Jackson. These ablations may allow for a better centered hyperopic shape to be created on the cornea, along with compensation for existing higher order aberrations within the patient's visual system. Figure 3-17 is an example of a wavefront ablation pattern.

Summary

In a 2002 survey conducted by Dr. David Leaming with members of the American Society of Cataract and Refractive Surgery, respondents were asked to give their recommendations for refractive surgery on various refractive candidates. The results are summarized in Table 3-1.

Table 3-1

Refractive Surgery Procedure Recommendations for a 45-year-old patient, From the 2002 ASCRS Leaming Study[102]

Refractive Error	*No Surgery*	*PRK*	*LASIK*	*LASEK*	*LTK*	*CLE*	*Wait*
+1.0D	24%	1%	46%	1%	14%	0.8%	13%
+3.0D	8%	1%	64%	1%	5%	5%	16%
+5.0D	13%	1%	18%	0.3%	1%	26%	41%

These results show that, as of 2002, LASIK has become the predominant procedure for the correction of low and moderate hyperopia, while clear lens exchange is preferred for higher levels of hyperopia. Approximately one-third of surgeons would delay or not operate on low levels of hyperopia, while over half of surgeons would delay or not operate on high levels of hyperopia.

This chapter has reviewed the numerous surgical techniques, attempted over the last 100 years to treat hyperopia and presbyopia. A number of procedures have been tried and abandoned due to a variety of problems. The study of these past investigations and failures is very valuable in choosing the best approaches to this problem and much research remains to be done.

References

1. Casebeer JC. Hyperopia. In Roy FH, ed. *Master Techniques in Ophthalmic Surgery*. Philadelphia: Williams & Wilkins Co; 1995.
2. Bores LD. *Refractive Eye Surgery*. Boston: Blackwell Scientific Publications; 1993.
3. Casebeer JC, Phillips SG. Hexagonal keratotomy: an historical review an assessment of 46 cases. *Ophthalmology Clinics of North America*. 1992;5(4):727-744.
4. Waring GO. Development and classification of refractive surgical procedures. In: Waring GO, ed. *Refractive Keratotomy for Myopia and Astigmatism*. St. Louis: Mosby-Yearbook;1992;145.
5. Mendez A. *Hyperopia Correction With Hexagonal Keratotomy*. Presented at the Keratorefractive Society Symposium, San Francisco; 1985.
6. Gilbert ML, Roth AS, Friedlander MH. Corneal flattening by shallow circular trephination in human eye bank eyes. *Refractive Corneal Surgery*. 1990;6:113.
7. Yamashita T, Gaster R. *Experimental Hyperopia Correction I and Experimental Hyperopia Correction II*. Presented at Keratorefractive Society Symposium, Chicago; 1983.
8. Thornton SP. Astigmatic keratotomy: a review of basic concepts with case reports. *J Cataract Refract Surg*. 1990;16:430.
9. Seiler T. Biomechanics of transverse incisions of the cornea. In: Waring G, ed. *Refractive Keratotomy for Myopia and Astigmatism*. St. Louis: Mosby-Year Book; 1992;863.
10. Casebeer JC, ed. *A System of Precise, Predictable Keratorefractive Surgery*. Course Manual, Flagstaff, AZ; 1992.
11. Grady SJ. Hexagonal keratotomy for corneal steepening. *Ophthalmic Surgery*. 1988;19:622.
12. Jensen RP. Experience with hexagonal keratotomy. *J Cataract Refract Surg*. 1988;14:580.
13. Neumann AC, McCarty GR. Hexagonal keratotomy for correction of low myopia: preliminary results of a prospective study. *J Cataract Refract Surg*. 1988;14: 265-269.
14. Yamashita T, Schneider MD, Fuerst, DJ, Pearce WJ. Hexagonal keratotomy reduces hyperopia after radial keratotomy in rabbits. *J Refract Surg*. 1986; 2:261-264.
15. Yamashita T, Gaster R. *Experimental Hyperopia Correction I and Experimental Hyperopia Correction II*. Presented at Keratorefractive Society Symposium, Chicago; 1983.
16. Gills J. Trephination in combination with radial keratotomy for myopia. In: R Schacher et al, eds. *Radial Keratotomy*. LAL: Dennison; 1980.
17. Mendez A. *Advances in the Hyperopia Correction With Hexagonal Keratotomy*. Presented at American Society of Cataract and Refractive Surgery meeting. Los Angeles; 1996.
18. Akiyama K, Shibata M, Kanai A, et al. Development of radial keratotomy in Japan, 1939-1960. In: Waring GO, ed. *Refractive Keratotomy for Myopia and Astigmatism*. St. Louis: Mosby; 1992;179.
19. Mendez A. *Hyperopia Reduction With Hexagonal Keratotomy*. Presented at the Keratorefractive Society Symposium; 1988.
20. Neumann AC, McCarty GR, Copello B, et al. Enhanced accuracy as necessary for refractive surgery instrumentation. *J Cataract Refract Surg*. 1989;15:220.
21. Basuk WL, Zisman M, Waring GO, et al. Complications of hexagonal keratotomy. *Am J Ophthalmol*. 1994;117:37-49.
22. Vinger PF, Mieler WR, Oestreicher JM, Easterbrook M. Ruptured globes following radial and hexagonal keratotomy surgery. *Arch Ophthalmol*. 1996;114(2):129-34.

23. McDonnell PJ, Jean JS, Schanzlin DJ. Globe rupture from blunt trauma after hexagonal keratotomy. *Am J Ophthalmol.* 1987:103:241-2.
24. Parmley VC. Ruptured globes following radial and hexagonal keratotomy surgery. *Arch Ophthalmol.* 1996;114(2): 129-134.
25. Jensen RP. Experience with hexagonal keratotomy (letter). *J Cataract Refract Surg.* 1988;14:580.
26. Jensen RP. Hexagonal keratotomy: clinical experience with 483 eyes. *International Ophthalmology Clinics.* 1991;31: 69.
27. Gilbert ML, Friedlander MH, Granet N. Corneal Steepening in human eye bank eyes by combined and transverse keratotomy. *Refractive Corneal Surgery.* 1990; 6:126-30.
28. Nordan LT, Maxwell WA. Avoid both keratotomy with small optical zones and hexagonal keratotomy. *Refractive Corneal Surgery.* 1992;8:331.
29. Grandon SC, Sanders DR, Anello RD, et al. Clinical evaluation of hexagonal keratotomy for the treatment of primary hyperopia. *J Cataract Refract Surg.* 1995;21:140-149.
30. Hollis S. Hexagonal keratotomy. In: Rozakis GW (ed). *Refractive Lamellar Keratoplasty.* Thorofare, NJ: SLACK Incorporated; 1994;84.
31. Werblin TP. Hexagonal keratotomy-should we still be trying? *J Refract Surg.* Mar-Apr 1997; 3(2):128.
32. Ruiz LA. *Lamellar Keratectomy for Hyperopia.* Dallas: Keratorefractive Society; 1987.
33. Casebeer JC. Hyperopia. In: Roy FH, ed. *Master Techniques in Ophthalmic Surgery.* Williams & Wilkins Co; 1995;972-975.
34. Schanzlin DJ, Jester JV, Eunduck K. Cryolathe corneal injury. *Cornea.* 1983;2:51-68.
35. Hollis S. Hyperopic lamellar keratoplasty. In: Rozakis GW, ed. *Refractive Lamellar Keratoplasty.* Thorofare, NJ: SLACK Incorporated; 1994.
36. Casebeer JC, Slade SG, Dybbs A, Mahanti RL. Intraoperative pachymetry during automated lamellar keratoplasty: a preliminary report. *J Refract Corneal Surg.* 1994 Jan-Feb;10(1):41-4.
37. Kezirian GM, Gremillion CM. Automated lamellar keratoplasty for the correction of hyperopia. *J Cataract Refract Surg.* 1995 Jul;21(4):386-92.
38. Hollis S. Hyperopic lamellar keratoplasty. In: Rozakis GW, ed. *Refractive Lamellar Keratoplasty.* Thorofare, NJ: SLACK Incorporated; 1994.
39. Manche EE, Judge A, Maloney RK. Lamellar keratoplasty for hyperopia. *J Refract Surg.* 1996 Jan-Feb;12(1):42-9.
40. Casebeer JC. New nomogram for lamellar keratoplasty for hyperopia. *J Refract Surg.* 1996 Jul-Aug;12:565.
41. Ghiselli G, Manche EE, Maloney RK. Factors influencing the outcome of hyperopic lamellar keratoplasty. *J Cataract Refract Surg.* 1998 Jan;24(1):35-41.
42. Ansari E, Morrell AJ, Sahni K. Corneal perforation and decompensation after automated lamellar keratoplasty for hyperopia. *J Cataract Refract Surg.* 1997 Jan-Feb;23(1):134-6.
43. Kaufman HE, The correction of aphakia. *Am J Ophthalmol.* 1980;89:1-10.
44. Morgan KS, McDonald MB, Hiles DA, et al. The nationwide study of epikeratophakia for aphakia in children. *Am J Ophthalmol.* 1987;103:366-374.
45. Morgan KS, Stephenson GS, McDonald MB, Kaufman HE. Epikeratophakia in children. *Ophthalmology.* 1984;91:780-784.
46. Morgan KS, Asbell PA, McDonald MB, et al. Preliminary visual results of pediatric epikeratophakia. *Arch Ophthalmol.* 1983; 101:1540-1544.
47. Morgan KS, Arffa RC, Marvelli TL, Verity SM. Five year follow-up of epikeratophakia in children. *Ophthalmology.* 1986;93:423-432.
48. McDonald MB, Kaufman HE, Durrie DS, et al. Epikeratophakia for keratoconus. The nationwide study. *Arch Ophthalmol.* 1986;104:1294-1300.
49. Kaufman HE, Werblin TP. Epikeratophakia for the treatment of keratoconus. *Am J Ophthalmol;* 1982;93:342-347.
50. McDonald MB, Koenig SB, Safir A, Kaufman HE. Onlay lamellar keratoplasty for the treatment of keratoconus. *Am J Ophthalmol.* 1983;67:615-618.
51. Kaufman HE, McDonald MB. Refractive surgery for aphakia and myopia. *Trans Ophthalmology Soc UK.* 1984;104:43-47.
52. McDonald MB, Klyce SD, Suarez H, et al. Epikeratophakia for myopia correction. *Ophthalmology.* 1985;92:1417-1422.
53. Werblin TP, Kaufman HE, Friedlander MH, Sehon KL, McDonald MB, Granet NS. A prospective study for the use of hyperopic epikeratophakia grafts for the correction of aphakia in adults. *Ophthalmology.* 1981 Nov;88(11):1137-1140.
54. Dingeldein SA, McDonald MB. Epikeratophakia. *International Ophthalmology Clinics.* 1977;28(2):134-144.
55. Werblin TP, Kaufman HE, Freidlander MH, Granet NS. Epikeratophakia: the surgical correction of aphakia III, preliminary results of a prospective clinical trial. *Arch Ophthalmol.* 1981;99:1957-60.
56. Yamaguchi T, Koenig SB, Kimura T, et al. Histological study of epikeratophakia in primates. *Ophthalmic Surg.* 1984;15:230-235.
57. Goodman GL, Pfeiffer RL, Werblin TP. Failed epikeratoplasty for keratoconus. *Cornea.* 1986;5:29-34.
58. Tamaki K, Yamaguchi T, McDonald MB, Kaufman HE. Histological study of epikeratophakia tissue lenses for myopia removed from two patients. *Ophthalmology.* 1986;93:1502-1508.
59. Binder PS, Baumgartner SD, Fogle JA. Histology of a case of epikeratophakia (aphakic epikeratoplasty). *Arch Ophthalmol.* 1985;103:1357-1363.
60. AMO Keratolens Update. 1987:4(2).
61. Werblin TP, Kaufman HE, Friedlander Mh, MCDonald MB, Sehon K. Epikeratophakia: the surgical correction of aphakia. Update 1981. *Ophthalmology.* 1982;89:916.

62. Safir A, McDonald MB, Klyce SD, et al. The cornea press: restoring donor corneas to normal dimensions and hydration before cryolathing. *Ophthalmic Surg*. 1983;14:327-331.
63. Safir A, McDonald MB, Friedlander MH, et al. Compensating for thermally caused dimensional changes in the cryolathe. *Ophthalmic Surg*. 1984;15:306-309.
64. McDonald MB, Koenig SB, Safir A, et al. Epikeratophakia. The surgical correction of aphakia. Update 1982. *Ophthalmology*. 1983;90:668-672.
65. US patent #4, 662,881, granted May 5, 1987.
66. Ehrlich MI, Nordan LT. Epikeratophakia for the treatment of hyperopia. *J Cataract Refract Surg*. 1989;15:661-666.
67. Friedlander MH, Werblin TP, Kaufman He, Granet NS. Clinical results of keratophakia and keratomileusis. *Ophthalmology*. 1981;88(8):716-720.
68. Arffa RC, Busin M, Barron BA, et al. Epikeratophakia with commercially prepared tissue for the correction of aphakia in adults. *Arch Ophthalmol*. 1986;104:1294-1300.
69. McDonald MB, Kaufman HE, Aquavello JV, et al. The nationwide study of epikeratophakia for aphakia in adults. *Am J Ophthalmol*. 1987;103:358-365.
70. Lans LJ. Experimentelle Untersuchungen uber die Entstehung von Astigmatismus durch nicht-perforierende Conreawunden, Graefes Arch Clin Exp Ophthalmol 1898;45:117-152.
71. Aquavella J. Thermokeratoplasty. *Ophthalmic Surg*. 1976;4:39-48.
72. Gasset AR, Schaw EL, Kaufman HE, et al. Thermokeratoplasty. *Trans Am Acad Ophthalmol*. 1973; 77:441.
73. Kennas R, Dingle J. Thermokeratoplasty for keratoconus. *Ophthalmic Surg*. 1975;6:89-92.
74. Shaw EL, Gasset AR: Thermokeratoplasty (TKP) temperature profile. *Invest Ophthalmol Vis Sci*. 1974;13:181-186.
75. Gasset AR, Kaufman HE. Thermokeratoplasty in the treatment of keratoconus. *Am J Ophthalmol*. 1975;79:226-232.
76. Newmann AC, Sanders D, Raanan M, DeLuca M. Hyperopic thermokeratoplasty: clinical evaluation. *J Cataract Refract Surg*. 1991;17:830-8.
77. Seiler T, Matallana M, Bende T. Laser thermokeratoplasty by means of a pulsed holmium: YAG laser for hyperopic correction. *Refract Corneal Surg*. 1990;6:328.
78. Schachar RA. Radial thermokeratoplasty. *Refract Surg*. 1990;3:47.
79. Moreira H, Campos M, Sawusch MR, et al. Holmium laser thermokeratoplasty. *Ophthalmology*. 1993;100:752-61.
80. Seiler T, Matallana M, Bende T. Leserkoagulation der Hornhaut mit einem Holmium:YAG-Laser zur Hyperopiekorrektur. *Fortschr Ophthalmol*. 1991;88:121-4.
81. Durrie DS, Schumer DJ, Cavanaugh TB. Holmium: YAG laser thermokeratoplasty for hyperopia. *ᴶ Refract Corneal Surg*. 1994;10:S277-80.
82. Thompson VM, Seiler T, Durrie DS, Cavanaugh TB. Holmium:YAG laser thermokeratoplasty for hyperopia and astigmatism: an overview. *Refract Corneal Surg*. 1993;9:S134-7.
83. Vinciguerra P, Kohnen T, Azzolini M, et al. Radial and staggered treatment patterns to correct hyperopia using noncontact holmium:YAG laser theral keratoplasty. *J Cataract Refract Surg*. 1998;24:21-30.
84. McDonald MB, Hersh PS, Manche EE, et al. Conductive keratoplasty for the correction of low to moderate hyperopia: US clinical trial 1-year results of 355 eyes. *Ophthalmology*. 2002;109:1978-89.
85. Choyce DP. Intra-cameral and intra-corneal implants. A decade of personal experience. *Trans Ophthalmol Soc UK*. 1966;86:507-525.
86. Lane SS, Lindstrom RL. Polysulfone intracorneal lenses. *Int Ophthalmol Clin*. 1991;31:37-46.
87. Barraquer, JI. Queratoplastia refractive. *Estudios Inform Oftal Inst Barraquer*. 1949;10:2-21.
88. Knowles WF. Effect of intralamellar plastic membranes on corneal physiology. *Am J Ophthalmol*. 1961;51:1146-1156.
89. McCarey BE, Andrews DM. Refractive keratoplasty with intrastromal hydrogel lenticular implants. *Invest Oph Vis Sci*. 1981;21:107-115.
90. Fukala V. Surgical treatment of high degrees of myopia through aphakia. *Graefes Arch Ophthalmol*. 1890;36:230-244.
91. Lyle WA, Jin GJ. Clear lens extraction for the correction of high refractive error. *J Cataract Refract Surg*. 1994;20:273-276.
92. Obstbaum SA. Clear lens extraction for high myopia and high hyperopia. *J Cataract Refract Surg*. 1994;20:271.
93. Siganos DS, Siganos CS, Pallikaris IG. Clear lens extraction and intraocular lens implantation in normally sighted hyperopic eyes. *J Refract Corneal Surg*. 1994;10:117-124.
94. Bloomenstein MR, Dulaney DD, Barnet RW, et al. Posterior chamber phakic intraocular lens for moderate myopia and hyperopia. *Optometry*. 2002;73:435-46.
95. Alio JL, Mulet ME, Shalaby AM. Artisan phakic iris claw intraocular lens for high primary and secondary hyperopia. *J Refract Surg*. 2002;18:697-707.
96. Dick HB, Alio J, Bianchetti M. Toric phakic intraocular lens: European multicenter study. *Ophthalmology*. 2003;110:150-62
97. L'Esperance FA Jr. *Ophthalmic Lasers*. 2nd ed. St. Louis: Mosby-Year Book. 1989;892.
98. L'Esperance FA Jr, Warner JW, Telfair WB, et al. Excimer laser instrumentation and technique for human corneal surgery. *Arch Ophthalmol*. 1988;107:131-139.
99. Sher NA, Bowers RA, Zabel RW, et al. The clinical use of the 193 nm excimer laser in the treatment of corneal scars. *Arch Ophthalmol*. 1991;109:491-497.
100. Dausch D, Klein R, Schroder E. Excimer laser photorefractive keratectomy for hyperopia. *J Refract Corneal Surg*. 1993;9:20-28.
101. Dausch D, Landesz M. The Aesculap-Meditec excimer laser: results from Germany. In: Salz JJ, ed. *Corneal Laser Surgery*. St. Louis: Mosby; 1995.

102. Leaming, DV. Practice styles and preferences of ASCRS members-2001 survey. *J Cataract Refract Surg.* 2002;28:1681-1688
103. Salz JJ, Stevens CA. LASIK correction of spherical hyperopia, hyperopic astigmatism, and mixed astigmatism with the LADARVision excimer laser system. *Ophthalmology.* 2002;109:1647-56; discussion 57-8.
104. Lian J, Ye W, Zhou D, et al. Laser in situ keratomileusis for correction of hyperopia and hyperopic astigmatism with the Technolas 117C. *J Refract Surg.* 2002;18:435-8.
105. Ditzen K, Fiedler J, Pieger S. Laser in situ keratomileusis for hyperopia and hyperopic astigmatism using the Meditec MEL 70 spot scanner. *J Refract Surg.* 2002;18:430-4.
106. Pineda-Fernandez A, Rueda L, Huang D, et al. Laser in situ keratomileusis for hyperopia and hyperopic astigmatism with the Nidek EC-5000 Excimer laser. *J Refract Surg.* 2001;17:670-5.
107. el-Agha MS, Johnston EW, Bowman RW, et al. Excimer laser treatment of spherical hyperopia: PRK or LASIK? *Trans Am Ophthalmol Soc.* 2000;98:59-66; discussion -9.
108. Nagy ZZ, Munkacsy G, Popper M. Photorefractive keratectomy using the Meditec MEL 70 G-scan laser for hyperopia and hyperopic astigmatism. *J Refract Surg.* 2002;18:542-50.

Chapter Four

Preoperative Evaluation of the Prospective Hyperopic Refractive Surgery Patient

William Trattler, MD and James Salz, MD

Introduction

Surgical options for hyperopes have expanded over the last decade. Many of these surgical options have become more predictable and less risky than their predecessors (automated lamellar keratoplasty [ALK] or hexagonal keratotomy [HK]). However, even with these modern surgeries, there are serious risks associated with surgery. Selecting patients who are good candidates for surgery can reduce the chance of a poor surgical outcome. The goal of this chapter is to help provide a framework for a thorough evaluation of patients considering refractive surgery. It is important to understand that modern refractive surgery is a rapidly changing field, so it is imperative for readers to also follow the literature for breaking information that may impact patient selection.

Although myopic refractive surgery is dominated by the excimer laser, there are many other viable surgical options for hyperopes. Besides photoreactive keratotomy (PRK), laser-assisted epithelial keratectomy (LASEK), and laser-assisted in-situ keratomileusis (LASIK), surgeons can choose to perform laser thermokeratoplasty (LTK), conductive keratoplasty (CK), clear lens extraction (CLE), and phakic intraocular lenses (IOLs). Also, there are other surgeries under evaluation including the intracorneal lens.

Patient Evaluation

Determination of a patient's candidacy for surgery requires the active involvement of the surgeon, as the results of the preoperative testing are critical for determining which surgical option (if any) is best for the patient. Although the surgeon can delegate certain tests, it is important for the surgeon to be actively involved to ensure that testing is performed accurately. Throughout the preoperative evaluation, the exams performed will help identify patients with either absolute or relative contraindications to surgery.

The preoperative evaluation should also be an educational process for patients. Patients should be educated on the types of surgery available along with the limits of these surgeries and the risks involved with each surgery. Because every form of hyperopic refractive surgery has risks that range from mild to life altering, it is critical that patients have a complete understanding of the risks involved. For example, many studies on hyperopic LASIK report that even without a surgical complication, there is a 1% to 5% risk of loss of two lines of best corrected visual acuity (BCVA).[1,2] Also, it is important to identify patients who have unrealistic expectations or who are unwilling to accept any level of risk.

Patient Expectations/Goals

A thorough understanding of a patient's home and work environments is critical for determining whether a patient will benefit from hyperopic refractive surgery. Care should be taken to understand the reasons a patient desires refractive surgery and to make sure that these expectations are reasonable. In addition, patients need to be willing to accept a level of risk to reach their goals. If patients have unrealistic expectations or are unwilling to accept risk, then hyperopic refractive surgery may not be an option.

Ocular History

A thorough ocular history is a vital part of the preoperative evaluation. A variety of ocular conditions will alter the candidacy of patients considering refractive surgery. For example, patients with a history of ocular herpes simplex virus (HSV) may be poor candidates for refractive procedures on the cornea. The ocular history may also provide important information that will allow the surgeon to zero in on key preoperative tests. For example, patients with a history of contact lens intolerance may have significant dry eye, and thus be poor candidates for LASIK.

Ocular Infections

A controversial area in refractive surgery is the candidacy of patients with a history of ocular herpes. Animal studies by Dhaliwal have shown that the excimer laser can initiate the recurrence of HSV in the eye.[3] Dhaliwal has also shown that oral anti-viral agents can reduce but not eliminate the risk of recurrence of ocular HSV after excimer laser treatment.[4]

A number of reports have documented recurrence of ocular HSV following LASIK, PRK, and PTK.[5-7] Patients with a history of HSV may also have decreased corneal sensation, and when coupled with decreased corneal sensation following LASIK, may be at high risk for a serious complication. For example, Biser and Donnenfeld[8] have documented a series of patients with a history of ocular HSV who developed serious ocular complications, including corneal perforations, following LASIK. With this information, many refractive surgeons recommend against corneal refractive procedures (PRK/LASIK) in patients with a history of ocular HSV.

Although no HSV-related complications have been reported following LTK or CK in the peer-reviewed literature, one would expect that these corneal surgeries might also place a patient with previous ocular HSV at increased risk of a complication. Also, phakic IOL and clear lens extraction surgeries can potentially initiate a recurrence of HSV, so a thorough discussion of the potential risks should be presented to the patient.

History of Strabismus

Patients with a history of strabismus are of great concern to surgeons considering refractive surgery. Patients with a history of strabismus who have undergone successful eye muscle surgery in the past have been reported to develop a recurrence of their strabismus after LASIK.[9] Patients with diplopia due to ocular misalignment at the time of their preoperative evaluation should be informed that refractive surgery will not eliminate their need for prisms. Because eye muscle surgery can alter the corneal topography and refractive error, it is important for patients to consider having their strabismus corrected surgically prior to having refractive surgery.[10-12] Another concern for patients with a history of strabismus is that they may have a strong fixation preference for their dominant eye. This strong fixation preference may prevent a patient from being able to change fixation to their nondominant eye for reading following surgery for monovision.

Research has been performed to see whether hyperopic LASIK can help the ocular alignment of patients with accommodative esotropia. A recent study found that although the amount of esodeviation was reduced in 58% of patients following LASIK, it was impossible to determine preoperatively which patients would respond.[13] Therefore as a therapeutic tool, refractive surgery requires further evaluation to determine which patients with accommodative esotropia will obtain benefit.

Monocular Patients

Patients with significant amblyopia or other causes of poor vision in one eye should be considered less than optimal candidates for refractive surgery. Current methods of hyperopic refractive surgery have a low complication rate. However, a complication in the only "good" eye could jeopardize the ability of a patient to function a normal life. If a patient feels that he or she could potentially function with their "poor" eye in the case of serious complication in their good eye, then elective refractive surgery can be considered.

It is critical that monocular patients have the risks thoroughly explained, and even a trial of functioning with just the poor eye can be helpful for a patient to understand the potential consequences of a bad outcome.

History of Keloid Formation

Although a history of keloid formation was originally thought to be a risk factor for haze with PRK, various reports have confirmed that both LASIK and PRK can be performed in patients with a history of keloid formation.[14,15]

Contact Lens History

A complete contact lens history is vital to the preoperative evaluation. Many patients desire refractive surgery due to intolerance to their contact lenses. This group of patients requires careful evaluation of their dry eye state, as significant dry eyes before surgery may be a factor in considering intraocular or surface procedures rather than LASIK. One study reported that patients with significant dry eyes prior to surgery were much more likely to develop severe dry eyes after LASIK.[16]

The time that patients last wore their contact lenses is a critical question to ask on the preoperative exam. Both hard and soft contact lenses can significantly alter the corneal curvature and refraction of patients. Therefore, patients need to be advised that they must stop their use of contact lenses from weeks to months, depending on the type of contacts that they wear. For example, patients with rigid contact lenses can require many weeks to months for their corneas to relax into their natural state. During this process, it is important to perform serial examinations of the refraction and topography to document the point of stability. Patients who wear regular soft contact lenses generally need to be out of their contact lens for 1 to 2 weeks, while patients wearing soft toric contact lenses may require a few weeks for their corneal curvature and refraction to stabilize.

One important caveat for hard contact lens users is that their vision after LASIK may not be as crisp as they are used to. It is important to discuss this issue, as they may prefer methods of surgical correction that do not alter the cornea, such as phakic IOLs or clear lens extraction.

Presbyopia

Many patients considering hyperopic refractive surgery are over the age of 40. One common method for retaining near vision with refractive surgery is to target one eye for distance and the other eye for near (monovision). Because up to 20% of patients will not tolerate monovision, it is critical to perform a contact lens trial of monovision to determine whether the patient can adjust. Otherwise, patients may be subjected to surgery only to find out that they cannot adapt to monovision.

Another potential method for addressing presbyopia is the use of a multifocal IOL with clear lens extraction. In general, hyperopes tend to respond better to the array multifocal IOL (Allergan, Irvine, Calif) than myopes. However, some patients do not tolerate the multifocal lens, as it can cause bothersome nighttime visual symptoms. Therefore, extensive preoperative counseling is critical for patients considering multifocal IOLs.

Pregnancy/Breast Feeding

The altered hormonal levels that occur with pregnancy or during the postpartum period can significantly alter the refractive error. This hormonal alteration is prolonged in women who are breast-feeding. Therefore it is recommended to allow a few months after pregnancy or breast-feeding before determining the final refractive error that will be used in corrective surgery. Serial examinations that document stability are helpful at finding the point at which surgery can be performed.

High-Risk Activities

The alteration of the eye from refractive surgery can place a patient at risk of a complication in various high-risk activities. For example, boxers and martial artists should avoid LASIK due to the risk of a traumatic flap dislocation. PRK, CK, and LTK do not appear to structurally alter the strength of the eye. Phakic IOLs and clear lens extraction require an incision that can be the weak spot with direct trauma.

Medicines

Our knowledge into the types of medications that can affect the outcome of refractive surgery continues to evolve. Retinoic acid (Retina A [Johnson and Johnson, Raritan, NJ]) and oral antihistamines can be very drying to the eye, and can negatively impact the results of excimer laser treatments. Imitrex (GlaxoSmithKline, Philadelphia, Pa), a migraine medication, can cause corneal opacities and epithelial defects in dogs.[17] There is concern that Imitrex could affect corneal wound healing, so avoidance of this medication is recommended around the time of laser refractive surgery. Similar concerns have been raised about amiodarone, which can cause superficial corneal changes, possibly a problem with LASIK.

Medical Conditions

Diabetes, active autoimmune diseases (lupus, rheumatoid arthritis), and immunodeficiency states (HIV) can all potentially affect the outcome of refractive surgery. It is important to perform a complete medical history and determine whether there are any underlying conditions that could potentially affect the results of hyperopic refractive surgery.

Previous Radial Keratotomy

Radial keratotomy (RK), a popular form of refractive surgery for myopes in the 1980's, resulted in a large number of patients with secondary hyperopia. Numerous studies have looked at surface ablation and LASIK for post-RK hyperopes.[18-24] In general, these studies have found that although a large number of patients can have improvement of their hyperopia with these surgeries, the risk of a complication is higher in post-RK eyes as compared to virgin eyes. In particular, studies found that there was an increased risk of haze with surface ablation surgery while there was an increased risk of epithelial ingrowth and DLK following LASIK. Many surgeons report difficulty trying to lift the LASIK flap when attempting a LASIK enhancement on post-RK eyes.

Alternatively, intraocular surgeries may be a viable option on post-RK eyes. Thus the optimal refractive surgery for post-RK patients has yet to be determined.

Recent Refractive Surgery

A large group of patients undergoing hyperopic refractive surgery consists of those patients who have recently undergone myopic or hyperopic PRK/LASEK/LASIK but ended up on the hyperopic side. Although patients typically have high expectations and can be demanding of rapid visual rehabilitation, it is critical for surgeons to be patient and wait for refractive and topographic stability. Although 3 months can be a good target, there are many patients that take 6 months or longer to stabilize following their excimer laser surgeries. Therefore, it is important to determine that patients have reached stability, such as with two exams showing similar refractions and topographies a few weeks apart, before proceeding with additional refractive surgery.

Preoperative Examination

Visual Acuity

Uncorrected and corrected visual acuity should be measured. Patients with preoperative best-corrected visual acuity of 20/15 may be disappointed if their final visual acuity is 20/25. Therefore, it is important to determine whether patients preoperatively have 20/15 or better vision with their glasses/contacts.

It is also important that surgeons understand that although Snellen visual acuity is a useful way to measure the improvement of vision following refractive surgery, it is basically a test of high-contrast visual function. Many patients who have had refractive surgery may find that although they can read the 20/20 Snellen line, their quality of vision is in certain ways diminished. Further testing such as contrast sensitivity and wavefront measuring may be helpful in determining the true status of their postoperative vision.

Refraction

Refraction should be performed early in the preoperative exam before a patient has received drops or has had instruments touch the cornea. A cycloplegic refraction is essential to identify patients with latent ciliary hypertonus.

The level of hyperopia and hyperopic astigmatism is critical in the determination of which refractive surgery can be considered. LTK and CK are procedures designed for low degrees of hyperopia without astigmatism. PRK, LASEK, and LASIK are most effective with lower refractive errors. With increasing amounts of hyperopia, the LASIK success rate drops.[25] Many studies reveal a significant increase of loss of two or more lines of BCVA when treating patients with 5 or more diopters of hyperopia with LASIK.[26,27] Patients with higher degrees of hyperopia may benefit from clear lens extraction or phakic IOLs.

Because the refraction will dictate the magnitude of the refractive surgery, it is important to emphasize that the examiner should refrain from increasing minus lenses if no additional letters are read and should stress that the goal of refraction is to achieve the very least minus correction for best vision.

The vertex distance must also be measured carefully, because surgical alterations of the corneal refraction are necessarily performed at the corneal plane.

Contrast Sensitivity

Contrast sensitivity is a technique that can be used in addition to Snellen visual acuity to characterize a patient's visual function. A number of studies have shown that contrast sensitivity can be reduced following both PRK and LASIK.[28-32] These studies have shown that contrast sensitivity testing improves over 6 to 12 months after surgery, but there is slower recovery in patients with higher degrees of refractive correction.

Keratometry

Manual keratometry can be useful as part of the examination as the quality of the keratometric mires is a very sensitive indicator of irregular astigmatism both pre- and postoperatively. Many surgeons opt to use the corneal topography instead of the manual keratometry.

Computed Topography and Orbscan

Corneal topography is an important component of the preoperative evaluation, as there are a number of patients that will have completely normal preoperative exams except for the corneal topography. The corneal topography screens for corneal abnormalities, such as keratoconus, forme-fruste keratoconus, pellucid marginal degeneration, or other forms of irregular astigmatism (Figures 4-1A, B, C, D, and E). It is important to note that although patients with these ocular conditions are generally myopic, these conditions can occur in hyperopes. These corneal abnormalities are typically contraindications to excimer laser treatments.

The corneal topography provides information on the overall steepness of the cornea. This information is useful for determining whether a patient may be at risk for flap complications such as buttonholes (increased risk with steeper corneas) or free flaps (increased risk with flatter corneas).[33] Corneal topography along with the level of the preoperative level of hyperopia is important in determining whether a person will end up with an abnormally steep cornea, which can affect the quality of the postoperative visual acuity.

The Orbscan (Bausch & Lomb, Rochester, NY) is a very useful corneal topography unit, as it is able to measure both the anterior and posterior surfaces of the cornea, as well as provide corneal thickness information. Certain experts feel that the Orbscan's measurement of the "posterior float" is useful at screening patients who may be at risk for ectasia (see Figure 4-1B). However, there are currently no controlled studies that have determined the risk a person with an increased posterior float has for developing ectasia after LASIK.

Pupil Exam

Pupil size evaluation is critical to the evaluation of a patient for any form of refractive surgery. Large pupils are an important risk for postoperative night vision problems for patients of the same refractive error. These nighttime problems, which include glare, halos, and starbursts, can occur after excimer laser (LASIK, PRK) and intraocular (phakic IOL) surgeries.

Preoperative pupil testing provides the necessary information for a surgeon to advise a patient on their risks of visual quality parameters after PRK, LASEK, and LASIK. Hyperopic excimer laser treatments are performed by creating a steep area in the central cornea. The width of the optical zone created by hyperopic excimer laser treatments can be small, resulting in problems for patients with large pupils.

To provide patients with an understanding of their risk of nighttime vision problems, it is critical determine the natural maximum dilation of the pupil. Surgeons and patients should be aware that the pupil size is dynamic, and stress/anxiety can affect the measured size of the pupil.[34] Though there are a variety of methods to measure pupil size, the type of method used is not the critical issue.[35,36] The key issue is for the measurement to be performed in a pitch-black environment. Also, accurate measurement requires that the patient fixate at a distance target, because accommodation causes pupillary miosis.

A wide variety of instruments and techniques are available to measure the maximum dilation of the pupil in darkness. A simple technique is to use the pupil gauge of a Rosenbaum near vision card to measure the pupil size. This technique can be accurate if care is taken to shine a dim amount of illumination from the side so that the size of the pupil can be measured without the light influencing the pupil size. Another simple technique is to use the cobalt blue filter on the slit lamp and measure the pupil size by adjusting the slit beam length.[36] Examples of infrared pupil measuring devices are seen in Figures 4-2A, B, C, and D. Hand-held pupillometers, the Colvard pupillometer and Keeler pupillometer (Philadelphia, Pa), are also commonly used devices to measure the scotopoc pupil size (Figures 4-2A and B). These devices allow the user to view the pupil in pitch darkness. One important issue is that it is still possible to mismeasure the pupil with these devices if the pupillometer distance from the eye is too far or too near.

For those refractive surgeons looking for even more precision in their ability to measure the largest pupil size in darkness, there are a number of new devices that are currently available. These include the Procyon (Keeler) (Figures 4-2C and D) and the PowerRef II (PlusOptix, Germany). When patients with large pupils are identified, the surgeon must discuss in detail the risks of nighttime vision problems so that the patient can make an informed decision as to whether to undergo surgery. Patients should be informed that for the same pupil size, their risk of nighttime vision problems after excimer laser increases with higher levels of hyperopia (as the

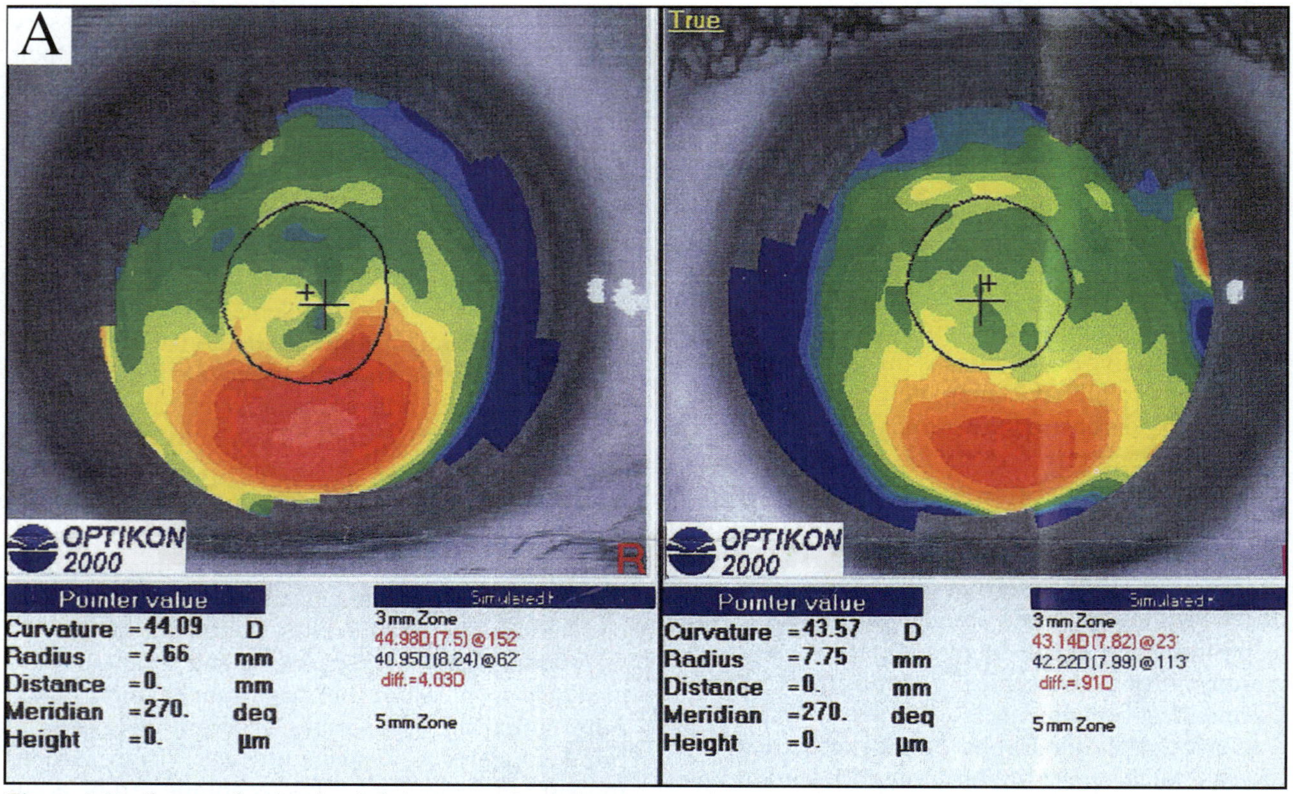

Figure 4-1A. Topography showing inferior steepening in keratoconus (courtesy of Patricia Kuster, MD).

Figure 4-1B. Orbscan showing elevated posterior float of patient with keratoconus.

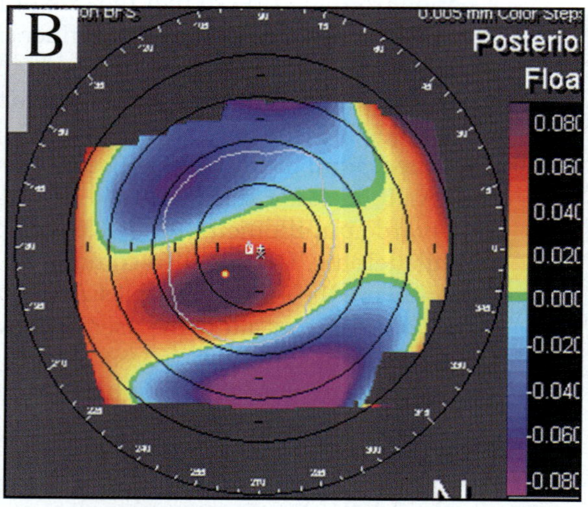

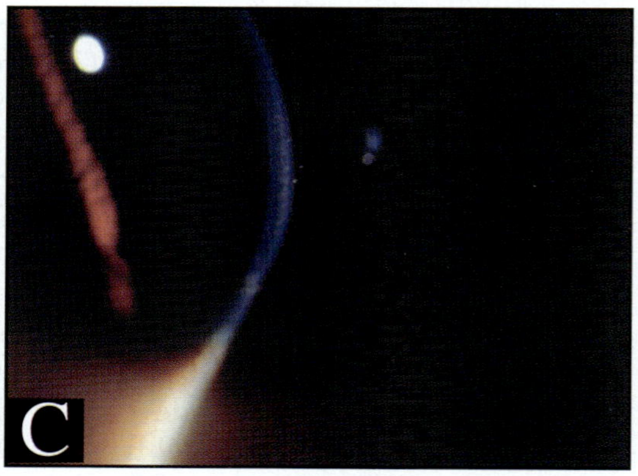

Figure 4-1C. Slit lamp photo of cornea in pellucid marginal degeneration showing corneal thinning (courtesy of Dr. David Hardten).

Figure 4-1D, E. Corneal image and topography of pellucid marginal degeneration (courtesy of Dr. David Hardten).

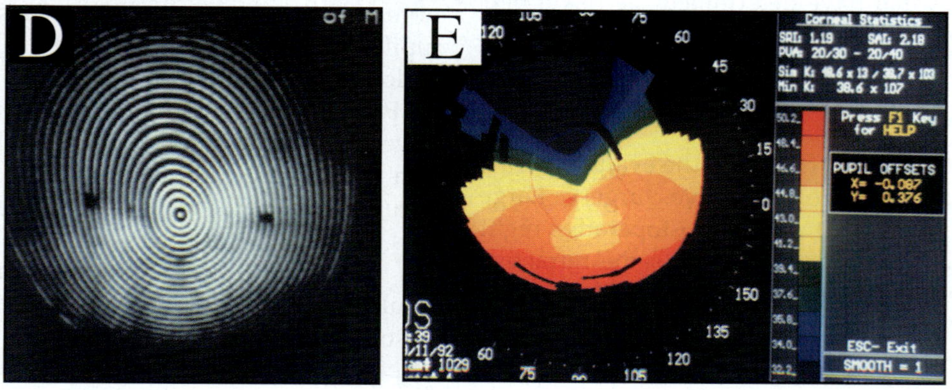

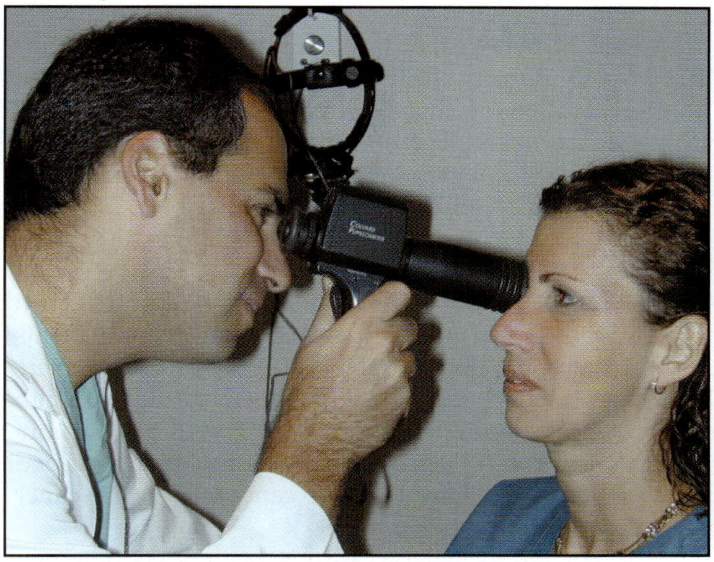

Figure 4-2A. Colvard pupillometer.

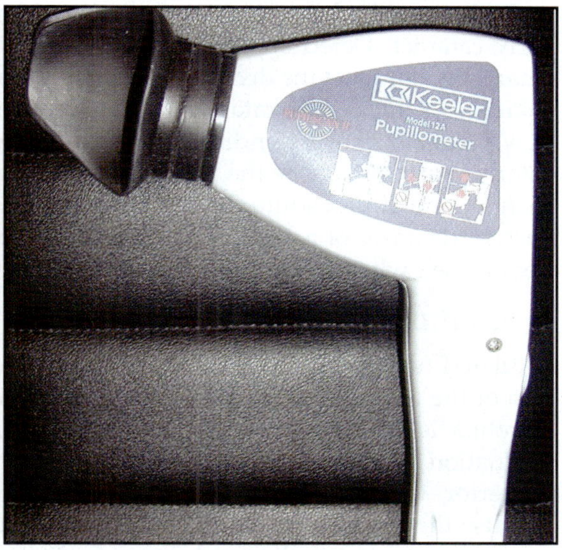

Figure 4-2B. Keeler pupillometer.

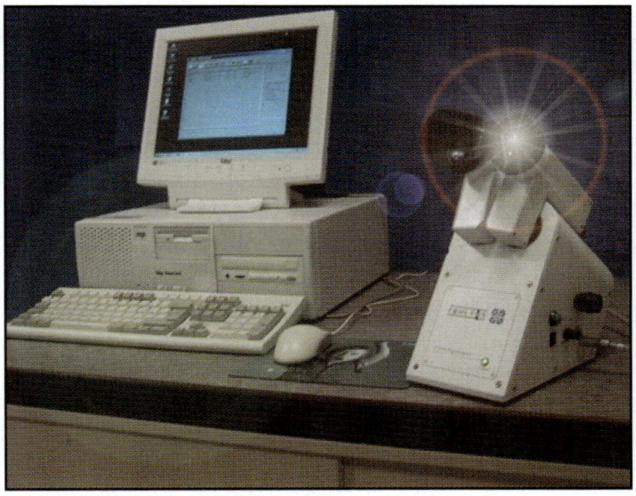

Figure 4-2C. Procyan pupillometer.

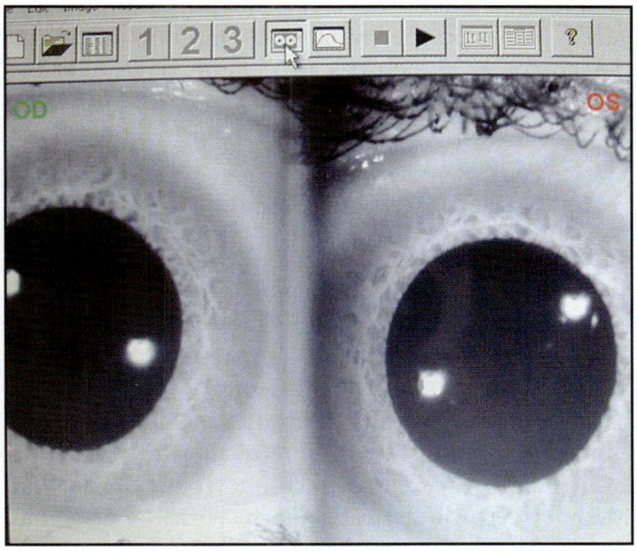

Figure 4-2D. Procyan pupillometer (pupil view).

optical zones created will be smaller). Patients can be offered surgery one eye at a time, so that the patient can determine whether the degree of postoperative visual problems is acceptable.

For patients considering intraocular surgery, the pupil size is critical to determining whether the edge of the optic of the IOL is smaller than the nighttime pupil size, as exposure of the optic edge can cause significant nighttime visual symptoms. Although current phakic IOLs for hyperopia tend to have small optics, it is hoped that future versions will have larger optics that will allow patients with larger pupils to be potential candidates for this type of surgery.

Slit Lamp Examination

A thorough slit lamp evaluation of the anterior segment of the eye is a critical part of the preoperative evaluation. The presence of anterior basement membrane disease, stromal scarring, or vascularization can impact the type of refractive surgery chosen. Also, the presence of thinning of the cornea from conditions such as Terrien's degeneration, keratoconus, or pellucid degeneration can be a contraindication to corneal refractive surgery. Endothelial dysfunction, as evidenced by guttata, swelling of the cornea, and Descemet's membrane haze are warning signs that both intraocular and corneal surgery can place a patient at risk for postoperative corneal decompensation.[37] These patients should of course undergo further testing, such as with endothelial cell density measurements and pachymetry.

Evaluation of the crystalline lens may reveal an early cataract. Determination of the severity of the cataract will impact the decision making process. For example, a moderate cataract, which reduces the BCVA to 20/25 may indicate that early elective cataract surgery may be the preferred surgery rather than a corneal procedure. Because phakic IOLs can hasten the onset of a cataract, they should typically not be used when a significant cataract is present.

Fundus Examination

A dilated fundus examination that includes evaluation of the optic nerve, macula retina, and peripheral retina is an important part of the preoperative evaluation. Also, documentation of the presence of a posterior vitreous detachment (PVD) is helpful, because there are some claims that the suction from a microkeratome may be a risk factor for PVDs.

Even if no peripheral retinal problems are discovered in the hyperopic eye, it is still important to educate patients on the signs and symptoms of retinal detachments. Hyperopes in general have a lower risk of retinal detachments than myopes. However, intraocular surgery is a risk factor for retinal tears and detachments.

Tonometry

Any patient coming for an ophthalmic evaluation should have their intraocular pressure checked, because there are no symptoms for early open-angle glaucoma. When elevated intraocular pressure is identified preoperatively, the need for treatment must be evaluated. The level of intraocular pressure can influence the success of refractive surgery.[38,39] As well, many researchers have shown evidence that tonometry readings, particularly with the applanation method, can be significantly underestimated after excimer laser surgery as a result of the alteration of the curvature and/or thickness of the cornea.[40,41]

Pachymetry

Accurate ultrasonic pachymetry readings are essential in many forms of refractive surgeries—RK, AK, PRK, and LASIK. Pachymetry readings are important in patients who have had previous corneal surgery and are interested in more surgery. Patients with abnormally thin corneas (490 µm or less) should be advised that they might be at slightly higher risk of developing ectasia with LASIK. Although surface ablation may be an option for very thin corneas, the long-term risk for these patients is still unknown. Therefore, patients with thin corneas may be better candidates for intraocular surgery.

Abnormally thick corneas should have a careful evaluation of their endothelial cell density, as a decreased number of endothelial cells can lead to corneal decompensation following intraocular surgeries and LASIK.[37]

Endothelial Cell Evaluation

Routine endothelial cell evaluation has not been found to be clinically relevant for most patients undergoing laser refractive surgery. However, there are isolated reports of patients ending up with corneal decompensation after LASIK.[37] Therefore patients with Fuch's corneal dystrophy or damaged endothelium may be poor candidates for excimer laser procedures.

For intraocular procedures, healthy endothelium is critical. Candidates for phakic IOLs and clear lens extraction should have a careful evaluation of the endothelium by slit lamp or specular microscopy to make sure that they have sufficient endothelial functional reserve.

Anterior Chamber Depth

Patients considering a phakic IOL must have their anterior chamber depth measured to determine whether there is enough room for the IOL. If the anterior chamber depth is too small, the anterior chamber can be too crowded following the insertion of an IOL.

The anterior chamber depth is also an important measurement for Holladay II formula for IOL calculations in patients undergoing clear lens extraction.

Dry Eye Testing: Schirmer's Test and Tear Break-Up Testing

Dry eyes are one of the most commonly reported symptoms after LASIK. Studies have found that patients can experience dry eye problems after LASIK, with bothersome symptoms lasting well beyond 1 year.[42,43] Patients with symptoms and signs of preoperative dry eye are at higher risk of developing severe post-LASIK dry eye problems.[16] A Schirmer's test measures the quantity of lacrimal secretion over 5 minutes and is useful in diagnosing aqueous tear deficiency. A tear break up time measures the quality of the tear film. Lissamine green or rose bengal staining of the conjunctiva and cornea is a sensitive test for dry eye. Lissamine green is less irritating than rose bengal dye (Figure 4-3A, lissamine green staining, and Figure 4-3B, rose bengal staining).

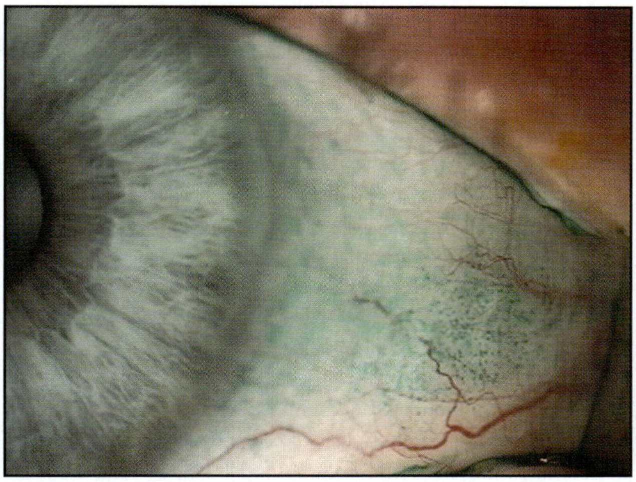

Figure 4-3A. Lissamine green staining bulbar conjunctiva (photo courtesy of Neal A. Sher, MD).

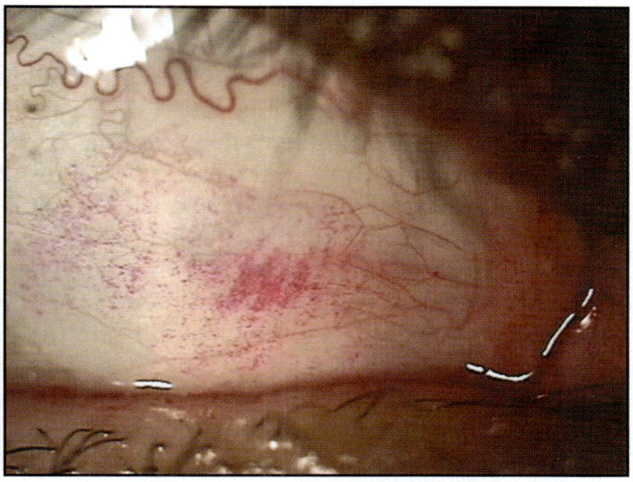

Figure 4-3B. Rose bengal staining bulbar conjunctiva (photo courtesy of Neal A. Sher, MD).

Patients with abnormal test results can be treated preoperatively with lubricants, punctual plugs, warm compresses, lid scrubs, and even Restasis (Allergan, Irvine, Calif) (topical cyclosporin), and later re-evaluated to see if scores improve. Otherwise, patients with abnormal scores are at higher risk of post-LASIK dry eye problems, and may want to consider other forms of refractive surgery (PRK, LASEK, LTK, CK, CLE, or phakic IOLs)

Other tests for dry eyes include the measurement of lactoferrin levels and tear osmosis.

Ocular Dominance Determination

Determination of ocular dominance is done preoperatively to help with monovision trials as well as to see which eye will be treated first when the refractive surgery is performed one eye at a time. If both eyes are to be corrected for distance, it is prudent to start with the nondominant eye to allow any needed adjustments to the treatment parameters of the second eye when only one eye will be treated.

One effective way for determining ocular dominance is to have the patient fixate on a distant object or large letter on the eye chart. The patient views the object while looking through a small aperture held at arm's length. The patient determines the aiming eye by either closing one eye or by bringing the aperture closer to the aiming eye. Once the dominant eye is determined, the surgeon can discuss with the patient whether there is a preference as to which eye should be treated first. Occasionally, the patient will prefer a specific eye such as when one eye is contact lens intolerant.

Wavefront Testing

The science of wavefront testing has finally arrived for practicing ophthalmologists, who are now able to employ this advanced information in a variety of ways. Wavefront measurements can be used during the preoperative evaluation as a screening device. Certain preoperative abnormalities, such as high spherical aberration, may be a contraindication to excimer laser surgery, since conventional LASIK and PRK can raise the overall spherical aberration. Spherical aberration is considered important, as it appears to be the underlying cause for many patients of night glare, halos, and ghosting.

Wavefront technology will hopefully improve the ability to reduce the amount of spherical aberration following LASIK. Wavefront-linked excimer lasers can potentially treat patients and lower (or minimally elevate) their overall spherical aberration. In the meantime, patients with elevated preoperative spherical aberration can consider non-corneal methods of refractive surgery, which hopefully will not raise their underlying aberrations.

Informed Consent

Informed consent is much more than a patient signing a consent form. Informed consent is a process that provides the patient with the information needed to make a determination as to whether to consider refractive surgery. All types of refractive surgery have risks that include the risk of blindness. The informed consent process enables the patient to determine whether the benefits of surgery outweigh the potential risks. This is especially important with refractive surgery, because patients have safe and effective options to surgery, including glasses and contact lenses.

The informed consent process can begin even before a patient arrives in the office. If a patient encounters an advertisement guaranteeing 20/20 vision or "throwing away your glasses," it can result in a patient underestimating the true risk of complications and overestimating the true chances of reaching 20/20. By falsely altering the patient's risk versus benefit thought process, a patient can end up electing to proceed with surgery less than fully informed.

One of the key aspects of the informed consent process is to carefully evaluate the patient and determine his or her particular risks for surgery. The preoperative exam is therefore a critical component of the informed consent process, as it will identify specific issues that will alter a patient's potential risk with surgery. For example, patients with very dry eyes, thin corneas, large pupils, and high refractive errors should be informed that their risks of postoperative problems may be higher than for the average person if they undergo refractive surgery. The preoperative exam thus is critical to determining whether a patient undergoing a particular procedure has factors that put him or her at higher risk for a particular intraoperative or postoperative problem.

Surgeons should be prepared for patients to have false expectations as to the success rate of refractive surgery. These expectations are typically generated by the significant amounts of positive advertisements in the media as well as the favorable reviews of the surgery from friends and families. Therefore, it is critical for the surgeon to fully inform the patient of the risks that come with refractive surgery and ensure that the patient's expectations are reasonable, because there is typically no underlying pathologic condition. Without proper informed consent, surgeons open themselves up to the risk of lawsuits in the event of an untoward complication.

Informed consent documents for various ophthalmic procedures, including all the major refractive surgery procedures can be downloaded free of charge from the Ophthalmic Mutual Insurance Company Web site (http://www.omic.com/resources/risk_man/forms.cfm).

Summary

In summary, the refractive surgeon is the key person to determine whether a patient is a good candidate for hyperopic refractive surgery by performing a complete history, detailed exam, and a careful discussion of the issues involved with surgery.

References

1. Salz JJ, Stevens CA, LADARVision LASIK Hyperopia Study Group. LASIK correction of spherical hyperopia, hyperopic astigmatism, and mixed astigmatism with the LADARVision excimer laser system. *Ophthalmology*. 2002 Sep;109(9):1647-56; discussion 1657-8.
2. Pineda-Fernandez A, Rueda L, Huang D, Nur J, Jaramillo J. Laser in situ keratomileusis for hyperopia and hyperopic astigmatism with the Nidek EC-5000 Excimer laser. *J Refract Surg*. 2001 Nov-Dec;17(6):670-5.
3. Dhaliwal DK, Romanowski EG, Yates KA, Hu D, Goldstein M, Gordon YJ. Experimental laser-assisted in situ keratomileusis induces the reactivation of latent herpes simplex virus. *Am J Ophthalmol*. 2001 Apr;131(4):506-7.
4. Dhaliwal DK, Romanowski EG, Yates KA, et al. Valacyclovir inhibition of recovery of ocular herpes simplex virus type 1 after experimental reactivation by laser in situ keratomileusis. *J Cataract Refract Surg*. 2001 Aug;27(8):1288-93.
5. Davidorf JM. Herpes simplex keratitis after LASIK. *J Refract Surg*. 1998 Nov-Dec;14(6):667.
6. Pepose JS, Laycock KA, Miller JK, et al. Reactivation of latent herpes simplex virus by excimer laser photokeratectomy. *Am J Ophthalmol*. 1992 Jul 15;114(1):45-50.
7. Vrabec MP, Anderson JA, Rock ME, et al. Electron microscopic findings in a cornea with recurrence of herpes simplex keratitis after excimer laser phototherapeutic keratectomy. *CLAO J*. 1994 Jan;20(1):41-4.
8. Biser SA, Perry HD, Donnenfeld ED, at al. *Herpes simplex keratitis following LASIK*. Presented at the ASCRS annual meeting, Philadelphia, June 2, 2002.
9. Schuler E, Silverberg M, Beade P, Moadel K. Decompensated strabismus after laser in situ keratomileusis, *J Cataract Refract Surg*. 1999 Nov;25(11):1552-3. *Ophthalmology*. 2002 Jun;109(6):1148-53.
10. Hainsworth DP, Bierly JR, Schmeisser ET, Baker RS. Corneal topographic changes after extraocular muscle surgery. *J AAPOS*. 1999 Apr;3(2):80-6.
11. Preslan MW, Cioffi G, Min YI. Refractive error changes following strabismus surgery. *J Pediatr Ophthalmol Strabismus*. 1992 Sep-Oct;29(5):300-4.
12. Denis D, Bardot J, Volot F, Saracco JB, Maumenee IH. Effects of strabismus surgery on refraction in children. *Ophthalmologica*. 1995;209(3):136-40.
13. Stidham DB, Borissova O, Borissov V, Prager TC. Effect of hyperopic laser in situ keratomileusis on ocular alignment and stereopsis in patients with accommodative esotropia. *Ophthalmology*. 2002 Jun;109(6):1148-53.
14. Tanzer DJ, Isfahani A, Schallhorn SC, LaBree LD, McDonnell PJ. Photorefractive keratectomy in African Americans including those with known dermatologic keloid formation. *Am J Ophthalmol*. 1998 Nov;126(5):625-9.
15. Epstein, R. Results of Internet poll on outcome of LASIK in keloid formers. *J Refract Surg*. 2000 May-Jun;16(3):380-1.

16. Toda I, Asano-Kato N, Hori-Komai Y, Tsubota K. Laser-assisted in-situ keratomileusis for patients with dry eye. *Arch Ophthalmol*. 2002;120:1024-1028.
17. *Physician's Desk Reference*. 2000;54:1204-1205.
18. Francesconi CM, Nose RA, Nose W. Hyperopic laser-assisted in-situ keratomileusis for radial keratotomy induced hyperopia. *Ophthalmology*. 2002 Mar;109(3):602-5.
19. Clausse MA, Boutros G, Khanjian G, Wagner C, Garabet AL. A retrospective study of laser in-situ keratomileusis after radial keratotomy. *J Refract Surg*. 2001 Mar-Apr;17(2 Suppl):S20.
20. Portellinha W, Nakano K, Oliveira M, Simocelli R. Laser in situ keratomileusis for overcorrection after radial keratotomy. *J Refract Surg*. 2000;16 (suppl):S253-S256.
21. Probst LE, Machat JJ. Conservative photorefractive keratectomy for residual myopia following radial keratotomy. *Can J Ophthalmol*. 1997 Feb;32(1):25-30.
22. Gimbel HV, Sun R, Chin PK, van Westenbrugge J. Excimer laser photorefractive keratectomy for residual myopia after radial keratotomy. *J Cataract Refract Surg*. 1996 Sep;22(7):901-5.
23. Nordan LT, Binder PS, Kassar BS, Heitzmann J. Photorefractive keratectomy to treat myopia and astigmatism after radial keratotomy and penetrating keratoplasty. *J Refract Surg*. 1997 Aug;13(5 Suppl):S456.
24. Venter JA. Photorefractive keratectomy for hyperopia after radial keratotomy. *J Refract Surg*. 1997 Aug;13(5 Suppl): S456.
25. Cobo-Soriano R, Llovet F, Gonzalez-Lopez F, Domingo B, Gomez-Sanz F, Baviera J. Factors that influence outcomes of hyperopic laser in situ keratomileusis. *J Cataract Refract Surg*. 2002 Sep;28(9):1530-8.
26. Choi R, Wilson S. Hyperopic laser in-situ keratomileusis. *Cornea*. 2001;20(4):388-393.
27. Lindstrom RL, Hardten DR, Houtman DM, et al. Six month results of hyperopic and astigmatic LASIK in eyes with primary and secondary hyperopia. *Trans Am Ophthalmol Soc*. 1999;97:241-60.
28. Nagy ZZ, Munkacsy G, Krueger RR. Changes in mesopic vision after photorefractive keratectomy for myopia. *J Refract Surg*. 2002 May-Jun;18(3):249-52.
29. Montes-Mico R, Charman WN. Mesopic contrast sensitivity function after excimer laser photorefractive keratectomy. *J Refract Surg*. 2002 Jan-Feb;18(1):9-13.
30. Chan JW, Edwards MH, Woo GC, Woo VC. Contrast sensitivity after laser in situ keratomileusis one-year follow-up. *J Cataract Refract Surg*. 2002 Oct;28(10):1774-9.
31. Nakamura K, Bissen-Miyajima H, Toda I, Hori Y, Tsubota K. Effect of laser in situ keratomileusis correction on contrast visual acuity. *J Cataract Refract Surg*. 2001 Mar;27(3):357-61.
32. Stevens JD, Ficker LA. Results of photorefractive keratectomy for hyperopia using the VISX star excimer laser system. *J Refract Surg*. 2002 Jan-Feb;18(1):30-6.
33. Gimbel, HV, Penno, EEA. *LASIK Complications: Prevention and Management*. Thorofare, NJ: SLACK Incorporated; 1998; 54-57.
34. Loewenfeld IE. Anatomy and physiology. In: Loewenfeld IE, Lowenstein O, eds. *The Pupil: Anatomy, Physiology, and Clinical Applications*. Iowa City: Iowa State University Press; 1993; 498-510.
35. Frauenfelder FT. *Drug Induced Ocular Side Effects and Drug Interaction*. 2nd ed. Philadelphia: Lea & Febiqer; 1989.
36. Starck T, Liu Y, Prewett AL, G Curup L. Comparison of scotopic pupil measurement with slitlamp-based cobalt blue light and infrared video-based system. *J Cataract Refract Surg*. 2002 Nov;28(11):1952-6.
37. Vroman DT, Solomon KD, Holzer MP, Peng Q, Apple DJ, Bowie EM. Endothelial decompensation after laser in situ keratomileusis. *J Cataract Refract Surg*. 2002 Nov; 28(11):2045-9.
38. Feldman ST, et al. The effect of increased intraocular pressure on visual acuity and corneal curvature after radial keratotomy. *Am J Ophthalmol*. 1989;108:126-129.
39. Whitacre MM, Stein RA, Hassanein K. The effect of corneal thickness on applanation tonometry. *Am J Ophthalmol*. 1993 May 15;115(5):592-6.
40. Simon G, Small RH, Ren Q, Parel JM. Effect of corneal hydration on Goldmann applanation tonometry and corneal topography. *Refract Corneal Surg*. 1993 Mar-Apr;9(2):110-7.
41. Mardelli PG, Piebenga LW, Whitacre MM, Siegmund KD. The effect of excimer laser photorefractive keratectomy on intraocular pressure measurements using the Goldmann applanation tonometer. *Ophthalmology*. 1997; June 104 (6): 945-8; discussion 949.
42. Battat, L, Macri, A, Dursun, D, Pflugfelder, S. Effects of laser in situ keratomileusis on tear production, clearance, and the ocular surface. *Ophthalmology*. 2001;108:1230-1235.
43. Albietz JM, Lenton LM, McLennan SG. Effect of laser in situ keratomileusis for hyperopia on tear film and ocular surface. *J Refract Surg*. 2002 Mar-Apr;18(2):113-123.

Chapter Five

Contact Lens Use for Hyperopia

Gayla Rowland, MD and Charles B. Slonim, MD, FACS

Hard contact lenses made of polymethylmethacrylate (PMMA) were the first contact lenses introduced into the US market in the early 1950's. Bausch & Lomb (Rochester, NY) introduced the first soft hydrogel lenses in 1971. By the early 1980's gas permeable acrylate materials began to dominate the rigid lens market. Lenses made of pure silicone were available in mid-1980's. Although not popular in the general contact lens practice due to their poor wettability, silicone lenses are still used in the treatment of aphakia in children because of their superior oxygen permeability. The highly oxygen-permeable, silicone hydrogel lenses were introduced in 1999. These lenses combined the best features of both the soft hydrogel and silicone lenses into one material.

Prior to the development of refractive surgical techniques for hyperopia, the only options for refractive correction were spectacles or contact lenses in the phakic individual and spectacles, contact lenses or intraocular lenses (IOLs) in the aphakic individual. Correction of a phakic infant or child was usually done with spectacles due to the reliability of the correction fixed in a frame and the lack of dependency on an adult to insert a contact lens into a child's eye. Aphakic children were frequently fitted in silicone contact lenses.

Children with accommodative esotropia typically require bifocal spectacles to prevent the eyes from converging at both distance and near viewing lengths. When the pre-presbyopic hyperope develops asthenopic symptoms of eye fatigue and blurred vision, they typically seek out the help of an eyecare professional. Having never worn spectacles in the past, these hyperopes frequently dislike wearing spectacles and quickly inquire about the possibility of wearing contact lenses.

There are a number of reasons why the hyperopic patient may want to wear contact lenses. Contact lenses have a distinct optical advantage for some patients in addition to the cosmetic benefit and the convenience of not having to wear glasses. Contacts offer the advantage of a larger corrected field of vision than spectacles and lack of distortion when looking through the peripheral portion of the lens.[1]

The hyperopic or "farsighted" eye is either anatomically too short in its axial length or does not possess sufficient refractive power to bring images into focus sharply on the retina.[2] In the hyperopic eye, light is focused at a point behind the retina, or at the secondary focal point.[3] The crystalline lens has the inherent ability to increase its refractive power and bring this focal point from behind the retina onto the retina. This ability is referred to as "accommodation" or "focusing."

The emmetropic adult is typically born with a hyperopic (ie, small axial length) eye. The tremendous accommodative power of an infant or child can easily compensate for small to moderate amounts of hyperopic refractive error. The greater the hyperopic refractive error, the greater the accommodative effort needed to bring a distant object into focus. Large accommodative efforts typically cause a simultaneous convergence of the eyes. This convergence or esotropia is frequently the first sign of moderate to high hyperopia in an infant or child (ie, accommodative esotropia).

Hyperopes without presbyopia constantly accommodate to bring distant objects into focus onto their retinas. They may go for many years without visual complaints. They are commonly referred to as "latent" hyperopes. As they lose their accommodative ability with the onset of presbyopia, the farsightedness becomes "manifested." It is not uncommon for the latent hyperope to become symptomatic in their early to mid-thirties. Some hyperopes may not have the accommodative power needed for a greater amount of hyperopia. These persons will manifest their hyperopic refractive error earlier than others. Correction of their hyperopic refractive error with contact lenses or spectacles frequently eliminates these symptoms.

The loss of the crystalline lens (aphakia) creates a relatively high hyperopic refractive error requiring correction with spectacles, contacts lenses or intraocular lenses. Aphakia is typically the most severe form of refractive hyperopia that the eyecare professional has to deal with. When the insertion of intraocular lenses during cataract surgery became the standard of care in the early 1980's, the numbers of aphakic patients has diminished considerably. Secondary intraocular lens implantation into aphakic patients has further lowered the aphakic population in the United States.

The refractive correction of a hyperopic eye can be provided by placing a convex or converging "plus" lens in front of the eye.[4] By converging the light rays before they reach the cornea, the focus point is moved forward onto the retina instead of behind the retina. Correcting the hyperopia of a young patient with accommodative esotropia frequently relaxes the convergence of the eyes and reduces, sometimes eliminating, the esotropia. This can be accomplished with contact lenses as well as with spectacles.

Latent hyperopes, on the other hand, who have never worn corrective lenses of any sort, may not accept the "total" amount of correction necessary to correct their hyperopic refractive error. A pre-presbyopic patient may not tolerate the "full" correction if they have become accustomed to their "accommodative" effort for focusing on distant objects. Frequently, only a portion of the total refractive error is given to the patient in some form of a corrective lens (ie, contact lens or spectacle). Pre-presbyopic patients typically require a cycloplegic refraction to determine the full refractive error followed by a post-cycloplegic refraction to determine the amount of correction that the patient will tolerate.

Aniseikonia is a difference in perceived image size in the two eyes resulting in asthenopic symptoms and distortions of binocular space perception.[5] Aniseikonia induced by a strong prescription in only one eye (eg, in unilateral aphakic correction) is also minimized by contact lenses. Because the lens is moved closer to the cornea (ie, reducing vertex distance), the magnification created by a convex spectacle lens is markedly reduced and almost eliminated.

The perceived image size is a product of both the image size on the retina and mapping of photoreceptors through the visual pathways all the way to the occipital cortex.[1] The latter can be affected by the space between the retinal photoreceptors. In axial myopia, the photoreceptors are further apart. In axial hyperopia, they are closer together. Shortening the vertex distance decreases the magnification created by a plus (convex) lens and decreases the minification of image size by a minus (concave) lens. contact lenses can improve aniseikonia induced by anisometropic correction by minimizing this vertex distance. The actual effect on image size is directly influenced by the magnitude of the refractive error.

Another advantage of a contact lens used in this regard is elimination of induced optical anisophoria when looking through the non-axial portion of the lens. Anisophoria is caused by the prismatic effect of the spectacles when there is a difference in the correction between the two eyes. Optical anisophoria can also lead to distortions of space perceptions and to asthenopic symptoms.[6] For example, a plus (convex) lens causes a relative magnification of image size. Structurally, it represents two back-to-back, base-in prisms with the bases aligned down the central visual axis. When viewing through a peripheral portion of a plus lens in either right or left gaze, the lens' prismatic effect will cause images to be displaced more peripherally.

In the case of bilateral axial myopia and unilateral aphakia, wearing a contact lens in the phakic eye also can further minimize residual aniseikonia. The contact lens increases the image size by reducing the minification effect compared to myopic spectacles. In pre-existing hyperopia, however, the magnification in the aphakic eye is reduced by the contact lens.

To further reduce aniseikonia, the phakic hyperopic eye can be corrected by increasing the vertex distance with glasses to maximize the image size.

The vertex distance is the distance between the correcting lens and the front of the cornea.[2] The "spectacle lens plane" is the plane in which the lens is worn. The position of this plane may vary depending upon factors such as the patient's facial anatomy, the design of the frame of the glasses, and how the patient prefers to wear the glasses. There can be a significant change in lens power for a relatively small change in distance. Smaller power lenses are less affected by the vertex distance and are often small enough to be disregarded. When refractions are measured with a phoropter, the vertex distance present between the phoropter and the cornea must be taken into account when converting to a contact lens prescription where the vertex distance is virtually zero.

No single style or design of contact lens will fit all hyperopic patients. Due to marketing concerns, most contact lens manufacturers produce their hyperopic parameters for a specific design of lens sometime after their myopic parameters are released. Currently, the hyperopic patient has available virtually the same variety of contact lenses as does the myopic patient. Hyperopic parameters are available in disposable lenses, toric lenses, multifocal lenses and even tinted and cosmetic lenses.

The fitting of a contact lens on a hyperopic patient does not require special techniques, considerations or skills than those required for the myopic patient. From a fitting standpoint, the hyperopic cornea is slightly flatter on average than a myopic cornea. Soft contact lens fitting sets with hyperopic parameters generally come with slightly flatter base curves. Flatter corneal surfaces can also act on lens movement, especially with rigid lens fits. The flatter the corneal surface, the more difficult it is to get a rigid lens to fit in the center of the cornea. Fitting gas permeable lenses with larger diameters under the upper lid allows the upper lid to hold and support the lens between and during blinks. Occasionally the edge of the lens requires modification in order to help the lid hold the lens up. Creating a myoflange edge puts a base out prism at the periphery of the lens. This thickened lens edge makes it easier for the lid to hold the lens up.

There are basically two major classes of contact lenses: soft and rigid. Rigid lenses can be further subdivided into hard lenses made of PMMA and gas permeable lenses made of a variety of both silicone and fluorosilicone acrylate polymers. Each class of lens has its own set of advantages and disadvantages.

Rigid Lenses

Rigid lenses are initially uncomfortable and require a period of adaptation. Soft lenses are more comfortable initially and require a very little, if any, period of adaptation.

Of the 35 million US contact lens wearers in 2001, 87% wore soft lenses and 13% wore rigid lenses (down from 17% in 1998). Rigid gas permeable (RGP) lenses now account for almost all rigid lenses prescribed in the United States. According to Health Products Research (HPR, West Trenton, NJ) data, RGP lenses accounted for 7.6% of the 14.3 million "new fit/refit" patient visits in 2001, while soft lenses accounted for 92.3% of new fit/refits last year.[7]

The PMMA contact lens has two main advantages: durability and superior optical quality. PMMA lenses are fairly scratch and deposit resistant. They rarely change their physical parameters (warp) over time. Their parameters can be changed or modified by office personnel with modification equipment frequently found in the office of a contact lens practice. The optical quality of PMMA is superior to all other contact lens materials. Crisp vision is constant during, before, and after blinking. Hyperopic powers have always been available in PMMA.

The main problem with PMMA lenses is that they are impermeable to oxygen and have the potential to cause corneal hypoxia. Lens-induced corneal edema creates the symptom of spectacle blur. This blur represents the change in vision that occurs from the time that the patient removes their contact lens from their cornea to the time their vision with spectacles returns to normal. In order to prevent corneal hypoxia, PMMA lenses are fit small. This enhances their movement on the cornea, which allows for more tear flow to oxygenate the cornea.

Gas permeable lenses include a variety of plastic polymers that are physically more flexible than PMMA lenses but, more importantly, these materials allow oxygen to permeate the lens. These lenses do not depend on blinking as the sole source of oxygen for the cornea. These lenses can be made larger for better stability and have the advantage of being more comfortable than PMMA lenses. Hyperopic gas permeable lenses are available in toric, bitoric, bifocal, and multifocal designs. Unfortunately, these materials are easily prone to scratches and surface deposits. Over time, gas permeable lenses can warp, which changes their physical parameters. Because of their flexibility on the ocular surface, they can change their curvature during blink over an aspheric cornea or one with a moderate to severe amount of astigmatism. This curvature change during each blink is known as vaulting.

Soft Lenses

Soft lenses are considered significantly more comfortable than rigid lenses. These hydrogel polymer plastics contain various quantities of water, which makes these lenses oxygen permeable and very comfortable. Soft lenses require virtually no adaptation—even on new patients who have never worn a lens before. These flexible contact lenses are less successful in correcting higher amounts of cylinder. Soft toric contact lenses correct the astigmatic error by maintaining a specific rotational orientation. Rotational misalignment with larger amounts of astigmatism can cause significant visual distortions.

Soft lenses are available in a variety of extended wear, daily wear, tinted, costume, and therapeutic designs. The currently available toric, bifocal, and multifocal designs, in a variety of hyperopic powers have successfully been fitted on many new patients who thought they would never be able to find a contact lens that met their refractive needs.

Lenses are produced by a number of manufacturers in a wide range of hyperopic powers. Daily and extended wear soft lenses are available up to +20.00 D (eg, Durasoft 2 Clear MTO [Ciba Vision, Duluth, Ga], Hydrasoft DW Sphere [Cooper Vision, Irvine, Calif]). Disposable lenses (eg, Soflens One Day [Bausch and Lomb, Rochester, NY], 1-Day Acuvue [Johnson and Johnson, Jacksonville, Fla], Focus Dailies [Ciba Vision]) are available up to +6.00 D of spherical correction. Astigmatic correction is available in soft lenses up to -10.00 D of cylinder with up to +20.00 of sphere (eg, Hydrasoft Toric Div IV DW [Cooper Vision]).

Soft bifocal lenses are produced in conventional wear, disposable wear and daily disposable wear. Spherical powers up to +6.00 D and add powers up to +2.50 D are available (eg, Sunsoft Additions [Albuquerque, NM], Acuvue Bifocals [Johnson and Johnson]).

With this range of hyperopic parameters in both the rigid and soft lens materials, there are very few patients who are unable to find a lens with their refractive needs. It is the responsibility of the patient to seek out this non-surgical, time-honored method of vision correction prior to a surgical correction. It is the responsibility of the refractive surgeon to inform each potential hyperopic refractive patient that the wearing of contact lenses is a reasonable alternative treatment of hyperopic correction.

References

1. Miller et al. Optics, refraction, and contact lenses: Section 3. In: Liesegang MD, Deutsch TA, Grand MG, eds. *Basic and Clinical Science Course 2001-2002*. San Francisco, Calif: The Foundation of the American Academy of Ophthalmology; 2001:117-122,172-199.
2. Rubin ML. *Optics for Clinicians*. Gainesville, Fla: Triad Scientific Publishers; 1974:138-145.
3. Yanoff M. *Ophthalmology*. 1st ed. St. Louis: Mosby International; 1999:2.8,2.11,3.1.
4. Milder B, Rubin ML. *The Fine Art of Prescribing Glasses Without Making a Spectacle of Yourself*. Gainesville, Fla: Triad Scientific Publishers; 1978:5-17,276-296.
5. Enoch JM. Management of aniseikonia after IOL implantation or refractive surgery. *J Refract Surg*. 1997;13:79-82
6. *Vision Science III - Ocular Motility and Binocular Vision—Lecture 16—Aniseikonia I*. Available at: http://arapaho.nsuok.edu/-salmonto/VSIII_/Lecture16.doc. Accessed February 9, 2003.
7. *OptiStock Market Watch. Contact Lens Market: Specialty Lenses and Favorable Demographics Are Driving Growth Worldwide*. Contact Lens Report; November 2002.

Section Two

Hyperopia Surgery Using the Excimer Laser (PRK, LASEK, and LASIK)

Chapter Six

PRK AND LASEK FOR HYPEROPIA: TECHNIQUES, POSTOPERATIVE MANAGEMENT, AND RESULTS

Robin F. Beran, MD, FACS

INTRODUCTION

The ability to surgically alter the shape of the cornea for the correction of hyperopia and hyperopic astigmatism has presented much greater challenges for refractive surgeons than that same ability to correct myopia. Using the excimer laser to simply flatten the central cornea with the removal of stromal tissue is easier than trying to steepen it by the removal of mid-peripheral tissue. The epithelium's capacity to thicken and fill in over the surgical stromal defect is more efficient peripherally than centrally.

As seen in Chapter 3, early attempts to correct hyperopic refractive errors with incisional keratotomy found limited success. There was a reduction in the degree of hyperopia; however, this was at the expense of corneal stability and an unacceptable high incidence of irregular astigmatism. These two problems along with its poor predictability were responsible for its demise.

In 1983 Dr. Stephen Trokel and Dr. Srinivasan's introduction of the excimer laser for use in corneal refractive surgery marked the beginning of corneal laser surgery. Dr. Seiler in 1985 performed photorefractive keratectomy (PRK) on a blind eye in Berlin, Germany. In May 1988, Dr. McDonald performed the first PRK on a sighted eye in the United States. Approval by the US Food and Drug Administration (FDA) of the United States for the treatment of myopia with PRK occurred in 1995. PRK treatment for 1 to 6 D of hyperopia with less than 1 D of astigmatism with the VISX laser was received in 1998, 3 years after the approval for myopia. At the time of the writing this chapter, the Technolas and Nidek lasers have not yet received FDA approval for use in hyperopia.

This chapter is intended to look at PRK and laser-assisted epithelial keratectomy (LASEK) for the correction of hyperopia and hyperopic astigmatism. The characteristics discussed about these two procedures will provide insight as to their comparison with the lamellar procedure, laser-assisted in-situ keratomileusis (LASIK). However, it is not the intent of this discussion to debate a superiority of surface ablation versus lamellar laser surgery. The advantages and disadvantages of PRK and LASEK are put forth to permit the reader to judge the merits of each. Through this critical analysis the reader should then be able to apply the philosophy of choosing the optimal procedure for each individual patient.

CURRENT TECHNIQUES

Presently, PRK and LASEK comprise the two acceptable forms of surface photoablation for the surgical correction of hyperopia and hyperopic astigmatism.

PRK is the original laser vision correction technique and its basic principles have changed very little since first developed in the mid to late 1980's. LASEK is a recent modification of PRK and debate continues as to its true differences from this original procedure. Dr. Massimo Camellin of Italy should be given the primary credit for its development and increase in popularity.[1] In 1996 Dr. Dimitri Azar utilized a similar procedure but did not promote its use and proposed advantages over PRK for the treatment of myopia.[2]

PRK

The procedural fundamentals for hyperopic PRK are very similar to those for myopic PRK. There are three basic operational stages: first, epithelial removal; second, tissue removal; and third, surface management.

Epithelial removal originally was performed as simple manual mechanical debridement with a blade or spatula. This technique works well except that the individual eye's epithelial adhesiveness can create some variability of surgical time among patients. Consistency in technique is an important aspect in achieving reliable and reproducible results. It continues to be an acceptable form for epithelial removal. A second form of mechanical removal is the use of an Amoil's brush. It decreases the time variability for this stage of the procedure; however, it also requires an increased procedural cost for each disposable brush.

Chemical removal of the epithelium is the other form of debridement used for hyperopic corrections. Most commonly a dilute solution (20% alcohol/ 80% balanced salt solution [BSS]) of 99% dehydrated alcohol is used for 1 minute of epithelial contact time.

Its application may be either with the solution placed into a reservoir of the appropriate diameter (9 to 10 mm) or it can be saturated on a disc-shaped surgical sponge. Solution contact time varies from 20 to 60 seconds. The epithelium is generally easily removed with a surgical sponge or blunt spatula. The advantage of chemical debridement is improving the ability to consistently control the duration of this surgical step. It is also very effective at complete removal of all the epithelial cells, leaving a very clean and smooth Bowman's layer. The disadvantage is using a toxic solution with the potential to damage collateral limbal and epithelial cells.

In myopic PRK, the epithelium may be removed with the laser beam itself. This is termed laser scrape. However, with the larger diameter ablation zone required for hyperopic treatments, it is not utilized for hyperopia. While broad beam lasers tend not to have a large enough diameter beam, scanning lasers require an excessive amount of time and energy, which are also undesirable.

The second stage of stromal tissue removal is obviously performed with the excimer laser and is in the shape of a donut. This permits the central cornea to steepen with the removal of this mid-peripheral stromal tissue. Biomechanical effects are often overlooked and certainly poorly understood.[3] Results have proven best with ablation parameters of either a 5-mm inner diameter and 8-mm outer diameter or a 6-mm inner and 9-mm outer diameter. Smaller inner diameters permit less tissue removal but are associated with poorer visual quality from the smaller optic zone as well as increased regression of the refractive effect.

The actual treatment ablation may be followed by a smoothing ablation. Some surgeons will use a masking solution or gel to assist in improving the quality of the surface. The true effects of this on regression and on the development of haze are still unproven.

Surface management after the ablation is essentially irrigation and drying of the surface followed by placement of a therapeutic soft contact lens (CTL). There has been interest in cooling the ablation bed after and even before the ablation to reduce thermal damage and hopefully reduce the incidence of haze. This can be with chilled BSS in a reservoir or simple irrigation over the corneal surface.

LASEK

The major difference in LASEK when compared to PRK is the management of the epithelium in preparation for the ablation. Instead of completely removing the entire epithelial layer as in PRK, in LASEK an epithelial flap is constructed. The original method has been through chemical denaturing of the epithelium and its adhesion to Bowman's layer. A 20% solution of 99% dehydrated alcohol with BSS or distilled water are the most popular choices. Sterile water can also be used as it is toxic to the epithelial cells. A contact time of 30 to 35 seconds seems to maximize the efficiency of removal but provides a minimum of epithelial cell toxicity. After this length of exposure time, the viability of any epithelial cells is negligible. Dr. Marguerite McDonald has used an alcohol-free technique with methylcellulose gel to create epithelial detachment.[4]

Mechanical construction of the epithelial flap with a special microkeratome has been developed by Dr. Ioannis Pallikaris. The effectiveness and results of these have yet to be established. Attempts to manip-

Table 6-1

Personality Characteristics to Consider

Level of understanding and knowledge about LVC	Expectations
Intelligence and comprehensive ability	Visual/Pain tolerance
Level of anxiety, fears, concerns, and confidence	Impatient, demanding, obsessive, or compulsive
Pleasant, friendly, considerate	Abrupt, abrasive, introverted

ulate a flap of virgin epithelium are complicated by the friability of the tissue. Dr. Eugene Gordon at Medjet (NJ) has developed the capability to create epithelial flaps with a waterjet microkeratome; however, he has found it necessary to denature the epithelium to a more gelatinous consistency to permit its manipulation.

The standard LASEK flap has been hinged, keeping with the same design as for LASIK. However, two different configurations have been designed and are promoted by their respective developers. Dr. Paolo Vinciguerra developed his "butterfly LASEK" technique.[5] Here a thin paracentral epithelial linear defect is created before applying the alcohol solution. The epithelium is then retracted in both the superior and inferior directions to denude the area for ablation. His claims are for better comfort and faster visual recovery due to a more rapid return of re-epithelialization. These benefits need to be confirmed by others before accepting any significant advantage over the standard LASEK technique.

In Dr. McDonald's gel-assisted technique the flap configuration is 4 limbus-based triangular flaps. Theoretically this will improve the re-epithelialization process by providing a larger surface area and accessibility for the centripetally migrating cells. Again, there is not any conclusive data to support a significant superiority of this technique, especially in light of the more difficult technical aspects associated with this procedure.

The actual ablation step is really no different than that for PRK. The epithelial hinge should be outside the ablation area. Protection of the flap itself is of less concern because new cells will most likely grow. A smoothing technique may be used if desired.

The flap is gently repositioned over the ablated area. A small amount of balanced saline or hypertonic saline solution may be used to make this easier. The flap has a tendency to stretch and the edges are simply overlapped. A therapeutic CTL is then placed.

Criteria for Patient Selection

Evaluation

It can be argued that the most important part of the refractive surgery process is the preoperative evaluation. The preoperative evaluation includes much more than just the physical aspect of the ophthalmologic examination. It encompasses all the contacts and communications the potential candidate has with the laser center staff and physicians. Identifying personality characteristics, expectations, and demeanor can all assist in the determination as to the individual's candidacy for laser vision correction. The greater the level of staff training and commitment, the more effective this process will be.

Tables 6-1 and 6-2 identify many of the characteristics that must be considered in the determination as to if surgery is indicated and which procedure is best. The initial patient contact is generally by phone and this is an excellent opportunity to begin to collect information. An experienced staff member will be looking for these characteristics in this preliminary conversation and document any pertinent impressions. The phone screening process for booking evaluations should be efficient at identifying only candidates because spending time on non-candidates has a cost to the practice. Many patients are confused and actually have problems not amendable to laser vision correction. The type of refractive error, stability of refraction, expectations, and age of the prospective candidate can usually be obtained quickly. Knowing the CTL wear history will make certain the patient is properly prepared for the examination. It is critical to maximize the efficiency of the preoperative assessment because patient to staff/physician time is limited. With the rise in malpractice litigation, one cannot afford to ignore any suspicious characteristics.

The physical examination begins with a standard complete medical history including previous medical problems, surgical procedures, medications, allergies, and pertinent family history. A thorough

Table 6-2

Lifestyle and Occupational Characteristics to Consider

Risk of Trauma to a Healing Eye

High Risk	*Low Risk*
Law enforcement	Golf
Military	Aerobic exercises
Firefighters/paramedics	Professional: Business,Legal
Martial arts	
Contact sports	
Racket sports	
Waterskiing	

High Risk of Infection to a Healing Eye

Healthcare worker
Agricultural worker

Occupational Visual Requirements

Pilot
Commercial driver
Photographer

Time Demands

Flexible
Accessibility for follow-up
Recovery time

CTL history is mandatory as well as the time of discontinued lens wear prior to testing.

Uncorrected and best-corrected visual acuities at distance and near should be documented. Both manifest and cycloplegic (1% cyclopentolate is recommended) refractions need to be determined. The stability of the candidate's refractive error must be established so checking old spectacles or records from past exams is required.

Undoubtedly in the future wavefront analysis will be performed.

The pupil size for light and dark-adapted states is measured, preferably with a standard device such as the Colvard pupillometer. In addition, pupillary reactions to light and the presence or absence of an afferent defect are checked.

Ocular dominance is determined.

Keratometry is measured quantitatively and qualitatively with the Bausch & Lomb (Rochester, NY) keratometer. The corneal topography and the corneal pachymetry are checked. If available, the Orbscan (Bausch & Lomb) is efficient in measuring both of these corneal characteristics simultaneously. In addition to the anterior corneal topography, the Orbscan will measure the posterior corneal surface.

Intraocular pressures are measured with the Goldmann applanation tonometer.

The lids, cornea, anterior chamber, iris, and lens are evaluated with slit lamp biomicroscopy. A qualitative determination of the tear film and tear meniscus are completed and a Schirmer's test may be necessary. The reliability, cost effectiveness, and true clinical value for the tear lysozyme test remains to be proven.

In dealing with hyperopic eyes, gonioscopy is mandatory in any eyes with suspiciously narrow angles on slit lamp examination. Because there may be a shift in the refractive error after laser iridotomy, the necessity for this procedure needs to be determined before PRK or LASEK.

At this point a mydriatic and cycloplegic solution is instilled. In my practice, the candidate watches the informed consent and patient education video while dilating. Then the examination is completed with the cycloplegic refraction and funduscopic evaluation.

Table 6-3

General Indications for H-PRK or H-LASEK

1. +1.00 to +6.00 DSE (diopters of spherical equivalent) at spectacle plane. For hyperopic astigmatism: cylinder is not to exceed 4.00 D and SE not to exceed +6.00 D.
2. Patient consent.
3. At least 21 years of age.
4. Less than 0.75 D difference between manifest and cyclopentolate refraction.
5. Refractive stability—patients whose hyperopia is progressing at a rate greater than 0.5 D per year should not be treated.

Table 6-4

General Contraindications

1. Patients with systemic medical conditions- collagen vascular, autoimmiune, or immunodeficiency diseases. (Caution should be exercised with those diseases likely to affect wound healing such as diabetes, atopy, and connective tissue disease.)
2. Women—pregnant or nursing.
3. Patients with keratoconus or other corneal ectatic/degenerative disease.
4. Patients taking medications:
   Isoretinoin (Accutane)
   Amiodarone hydrochloride (Cordarone)
   Sumitripan (Imitrex)
5. Patient with history of keloid formation.
6. Not recommended at this time in patients with *herpes simplex* or *herpes zoster* keratitis.

Indications and Contraindications

Appropriate patient selection is required in all refractive surgical procedures in order to achieve optimal results. The patient's consent is imperative and it is important to not forget that the final decision as to the choice of procedure is the patient's. It is the surgeon's responsibility and right not to perform the procedure if he or she determines it not to be in the patient's best interest. The presentation of the information necessary for the patient to make his or her informed decision may be confusing if care is not taken in the explanations. It is easiest and least confusing to present the information used to determine first if the patient is a good laser vision candidate, then to present that necessary to determine which procedure is preferred.

The general indications for hyperopic corrections are presented in Table 6-3 while the general contraindications are in Table 6-4. Additional specific considerations are also extremely important. Some of these are controversial and debated varying from surgeon to surgeon. The discussion of these factors does reflect the author's personal bias and approach in these considerations. They demonstrate the principle of maximizing long-term safety without sacrificing the ability to achieve the desired refractive result.

Surgery should not be considered unless the patient's hyperopia is symptomatic. These asymptomatic patients will most likely be younger (under 35 years) without significant complaints. Most will not be wearing corrective lenses.

The degree of hyperopia and hyperopic astigmatism is very important in determining the potential for candidacy. Optimal results are achieved for hyperopia of 1 to 4 D. For hyperopia between 4 to 6 D the results are less predictable and above 6 D, the patient is better served by a non-laser keratorefractive procedure. With many hyperopic corneas being smaller in diameter and having flatter anterior curvatures, it is not always possible to get a large enough and well-centered LASIK flap to permit unrestricted ablation of the entire 9-mm treatment zone. The greater the ablation, the more tissue that may be masked in the area of the hinge or outside the keratectomy bed. This can potentially affect the symmetry of the ablation. Consequently, there is a greater chance for undercorrection or induction of irregular astigmatism with the lamellar procedure than with surface treatment.

Candidacy is affected by the degree and quality of the anterior and posterior corneal curvatures. The calculated postoperative curvature should not be greater than 50 D. Steeper than this and the quality of vision is affected similar to having a central island and irregular astigmatism. Preoperative corneal curvatures less than 40 D can lead to smaller flap diameters as well as greater incidence of flap construction complications if LASIK is utilized. Therefore these ocular factors make surface ablation the preferred procedures.

The quality of both curvatures may reflect an underlying corneal problem such as keratoconus. Certainly in dealing with hyperopic eyes, this is going to be an unusual finding.

Controversy does revolve around what safety standards should be used for corneal thickness. The safety standards chosen will determine both if surgery should be performed and which procedure; surface ablative or lamellar, should be selected. A preoperative corneal thickness of 500 µm is a reasonable minimum level to permit safe LASIK flap construction without weakening the corneal structure. For a LASIK flap thickness of less than 180 µm this seems to be an acceptable standard. To maintain the integrity of the corneal structure a conservative limit of 300 µm of residual posterior corneal stroma is prudent. A number of refractive surgeons will go down to 250 µm as their minimum. Therefore, corneas not within these limits should be better PRK or LASEK candidates. For these two procedures, leaving somewhere between a total postoperative thickness of 350 to 400 µm is suggested. The precise amount of tissue necessary is not known, and the inability to measure the quality of the tissue itself also hinders this determination. Not being able to measure the strength of the tissue itself means that more conservative levels for thickness must be utilized.

Another debated issue is in regards to scotopic pupil size and its association with increased glare and halo effects. A higher incidence of low-contrast and scotopic vision symptoms have been attributed to large scotopic papillary diameters (those larger than the diameter of the ablation zone). However, a recent study by Dr. Steven Schallhorn doesn't demonstrate this direct relationship,[6] at least in myopic eyes. This may or not be applicable to hyperopic eyes, and the author is not aware of any prospective study for hyperopic eyes. Wavefront analysis may help to identify how higher order aberrations may influence scotopic visual side effects.

The presence of an eccentric pupil may play a part in the choice of procedure. If a well-centered LASIK flap cannot be constructed, then surface ablation is the best alternative to ensure a complete, symmetrical ablation.

Surface ablation may be preferred for eyes in which the excessive transient pressure elevation induced by the LASIK fixation ring might affect the vitreous, retina, or optic nerve. Questions still exist as to whether or not problems such as central retina vein occlusion, glaucomatous optic atrophy, or ischemic optic neuropathy could be precipitated or aggravated with LASIK. Lattice degeneration and an increased risk for retinal detachment are less likely in hyperopic than myopic eyes; but again, PRK or LASEK may be the preferred procedure to avoid the pressure elevation, which might shift the vitreous. Eyes that have had a scleral buckling procedure frequently do not permit adequate fixation of the LASIK ring and necessitate a surface procedure.

Because symptomatic hyperopes tend to be older, many present with early lenticular opacification. Once presbyopia has occurred and any lens opacification has begun to affect visual functioning, the potential advantages of lens extraction and intraocular lens implantation must be considered as an alternative to laser vision correction. The quality of vision is most certainly superior with lens removal an IOL implantation than with keratorefractive surgery. This is especially true in the higher hyperopes with greater than 6 D of correction. Patients easily understand that it is preferable to perform cataract surgery a little earlier than to undergo laser surgery only to need cataract surgery a year or so later.

Finally, once all these anatomical and specific ocular features have been identified, they should be considered in context with the personal and lifestyle characteristics of the individual patient to make appropriate recommendations as to the preferred procedures. The final decision or recommendation should have both short- and long-term safety as its foundation. The patient is responsible for the final decision. The choice of procedure is based on honest and accurate information provided by the surgeon and staff. In some cases the surgeon's concerns may be overruled by the patient's desires. This is where it may be necessary for the surgeon to decide if he or she feels comfortable proceeding with the patient's choice.

Preoperative Management

Preoperative management of the hyperopic patient certainly includes identifying and applying all the considerations discussed in the previous section. In addition to these concerns, there are the following specific considerations, which will assist in achieving the most successful outcomes.

Overly nervous or anxious patients may benefit from additional education. Viewing other patients' surgeries should be offered as an option, for it may significantly reduce their fears. Occasionally, a preoperative anxiolytic medication will be given either the night before or the day of surgery. Caution must be exercised so as not to sedate too heavily and affect the patient's concentration and fixation ability.

The two most common problems needing preoperative treatment are lid disease and tear dysfunction. Marginal blepharitis should be classified as staphylococcal, seborrheic, meibomian gland dysfunction, or mixed. The appropriate treatment should be instituted and the problem improved before proceeding with surgery. Although oral tetracycline is useful in improving meibomian gland dysfunction, the possible effects of its increased photosensitivity response on the excimer's ablation profile are uncertain.

Dry eye disease is determined to be either qualitative or quantitative in nature. Quantitative is managed with artificial tears, lubricants, and punctal occlusion. Lubricants and possibly oral fatty acid supplements may be considered.

Atopic eyes should be quiet prior to the procedure. A topical steroid may be used for a day or so preoperatively to reduce the potential for diffuse lamellar keratitis.

Many surgeons prefer a prophylactic topical antibiotic for 1 to 3 days prior to surgery. The effectiveness of this practice and its possible contribution to bacterial resistance are still in question. A fluoroquinolone seems to be the most common choice among refractive surgeons.

Surgical Techniques

Anesthesia

The anesthesia used is the same for both procedures. A topical anesthetic solution such as proparacaine or tetracaine is sufficient. The administration of a mild oral sedative such as Valium (Roche, Switzerland) can be beneficial, not only for the operation itself, but also for the comfort of the patient in the early postoperative period. Excessive sedation is undesirable as patient cooperation is mandatory to insure excellent patient fixation.

Procedure

Preoperative Considerations

Proper informed consent is obtained for the specific procedure, LASEK or PRK.

A topical fluoroquinolone is routinely prescribed 4 times daily starting the day prior to surgery. Thirty minutes prior to surgery a topical anesthetic, topical fluoroquinolone, and topical nonsteroidal anti-inflammatory agent are instilled. Oral Valium is offered on an individual basis.

Operative Techniques

PRK

1. The patient is properly positioned under the operating microscope of the laser unit.
2. A hair bonnet is placed and a 4x4 gauze pad is placed on each side to absorb tears and solutions. An opaque eye shield is taped over the non-operated eye or the lids are simply taped.
3. Additional topical anesthetic and an adjustable, bladed lid speculum are placed.
4. The patient is briefly instructed on the fixation process and the sights, sounds, and smells of the procedure.
5. The epithelium is removed by preferred method.
   - Manual—Debridement of 9 to 10 mm with a spatula, 69 Beaver blade, or Amoil brush.
   - Alcohol—Alcohol maybe applied to loosen the epithelium, which is then easily removed with a surgical spear. A 9.5 to 10 mm reservoir is centered and then filled with 20% alcohol/BSS solution for 30 to 60 seconds. The solution removed with a surgical spear and the corneal surface irrigated with chilled BSS.
6. The desired hyperopic and astigmatic ablation is then performed.
7. The surface is irrigated with chilled BSS and wiped gently with a surgical spear.
8. A soft contact is then placed.
9. Lid speculum is removed.

LASEK

1. The patient is positioned under the operating microscope of the laser unit.
2. A hair bonnet is placed and a 4x4 gauze pad is placed on each side to absorb tears and solutions. An opaque eye shield is taped over the non-operated eye or the lids simply taped shut.

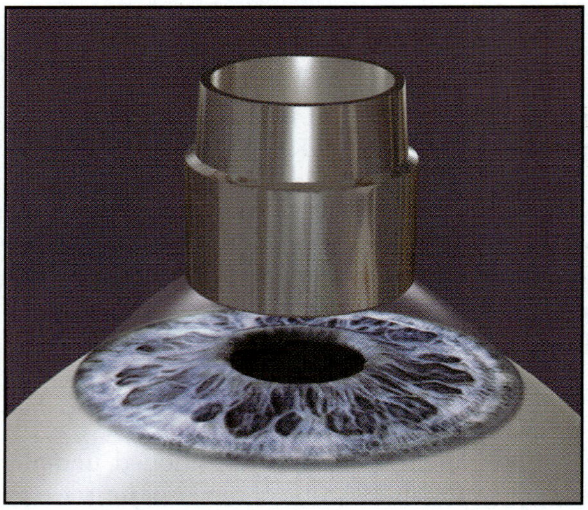

Figure 6-1A. The appropriate diameter sharp, modified disposable trephine (a non-disposable trephine may be preferred) is placed and centered on the pupil and slowly rotated 10 to 15 degrees in both clockwise and counterclockwise directions to create a full thickness epithelial incision. (Courtesy of Thomas Claringbold, DO.)

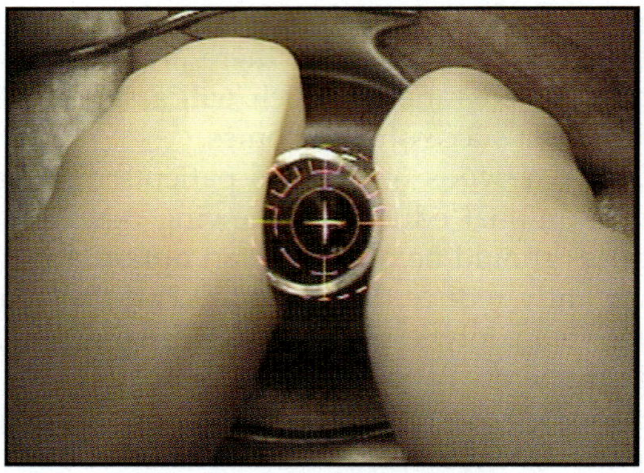

Figure 6-1B. Photo of Figure 6-1A.

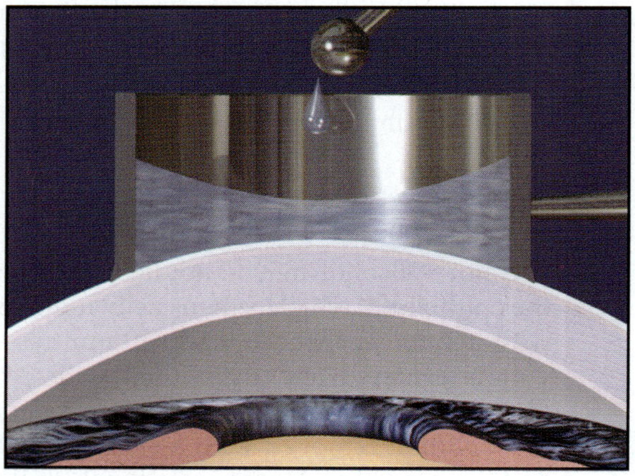

Figure 6-2A. The 20% ETOH/BSS solution is injected into the reservoir with a metal cannula and glass syringe. (Courtesy of Thomas Claringbold, DO.)

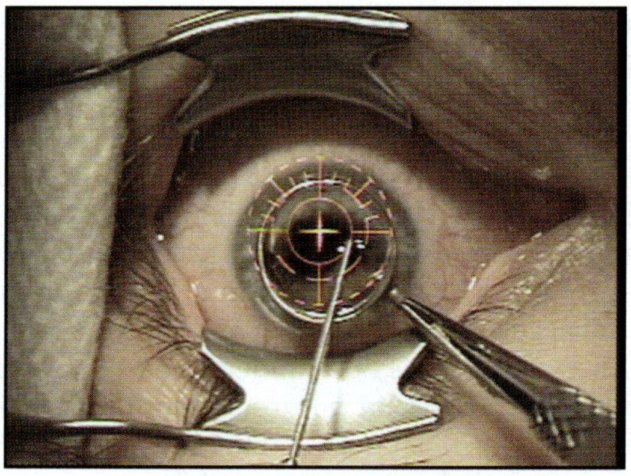

Figure 6-2B. Photo of Figure 6-2A.

3. Additional topical anesthetic and an adjustable, bladed lid speculum are placed.
4. The appropriate diameter sharp, modified disposable trephine (a non-disposable trephine may be preferred) is placed and centered on the pupil, held between both right and left index fingers. Firm but gentle pressure is placed onto the cornea and the trephine slowly rotated 10 to 15 degrees in both clockwise and counterclockwise directions. A full thickness epithelial incision is desired. Even with a sharp edge this can be accomplished without significantly penetrating or damaging Bowman's layer (Figures 6-1A and B).
5. The alcohol reservoir 0.5 mm larger than the trephine is placed very firmly onto the cornea. It is centered about the trephination incision. The patient should be reminded to keep both eyes open (if not taped) and directed to gaze straight ahead.
6. The 20% ETOH/BSS solution is injected into the reservoir with a metal cannula and glass syringe. The contact time is 30 seconds for routine cases. If the solution leaks out the eye should be immediately irrigated with BSS and the fornices dried with a surgical spear. The reservoir and ETOH/BSS solution are then reapplied for another 20 to 30 seconds (Figures 6-2A and B).
7. An Intac's pocket hook is used to test and free the edge of the epithelial flap (Figures 6-3A and B). If detachment does not occur easily then one should reapply the EOTH/BSS solution. It is possible to get evaporation of the EOTH or a denatured vial, so always try a fresh solution using a new vial of EOTH.
8. The microhoe is then used to slide back the epithelial flap. It is folded back on itself to the

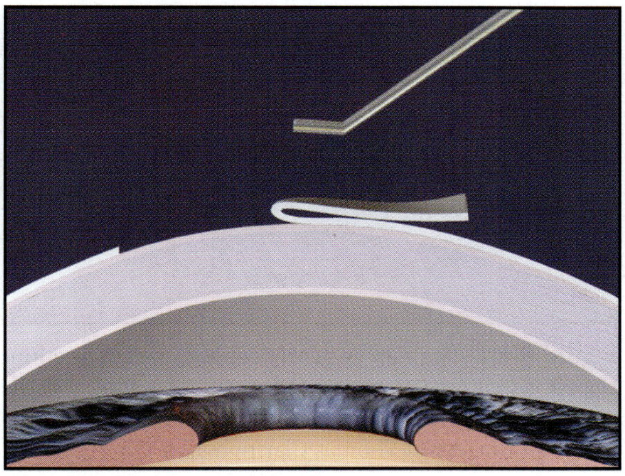

Figure 6-3A. Schematic of a pocket hook from the Intac's procedure. Used to test and free the edge of the epithelial flap. (Courtesy of Thomas Claringbold, DO.)

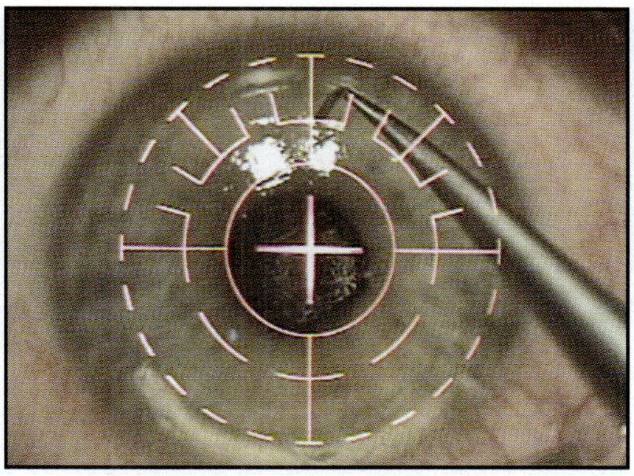

Figure 6-3B. Photo of 6-3A.

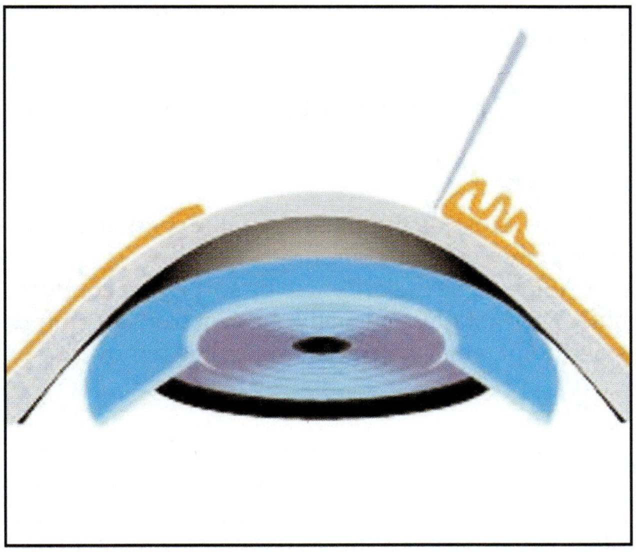

Figure 6-4A. The microhoe is then used to slide back the epithelial flap. It is folded back on itself to the superior aspect of the hinge.

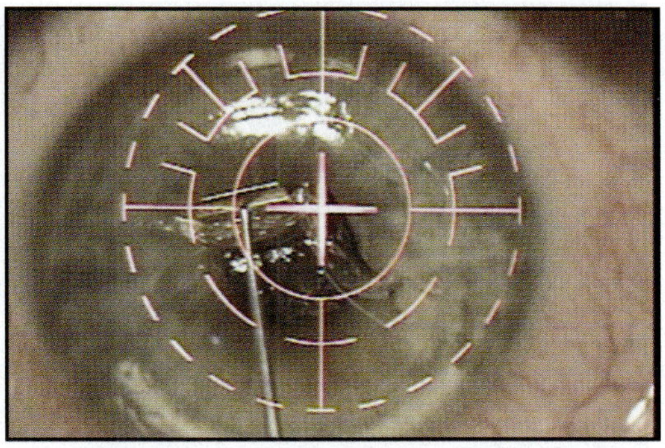

Figure 6-4B. Photo of 6-4A.

superior aspect of the hinge. It is not uncommon in the larger, hyperopic flaps to have a free flap (Figures 6-4A and 6-4B).

9. The laser ablation is then performed (Figure 6-5). The nomogram adjustment is similar to that for PRK. It is recommended when starting out to use this adjustment and modify it according to the results. This is in contrast to LASEK for myopia where the adjustment is closer to one's LASIK nomogram than that for PRK.
10. The flap is then gently repositioned. The blunt tipped instrument is moistened in the tear film and the epithelium is then unfolded and pushed inferiorly. If a free cap occurs then counter traction superiorly at the edge permits it to be nicely repositioned. Since realignment of the flap is not important, epithelial markings are not necessary (Figures 6-6A and 6-6B).
11. A drop or 2 of Muro 128 (Bausch & Lomb, Rochester, NY) solution is then placed on the epithelial flap. A Bausch & Lomb Purevision (14.2-mm diameter and 8.6-mm base curve) or Biomedics 55 (Ocular Sciences, Concord, Calif) (14.2-mm and 8.6-mm base curve) is placed.
12. The speculum is removed and gentle pressure with the 4x4 gauze pad placed on the closed lid to stabilize the contact.

Postoperative Evaluation and Management

It is definitely true that the postoperative management of laser vision correction patients is critical, not only to surgical success but also patient satisfaction. Patient education is paramount and cannot be stressed enough. The general expectations of the nature of the visual recovery, potential discomfort,

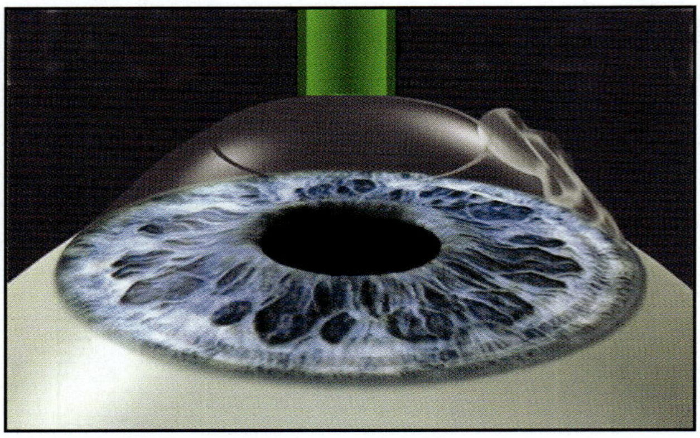

Figure 6-5. The laser ablation is performed.

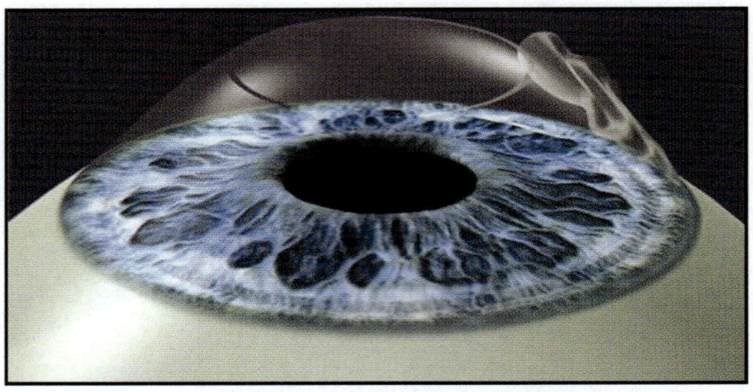

Figure 6-6A. The flap is gently repositioned. The blunt tipped instrument is moistened in the tear film and the epithelium is unfolded and pushed inferiorly. Soft CTL is placed. (Courtesy of Thomas Claringbold, DO.)

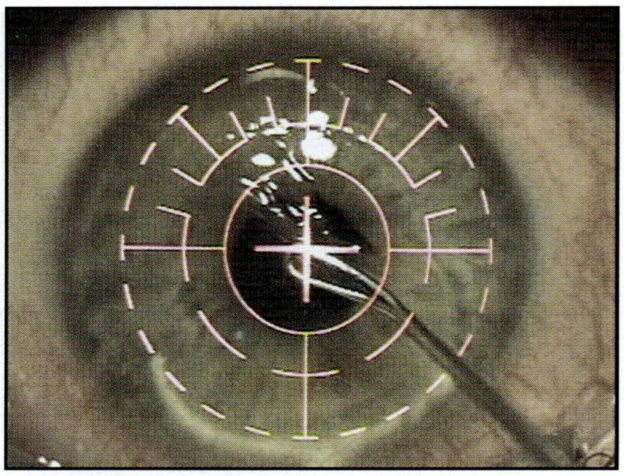

Figure 6-6B. Photo of Figure 6-6A.

and realistic final visual result must be understood. Especially with surface ablative procedures where there can be a significant amount of pain and a prolonged visual recovery. These patients will interact with LASIK patients and it is essential that they are able to comprehend why their postoperative experience was different.

Immediate Postoperative Period

PRK and LASEK

A drop each of the antibiotic, steroid, and nonsteroidal anti-inflammatory drugs such as Diclofenac (Voltaren, Novartis, East Hanover, NJ) or Acular PF (Ketorolac, Allergan, Irvine, Calif) are instilled. A less potent steroid such as fluoromethalone is used for surface ablation. Clear shields or sunglasses are worn for protection. Oral pain medications are always prescribed for these two procedures. Patient instructions are to go home, take a nap, and instill the medication drops every 4 hours. The patients are given a preservative-free non-steroidal. They are to use preservative-free artificial tears as necessary. An oral sleeping pill is given to take home at the patient's discretion.

Postoperative Day 1

Comfort

PRK—Most of the patients will experience only mild to moderate discomfort.

LASEK—The majority will be surprising comfortable. The first day is usually the best from a comfort standpoint, at least until the contact is removed.

Vision

PRK—Vision will range from 20/25 to 20/400. With hyperopic correction it is not unusual for the patients to remark that they can see better at near. Most will experience this initial myopic over correction.

LASEK—About 25% will have relatively decent vision especially at near. Fifty percent will have fair vision and the other 25% will have poor vision in the 20/100 to 20/400 range even at near.

Examination

External

PRK—The lids are normally quiet without significant edema or erythema. If lid edema is present it is generally mild and due to excessive blepharospasm against the lid speculum. Other causes such as a tight CTL, reaction to medication, or the rare possibility of an infectious process must be considered and eliminated.

LASEK—Same as PRK.

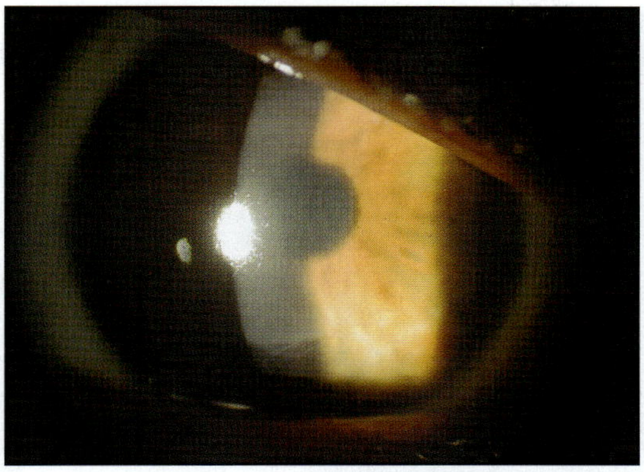

Figure 6-7. Postoperative appearance of eye 24 hours post LASEK. (Courtesy of William B. Trattler, MD.)

Slit Lamp Exam (SLE)

PRK

Conjunctiva—Most demonstrate none to mild injection. Diffuse injection is less specific as to the etiology, while localized limbal injection suggests a tight CTL with associated hypoxia. Generalized injection may indicate absence of the contact, hypoxia from a tight lens, adverse reaction to medication, or infection.

Cornea—The CTL should be well centered and show minimal movement. A small percentage will reveal mild stromal edema with or without folds. A large epithelial defect will be present. The anterior stromal surface should be clear. Careful attention should be given to the presence of any early infiltrates.

LASEK

Conjunctiva—Same as PRK.

Cornea—The CTL should be centered and without significant movement. The epithelial flap will range from completely clear and normal appearance to edematous. The overlying edges of the flap are almost always edematous and slight opaque. Figure 6-7 shows a typical postoperative appearance of LASEK on first postoperative day.

Management

PRK

1. Continue topical antibiotic QID. (fluoroquinolone).
2. Continue topical steroid QID. (Fluoromethalone 0.1% or equivalent). If moderate to severe inflammation occurs, the patient should increase it to 6 or 8 times a day.
3. Consider discontinuing the topical nonsteroidal anti-inflammatory drug at this time if insignificant discomfort or absence of inflammation. Recommend using individual dosage units of Acular PF and limit the number so that the patient will not inadvertently use it incorrectly. An increasing frequency of sterile infiltrate is seen the longer the nonsteroidal drug is used. Administration for the first 24 hours seems adequate in the majority of eyes to maintain comfort.
4. Non-preserved artificial tears frequently to maintain hydration of CTL.
5. Cool compresses as necessary for pain or lid reaction. It is important to minimize the weight of the compress as well as to avoid tap water from entering the eye.
6. Oral nonsteroidal drug such as ibuprofen for mild discomfort. Darvocet (Eli Lilly, Indianapolis, Ind) or Vicoprofen (Knoll, Whippahy, NJ) for moderate to severe pain. In most extreme cases use a stronger narcotic such as Mepergan Fortis (Wyeth, Madison, NJ).
7. Shields at bedtime.
8. Activity as common sense dictates. Avoid swimming or hot tubs for 3 to 4 weeks.
9. Reassure patient not to be concerned about vision at this point. It is normal to have better near acuity than distance.

LASEK

1. Essentially the same as PRK.
2. Change contact only if absolutely necessary. At this point even careful removal of the flap may loosen and likely result in loss of the epithelial flap.

Follow-Up

PRK

Routinely scheduled for 2 days but see in one if any concerns.

LASEK

Same as PRK.

Postoperative Days 2 through 10

It is imperative that patients understand the significant individual variability in the nature of the healing response. Although most recoveries are similar for all of the procedures, patients should be prepared for an extreme response and constant reassurance should be given. In this manner one can assist these patients through a difficult and slow recovery. The

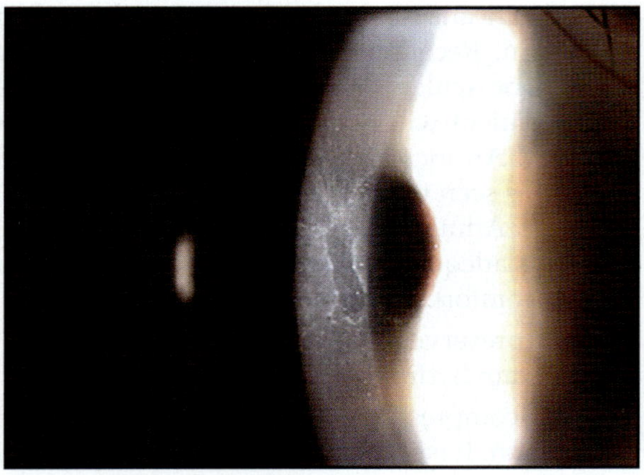

Figure 6-8 Postoperative appearance of eye 48 hours after PRK. Small remaining central defect. Additional 24 hours of healing time suggested before removing CTL. (Courtesy of Neal A. Sher, MD.)

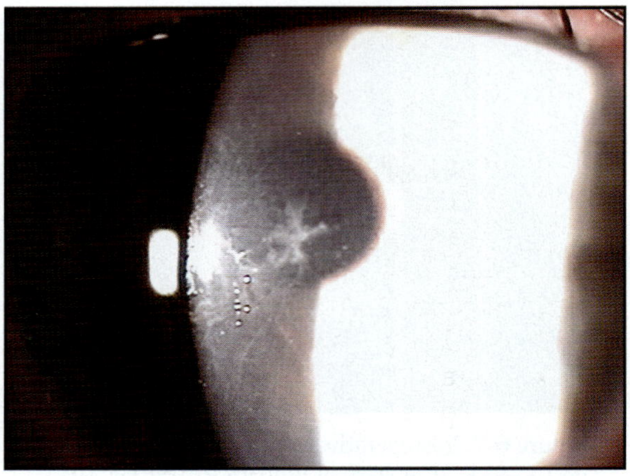

Figure 6-9. Postoperative appearance of eye 72 hours after PRK. Epithelium almost totally intact with central vortex whorl. (Courtesy of Neal A. Sher, MD.)

difference between the postoperative course for surface ablative procedures and LASIK cannot be emphasized enough. Despite even the best patient education, it is always amazing how many patients still ask in this early period, "Is this the best I'm going to see?" or "Is my vision going to improve?"

Comfort

PRK

Comfort for the hyperopic treatments tends to be better than for myopic treatments. This would certainly seem to be opposite what one would expect, because the epithelial defect and ablation area is larger than that for a myopic ablation. The author's personal experience is that severe pain is less common in hyperopic ablations. A tight CTL, hypoxia, poor tear function, adverse reaction to medications, and simply the wound healing response may all contribute to the discomfort.

LASEK

Comfort generally continues to be good. Just as in PRK, hyperopic LASEK cases demonstrate less discomfort than myopic ones.

Vision

PRK

Vision ranges from fair to poor. Expect considerable improvement 24 to 48 hours after the contact is removed and the epithelium is intact.

LASEK

Vision will normally decrease as the epithelial flap is replaced by the new regenerating epithelial cells. Near vision continues to be better than distance in most cases. As with PRK, vision will normally improve 24 to 48 hours after the contact is removed and the surface is intact.

Examination

External

PRK—Lids should be normal.

LASEK—Same as PRK.

SLE

PRK

Conjunctiva—The conjunctiva is normally quiet. If present, the injection will usually be limbal and due to hypoxia from the CTL. A toxic or allergic reaction to the topical antibiotic is possible.

Cornea—The central aspect of the epithelial defect will be the last to heal (Figures 6-8 and 6-9). This normally takes about 4 to 6 days to a maximum of 6 to 8 days. A tight or dirty contact can cause hypoxia and a delay of re-epithelialization. Also, this may be the cause for stromal edema. Any infiltrates need to be identified as sterile or infectious.

LASEK

Conjunctiva—Same as PRK.

Cornea—The normalization of the epithelium can be monitored and judged by observation of the mottled appearance in the residual edematous cells of the original flap. As these cells slough and are replaced, this characteristic appearance disappears. The entire process may take a minimum of 4 to 5 days to a maximum of 6 to 8 days. As with PRK, stromal edema may indicate a tight or dirty contact. Infiltrates must be identified as to infectious or sterile.

Management

PRK

1. Replace the contact if tight or dirty and the epithelium not completely intact and able to tolerate lid movement. Any question as to the integrity and durability necessitates continued CTL wear. It is better to error on keeping the lens a day or two longer than to remove it too soon and have a break down with subsequent delay in recovery. On some occasions in which there is a persistent small defect, it may be best to pressure patch for 12 to 24 hours. The failure to heal may be due to hypoxic or mechanical stress from the contact.
2. The topical antibiotic should be continued until the epithelium is completely healed.
3. The topical steroid is continued QID. If epithelial healing is delayed then decrease or stop it temporarily to promote recovery. If inflammation present increase accordingly.
4. Discontinue the topical nonsteroidal anti-inflammatory if not already discontinued at day one. The longer its administration, the greater the chances for sterile infiltrates.
5. Frequent use of artificial tears. Additional dry eye management as discussed in preoperative management.
6. Cool compresses as necessary.
7. Continue oral anti-inflammatory drug as well as analgesic prn.
8. Shields at bedtime for 4 to 5 days.
9. Activity as condition dictates. Vision will be the primary reason for restricted activity. Temporary spectacles may be necessary to permit driving and can be prescribed as soon as epithelium normalized.
10. Reassurance as to slow visual recovery.

LASEK

1. Same as PRK.
2. When changing CTL one may need to carefully debride loose tags of the residual epithelial flap.

Follow-Up

PRK—Patients are routinely seen 1 to 2 weeks after the contact is removed and the epithelium is intact.

LASEK—Same as PRK.

Postoperative 2 to 4 Weeks

Comfort

PRK

By this time almost all patients are comfortable. Some tenderness to the touch is common and some may experience minor dry eye symptoms.

LASEK

Same as PRK.

Vision

PRK

Vision for most should be functional. Regression should be reducing consecutive myopia. Still may see irregular astigmatism due to re-organization of the epithelium.

LASEK

Same as PRK.

Examination

External

PRK—Normal.
LASEK—Normal.

SLE

PRK

Conjunctiva—Normal.

Cornea—Should be clear. Trace subepithelial haze may be seen. Significant haze at this time is extremely unusual.

LASEK

Conjunctiva—Normal.

Cornea—Similar to PRK. It is a little more common to notice anterior basement membrane changes.

Management

PRK

1. The administration of the topical steroid should be determined with respect to the patient's age, the degree of correction, haze, and postoperative refractive error. Hyperopic refractions dictate an increased frequency/potency of application. Significant consecutive myopia is treated with decreasing frequency/potency. A short term of CTL wear is occasionally appropriate to enhance regression. Controversy does exist as to the precise titration of effect possible, but clinically these principles seem effective.

2. Irregularity of the epithelium or anterior basement membrane changes should be managed with hypertonic saline ointment and/or solution.

LASEK

Same as PRK.

Follow-Up

PRK

Two to 3 months. This should be modified if still administering significant topical steroids in order to monitor intraocular pressure.

LASEK

Same as PRK.

Postoperative 2 to 4 Months

Comfort

PRK—Normal.

LASEK—Normal.

Vision

PRK—There will still be some degree of fluctuation. Expected postoperative side effects of glare and haloes should be improving.

LASEK—Same as PRK.

Examination

PRK

Conjunctiva—Normal.

Cornea—Most will be clear. Occasionally will see trace granular haze, but with less frequency than myopic ablations.

LASEK

Conjunctiva—Normal.

Cornea—Same as PRK.

Management

PRK

1. Continue the use of a topical steroid if concern regarding presence or development of haze or regression.
2. Monitor intraocular pressure if on topical steroid.
3. Dry eye management as indicated.
4. Hypertonic ointment or saline if anterior basement membrane changes or corneal erosions.
5. Spectacle or CTL correction for symptomatic residual refractive error.

LASEK

Same as PRK.

Follow-up

PRK—Two to 3 months if routine course. Sooner if on steroids or managing a specific problem.

LASEK—Same as PRK.

Postoperative 6 to 12 Months

PRK—Waiting for complete stabilization of the refraction and visual acuity to determine if an enhancement is necessary. Any late haze should be managed with topical steroids. If severe, then retreatment with mitomycin-C needs be considered.

LASEK—Same as PRK.

Surgical Results

One must exercise caution when interpreting and evaluating the results of PRK and LASEK for hyperopia. All the variables must be considered and the reported results taken in context. These variables range from the make and model of the excimer laser to the skill level and integrity of the surgeon. The rapid rates of procedural and technical advances make it very difficult if not impossible to meaningfully compare results.

It is normal for surgeons to have a bias as to the laser vision correction procedure they prefer. A number of factors in addition to the capacity to achieve satisfactory visual results are included in the creation of this bias. The technical difficulty, operative time, nature of postoperative care and desire of the patient are just a few of the numerous factors surgeons use to develop their procedure preference.

The visual results between hyperopic PRK and hyperopic LASEK appear comparable. The following study outcomes will help to support this. The choice between these two procedures is not as important as the decision as to whether to perform a surface ablation or lamellar procedure (LASIK). In making these decisions, the reason for selecting the procedure should be based on all pertinent factors while keeping the best visual result and long-term safety paramount.

PRK

The amount of information published regarding the correction of hyperopia and hyperopic astigmatism with PRK is considerably less than that for myopia and myopic astigmatism. Also, with the overwhelming popularity of LASIK most information available is from several years ago. This makes it more difficult to compare with LASEK results, which are based on the past 2 to 3 years and consequently utilizing laser technology upgrades not available in earlier years.

It is appropriate to begin with the results from the study which resulted in the FDA's Ophthalmic Device Advisory Panel's approval for hyperopic ablation with the VISX excimer laser, October, 1998.[7,8] This was a prospective, non-randomized, unmasked, multicenter study performed at 8 centers in the United States. One hundred and twenty-four eyes of 124 subjects with primary hyperopia were evaluated for 12 months after surgery. The mean preoperative sphere and cylinder were +2.28 SD 0.84 (range +0.38 to +4.00 D) and cylinder less than 1.00 D. The results were remarkably similar to those reported by other laser manufacturers for their units.

At 3 months, 55.9% and 80.8% of patients were within ±0.50 and ±1.00 D, respectively, of the intended correction. This improved to 74.1% and 90.5%, respectively at 6 months and 75.7% and 92.2% at 12 months. The uncorrected visual acuity (UCVA) was 20/20 or better in 53.3%, 20/40 or better in 96.0% at 6 months, and 63.9% and 94.8%, respectively, at 12 months. No eye ended up with a BCVA worse than 20/32.

VISX received FDA approval for hyperopic astigmatism 2 years later in October 2000. The study included eyes with a maximum spherical equivalent of +6.00 D with a range of the cylindrical component of +0.50 to +4.00 D. The range of the spherical component was +0.50 to +5.00 D. The visual and refractive results did not vary significantly from those for hyperopia alone. At 6 months 50.2% of the eyes were 20/20 or better and 96.5% were 20/40 or better.

Dr. Keith Williams of London reported on 52 eyes with spherical equipments of +1.00 to +6.00 D and cylindrical components of less than or equal to 1.50 D treated with the VISX laser. These results were comparable to those from the original VISX study. At six months 67% and 88% of the eyes, respectively were ±0.50 and ±1.00 D. By 12 months improvement for eyes within ±0.50 D was up to 79%. Visual acuity was 20/40 or better in 95.3% of the eyes at the 6-month evaluation. There was not any eye that lost best-corrected visual acuity. Only mild transient corneal haze was identified during the study.[9]

A report from 1998 by Dr. Bruce Jackson of Ottawa, Canada demonstrated excellent outcomes for 65 eyes of 38 patients. One to 4.00 D of spherical hyperopia was treated and at 1 year 80% were within ±0.50 D. Ninety-eight percent were within ±1.00 D. There was some regression noted from 1 to 6 months and one eye did develop clinically significant haze.[10]

It is interesting to compare these results obtained with the VISX laser to those reportedly achieved with the Technolas laser. In 1997, the results for hyperopia and hyperopic astigmatism on a Technolas 116 laser in a study of 45 eyes of 36 patients were evaluated over a 6-month postoperative period. The mean spherical equivalent was +3.33 SD 1.50 D (range +0.50 to +6.50 D) and the mean cylindrical equivalent 1.51 SD 1.39 D (range +0.50 to +5.00 D). Eighty-seven percent of all eyes were within ±1.00 D with a very small difference between HPRK (88%) and HPARK (85%). Only 38% of the eyes were 20/20 or better while 93% were 20/40 or better. Both still within reason as compared with the results with the VISX unit. The 6.7% of eyes that lost two or more lines of BCVA was higher than that from the other studies.[11]

Using the newer Technolas 217C laser, Dr. E Pacella showed (not surprisingly), much better outcomes than those from the 116. A higher mean spherical equivalent of 4.82 SD 2.11 D (range +1.00 to +7.75 D) and cylinder less than or equal to +0.50 D was treated. At 18 months 46.4% of eyes were 20/20 or better and 100% better than or equal to 20/32. None of the eyes lost two lines or more of best-corrected vision.[12]

Dr. Carones of Italy utilized the Alcon LADARVision laser in 2000 to evaluate 92 eyes of 57 patients. The mean spherical equivalent was +3.45 D (range +0.50 to +6.00 D) and the mean cylindrical equivalent 2.76 D. Eighty-two percent of the eyes were ±0.50 at 1 year. Visual acuity was 20/20 or better in 53% and 94% had better than or equal to 20/40. No eyes were reported to have lost BCVA.[13]

In conclusion, the results for visual acuity in the correction of hyperopia and hyperopic astigmatism are obviously not as good as those for myopia and myopic astigmatism. There also does not appear to be dramatically better outcomes for hyperopia alone than for hyperopic astigmatism and the results from the 3 lasers are also comparable.

LASEK

There is truly a paucity of data on the effectiveness of LASEK for hyperopia and hyperopic astigmatism. The author will present his data from clinical experience in treating these eyes over the past 2 years.

Of approximately 1500 LASEK procedures for all refractive errors, only 37 have been for primary hyperopia and hyperopic astigmatism. These 37 eyes were from 24 patients. The VISX Star 3 excimer laser was used, as was standard LASEK technique as described in the surgical technique section. This was a prospective evaluation and 6-month results are reported. There was 100% follow-up.

The average preoperative sphere and cylinder were +3.06 D (range +1.00 to +5.625 D) and 0.92 D (range 0.00 to 3.75 D), respectively. At 1 week the mean uncorrected visual acuity (UCVA) was 20/40. At three months, 84% and 92% of patients were within ±0.50 D and ±1.00 D of the intended correction. At 6 months this became 80% and 94%. At this 6-month period 95% of the eyes were 20/40 or better. Interestingly, for the 18 eyes in the high hyperopic group (spherical equivalent greater than or equal to +3.00 D), 78% were better than or equal to 20/20 and 100% 20/40 or better. There were no instances of clinically significant haze or loss of best-corrected vision. The lower success rate for lesser degrees of hyperopia is suspected to be due to a less aggressive nomogram. Further study is necessary to determine the appropriate treatment nomogram for all degrees of hyperopic refractive error.

Future Considerations

The surgical correction of hyperopia and hyperopic astigmatism by reshaping the anterior corneal surface with the excimer laser is safe and effective for a limited range of refractive error. A great deal more experience and investigation is necessary; however, before surgeons can better relate the optimal surgical procedural recommendations to their patients. Both surface ablation (PRK and LASEK) and lamellar (LASIK) procedures are comparable in their ability to achieve satisfactory visual results. Each of the techniques has its advantages and disadvantages that need to be analyzed and applied to the individual candidate in order to obtain the best chance for a safe successful visual result. One should first determine if surface ablation or LASIK is preferred, then one should decide whether PRK or LASEK is optimal.

It is hopeful that refinements in the laser equipment will assist in improving the level and consistency of the visual results. The development of wavefront technology is in its infancy. Certainly, this is even more so for hyperopia than for myopia. Hopefully, changes in the economic environment of medicine will not retard this progress. Surgeon and patients all are anxiously awaiting these future developments.

Conclusion

As the reader can conclude, it has not been clearly established that there is a consensus that either PRK or LASEK is the optimal form of surface ablation for hyperopic refractive errors. Although the author's outcomes for LASEK in the higher degrees (+3.00 D to +5.00 D) of hyperopic are better than those reported to this date for PRK, this alone is not enough to conclude LASEK the superior procedure. The low incidence of pain associated with hyperopic PRK does remove one of the major potential advantages that are seen for LASEK over PRK in myopia. Whether or not there is a difference in the development of postoperative corneal haze between the two surgeries is not known, but remains a potential advantage for LASEK based on data for myopic corrections. A study by Dr. S Wissing did demonstrate significantly less keratocyte loss with LASEK than PRK in a rabbit model and does provide early incite into a possible significant advantage for LASEK.[14]

Larger prospective studies comparing the two procedures in the same patient will be necessary to establish any significant differences, if any. Should these ultimately demonstrate little difference, then, at minimum, the development of LASEK will have forced refractive surgeons to reevaluate the use of surface ablation in appropriate cases.

References

1. Camellin M. LASEK. *Ocular Surgery News*. July 2000;14-17.
2. Ang R, Azar D. Laser epithelial keratomileusis. *Refractive Surgery Outlook*. Winter, 2001.
3. Grendahl MJ. LASIK/PRK Biomechanics, molecular biology, and physiology. *Aspen Ophthalmic Surgery Symposium*. March, 2001.
4. McDonald, MM. Gel-assisted LASEK. *EuroTimes*. March 2002.
5. Samalonis LB. LASEK techniques. *EyeWorld*. September 2002;31-32.
6. Schallhorn S. Pupil size irrelevant to post-LASIK complaints. *Ocular Surgery News*. March, 2002;24.
7. VISX. Photorefractive keratectomy. In: *VISX Star S2 Excimer Laser System. Professional Use Information*. VISX, Incorporated; 1996.
8. Smith SE. VISX hyperopic PRK results are good at 1 year. *Ocular Surgery News*. January 1999;32.
9. Williams DK. One-year results of laser vision correction for low to moderate hyperopia. *Ophthalmology*. 2000; 107(1):72-76
10. Jackson WB, Casson E, Hodge WG, Mintsioulis G, Agapitos PJ. Laser vision correction for low hyperopia. *Ophthalmology*. 1998;105(9):1727-1738.
11. Daya SM, Tappouni FR, Habib NE. Photorefractive keratectomy for hyperopia. *Ophthalmology*. 1997;104(11):1952-1958.
12. Pacella E, Abdolrahimzadeh S, Gabrieli CB. Excimer laser photorefractive keratectomy for hyperopia. *Ophthalmic Surgery and Lasers*. 2001;32(1):30-34.
13. Pop M, Payette Y. Photorefractive keratectomy versus laser in situ keratomileusis: a controlled study. *Ophthalmology*. 2000;107(1):251-257.
14. Ambrosio RJ, Periman LM. ARVO 2002 and *Review of Refractive Surgery*. October 2002;22.

Chapter Seven

Complications of PRK and LASEK for Hyperopia

Jason Stahl, MD and Daniel S. Durrie, MD

Introduction

Laser-assisted in-situ keratomileusis (LASIK) has been the dominant refractive procedure throughout the world for several years. However, the popularity of surface ablation has recently increased with the development of laser-assisted sub-epithelial keratectomy (LASEK). This resurgence of interest in surface ablation has paralleled the development of wavefront technology in refractive surgery. Wavefront testing has demonstrated that LASIK induces greater higher order aberrations than photorefractive keratectomy (PRK). The LASIK flap itself contributes to this increase in aberrations. Therefore, surface ablation techniques may be the ideal procedure for wavefront-guided custom excimer laser surgery. Unfortunately, many LASIK surgeons have a limited experience performing PRK and managing these patients postoperatively. PRK is a safe and effective treatment that has some unique complications with which LASIK surgeons may not be familiar. In this chapter, we describe complications that have been reported following hyperopic PRK.

Epithelial Healing

The creation of large corneal epithelial defects during hyperopic PRK raises concerns of epithelial healing problems. Corneal epithelial healing is usually complete between days 3 to 5 but delayed healing up to day 10 has been reported.[1-8] A delay in epithelial healing increases the risk of postoperative haze formation and prolongs the risk for development of infection keratitis.

Corneal epithelial surface irregularities are common during the early postoperative period following hyperopic PRK including: heaped epithelium, filaments, erosions, epithelial ridges, punctate epithelial erosions, and irregular, rough and/or loose epithelium.[2,7,8] Eyes with epithelial irregularities may exhibit a significant reduction in early postoperative uncorrected and best corrected vision. These epithelial irregularities typically resolve during the first few postoperative weeks with the help of topical lubricants but may persist up to 3 months.[2,7] Findings suggest epithelial irregularities persist longer in eyes treated for higher levels of hyperopia and in older patients.[2,8] As the epithelial irregularities resolve, an improvement in the vision usually follows. However, epithelial healing delays and/or irregularities influence corneal stromal healing that may result in persistent surface irregularities leading to prolonged loss of best corrected vision.[2] Because of these potential problems, rapid and complete re-epithelialization during the first week after surgery should be the goal in PRK surgery.

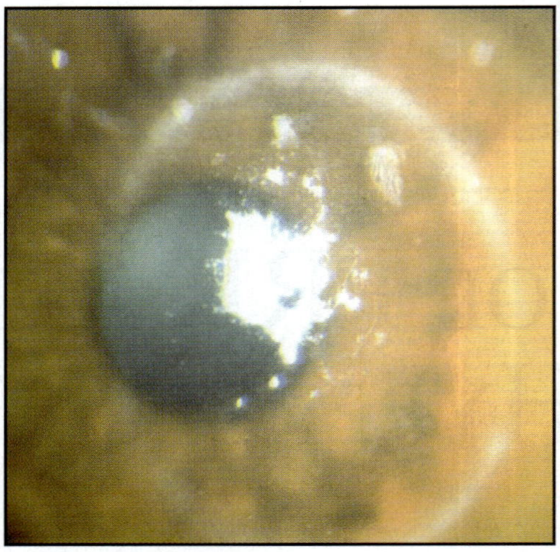

Figure 7-1. Sterile corneal infiltrate with immune ring following PRK, probably related to NSAIDs (courtesy of Neal A. Sher, MD).

Keratoconjunctivitis sicca (KCS) is a common cause of delayed epithelial healing after photorefractive keratectomy. Evidence of KCS should be sought during preoperative evaluation of refractive surgery patients. Analysis of the tear film includes visualization of the tear lake, staining of cornea and/or conjunctiva with rose bengal or fluorescein, Schirmer's testing of aqueous tear production, and tear lactoferrin testing. Aqueous deficiency should be treated preoperatively with artificial tears and lubricants and if necessary temporary or permanent punctal occlusion. Meibomian gland dysfunction (MGD) and blepharitis are commonly under-diagnosed disorders. MGD disrupts the tear film, increasing aqueous evaporation. Normal meibomian oils have a clear color and thin consistency. The oils should be expressed for evaluation by squeezing the lids with a cotton-tip applicator or a finger. If MGD is present, the eyelids are treated with the S-S-S eyelid hygiene technique of warm soaks, squeezing, and scrubbing. Oral doxycyline may also be employed to help thin the oils, thus improving the quality of the tear film.

Epithelial healing problems may also be caused by epithelial toxicity from eye drops. An eye undergoing PRK is typically exposed to: preoperative antibiotics, nonsteroidal anti-inflammatory drugs (NSAIDs) and anesthetics; intraoperative anesthetics, alcohol (to aid epithelial removal), and antibiotics; and postoperative antibiotics, steroids, NSAIDs, and artificial lubricants. Preservatives present in these topical agents are also capable of causing delayed epithelial healing. The judicious use of postoperative medications is especially important prior to closure of the epithelial defect. Preservative-free artificial lubricants are used at least until healthy epithelium is present.

Soft bandage contact lenses (CTLs) are typically used following PRK until re-epithelialization is complete. The proper fitting lens is important for patient comfort and epithelial healing. A tight lens reduces oxygen availability to the corneal epithelium that may contribute to delayed healing. Pain from tight-lens syndrome is another problem with a tight fitting lens. We have studied[9] CTLs following surface ablation and found that a properly fit non-ionic low- to medium-water content lens appears to offer the best chance for a successful immediate postoperative period following surface ablation. Our present choice of lens is the Bausch & Lomb (Rochester, NY) Soflens 66.

Sterile Infiltrates

Sterile corneal infiltrates following PRK were originally reported by surgeons in a multicenter clinical trial utilizing bandage CTLs and topical diclofenac, an NSAID, versus placebo to reduce postoperative pain.[10] While they reported corneal infiltrates in 3 (9%) of 32 patients, only 2 of the 3 eyes had been treated with diclofenac. Teal reported 30 cases of corneal infiltrates after PRK. All the patients were treated with NSAIDs (diclofenac or ketorolac) and bandage CTL except for one patient who had conventional patching postoperatively. Surveys of high volume PRK surgeons report the incidence of sterile corneal infiltrates to be one case per 200 to 300 eyes.[11,12]

The corneal subepithelial infiltrates typically occur on the first to third postoperative day and are associated with pain, decreased acuity, photophobia, and ciliary injection. Clinically, white subepithelial infiltrates are usually multiple (53%) but may be single (10%), diffuse (10%), satellite opacity (17%) or immune ring (10%).[11] Figure 7-1 demonstrates a sterile corneal infiltrate with immune ring following PRK. The infiltrates usually appear either within the ablation zone or just adjacent to the ablation zone with central (57%), inferior (27%), peripheral (4%), and superior (1%) locations being reported.[11] Permanent scarring resulting in reduced best corrected vision was the usual outcome.

The etiology of post-PRK sterile corneal infiltrates is unknown. Most surgeons presume an infectious etiology and treat with topical antibiotics.[11,12] However, no infectious etiology has been identified (no positive cultures).[11,12] Sterile corneal infiltrates are a well-known complication of soft CTL wear.

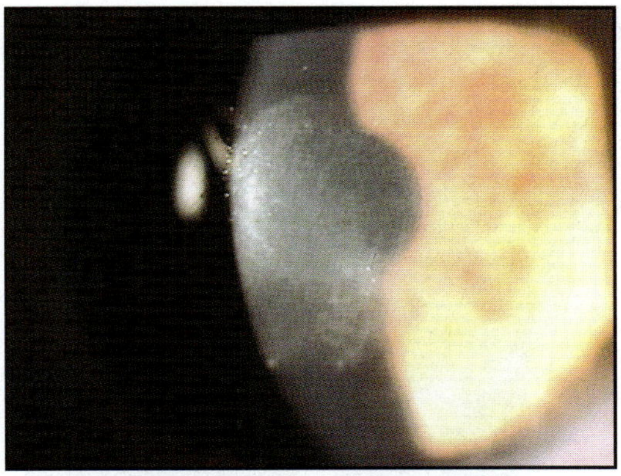

Figure 7-2. Infectious keratitis post-PRK, alpha *streptococci*, day 3.

However, subepithelial infiltrates following PRK have rarely been reported after conventional patching and NSAID use.[11] NSAIDs act by inhibiting the cyclo-oxygenase pathway, which may cause increased levels of arachidonic acid being shunted into the lipoxygenase pathway.[13] This pathway produces increased levels of leukotrienes and hydroxyeicosatetraenoic acid, which are chemoattractants for polymorphonuclear (PMN) cells, and increases leukocyte degranulation and oxygen free-radical formation.[14] Phillips[15] demonstrated an aggressive infiltration of PMNs into rabbit corneas treated with topical diclofenac alone following PRK. The administration of fluorometholone 0.1% has been shown to significantly reduce this response by inhibition of phospholipase A, preventing the conversion of membrane phospholipids to arachidonic acid. Sher[16] has reported no cases of sterile infiltrates following PRK when steroids were added along with the NSAIDs to the postoperative regime. Thus, the administration of topical NSAIDs without concomitant steroids before epithelial healing may be the etiology of sterile corneal infiltrates following PRK. However, an infectious etiology should always be ruled out when corneal infiltrates are seen following PRK.

Infectious Keratitis

Infectious keratitis is a rare complication of PRK. The incidence of this complication is unknown. A literature review found 15 cases of infectious keratitis following excimer laser PRK.[17-27] Most cases of infectious keratitis were diagnosed within 2 or 3 days postoperatively but one case was diagnosed on day seven[26] and another case 3 weeks[23] after PRK. Prompt treatment usually resulted in a good visual outcome. However, other cases have resulted in loss of vision due to endophthalmitis, corneal scaring, corneal thinning or scaring requiring penetrating keratoplasty, and glaucomatous optic neuropathy. The organisms identified are typically bacterial including *Staphylococcus aureus*,[26] *Staphylococcus epidermidis*,[24] methicillin-resistant *S. aureus*,[25] nonhemolytic *streptococci*[27] and *Pseudomonas aeruginosa*,[21] but one case of fungal keratitis with *Scopulariopsis* species has been reported.[23] Figure 7-2 is an example of an *alpha streptococci* infection day 3 after PRK.

A bandage CTL was used in almost all reported cases of infectious keratitis after PRK. The use of a bandage CTL following PRK is controversial. Bandage CTLs have been shown to significantly reduce postoperative pain after PRK.[22,28,29] Another benefit of a bandage CTL is faster epithelial healing following PRK[22] and traumatic corneal abrasions.[30] However, a bandage CTL may increase the risk of infection following PRK. Bandage lenses presumably interfere with the normal flushing activities of tears minimizing tear flow beneath the lens allowing cell debris and contaminants to collect over an exposed corneal stroma.

There are several important preventive measures surgeons should perform to reduce the risk of infection after PRK. Surgeons should evaluate the patient's eyelids, ocular surface, and lacrimal sac for possible sources of infection during the preoperative examination and treat these structures if needed before surgery. Performing surgery with aseptic techniques is extremely important for preventing infection. The use of preoperative, intraoperative, and postoperative prophylactic broad-spectrum antibiotics may reduce infections. Patients should be followed closely until the epithelium heals after PRK and educated on the importance of compliance with postoperative medication therapy.

Haze

Corneal subepithelial haze is a common finding following hyperopic PRK.[2,3,5-8,31,32,33] The haze is characteristically ring shaped corresponding to the hyperopic ablation pattern (Figure 7-3). Hyperopic ablations typically do not treat the central cornea therefore Bowman's layer remains intact leaving the central cornea clear. Most eyes develop haze 1 to 6 months following PRK. The haze typically fades with time as is seen in myopic PRK. The haze intensity tends to be related to the depth of ablation and is therefore more dense with higher hyperopic corrections.[2,31,32] This midperipheral haze usually has no effect on visual outcomes and studies typically

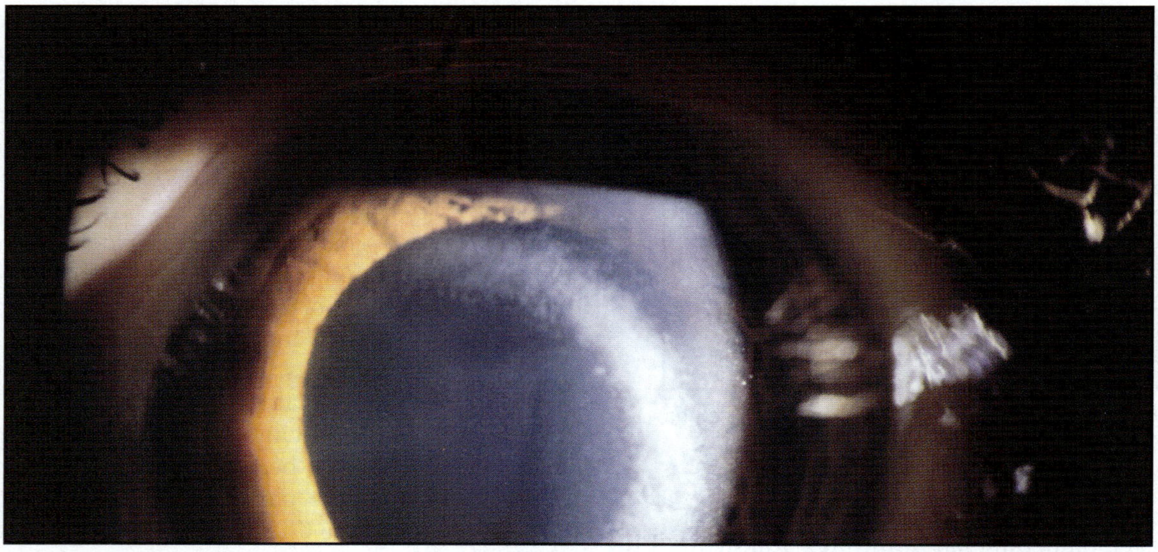

Figure 7-3. Characteristic mid-peripheral ring of haze following hyperopic PRK. (Courtesy of Edward Manche, MD.)

report no correlation between haze, best-corrected vision, or refractive regression.[6,8,32] However, a correlation between haze and regression of achieved correction has been reported.[31]

Induced Astigmatism

Surgically induced astigmatism following hyperopic PRK has been reported in several studies.[2-4,32,34] Vector analysis demonstrates the induced astigmatism tends to be aligned along the with-the-rule meridian.[32,34] Induced astigmatism may be seen more frequently with the correction of higher levels of hyperopia.[2]

The etiology of these astigmatic changes is not easy to explain. Slight decentration of the ablation may cause induced astigmatism. The newer generation excimer lasers utilize eye-tracking technology that helps center ablations. However, controversy exists over whether the hyperopic ablation should be centered over the pupil versus the visual axis. Another possible cause of induced astigmatism is asymmetrical corneal wound healing following PRK.

Our observation has been that procedures performed in the midperiphery of the cornea such as a hyperopic ablation have the tendency to magnify and make manifest any corneal asymmetry present at the location of treatment. Due to the fact that scanning-slit topographers such as the Orbscan (Bausch & Lomb, Rochester, NY) do not average values as it moves away from the corneal apex, we find its description of the midperipheral and peripheral cornea reliable. Figure 7-4A illustrates an example of a patient with a low degree of central asymmetry and significant peripheral astigmatism on anterior float. This patient demonstrates induced astigmatism at a predicable axis following hyperopic PRK (Figure 7-4B). In many patients with substantial peripheral asymmetry or significant higher order aberrations on wavefront testing, customized treatment is recommended.

Reactivation of Herpes Keratitis

Reactivation of latent herpes simplex virus by excimer laser PRK has been reported in humans.[35,36] Excimer laser ablation has also been demonstrated to trigger viral shedding and reactivation of herpetic keratitis in latently infected rabbits.[37,38] De-epithelialization alone was not sufficient to cause keratitis or viral reactivation. Prophylaxis with valacyclovir in rabbits decreased the recurrence rate in a dose-response fashion with no recurrences reported with 150 mg/kg/day.[38] Patients have also experienced reactivation of herpes keratitis after excimer laser phototherapeutic keratectomy.[39,40] Figure 7-5 shows a typical *h. simplex* dendritic figure. However, the cause-and-effect relationship between reactivation of herpetic keratitis and excimer ablation was cast in doubt when Fagerholm[39] found no significant difference between the incidence of reactivation of herpetic keratitis after PTK compared with the incidence

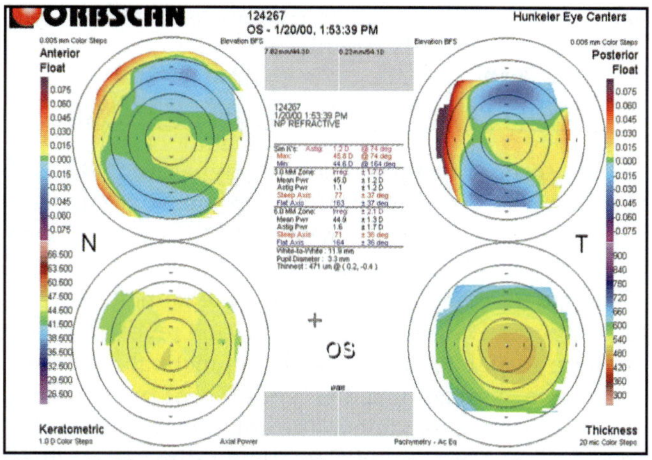

Figure 7-4A. Preoperative: The anterior float demonstrates peripheral astigmatism not manifested preoperatively. (Courtesy of Jason Stahl, MD.)

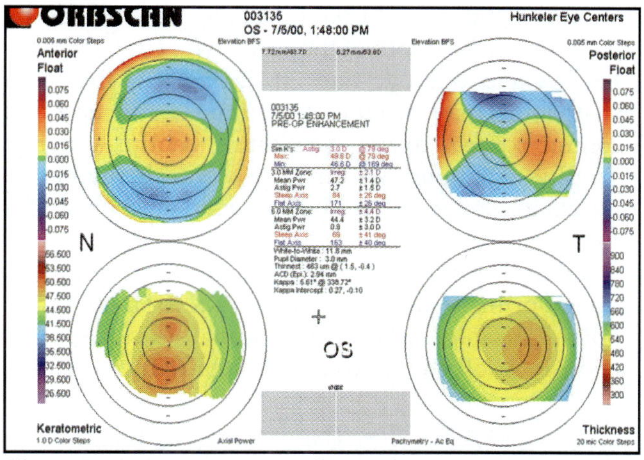

Figure 7-4B. Postoperative: Following hyperopic PRK, the anterior float appearance is as expected. However, the patient now manifests 2 diopters of WTR astigmatism consistent with that present in the periphery preoperatively. (Courtesy of Jason Stahl, MD.)

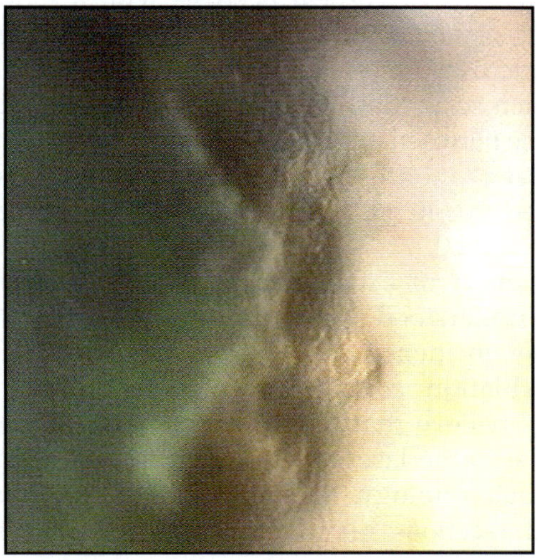

Figure 7-5. *Herpes simplex* dendritic figure.

prior to PTK. Beyer[41] has reported that corneal nerve disruption alone reactivates herpetic eye disease in latently infected rabbits. Although controversy exists has to whether exposure to excimer laser treatment reactivates latent herpes keratitis, we recommend prophylaxis with oral acyclovir for all patients with a history of ocular herpetic disease undergoing excimer laser treatment.

Apical Scarring

Sener[42] reported apical nodular subepithelial corneal scar occurring in 12 eyes of 6 patients that had undergone hyperopic PRK retreatment. The 5 men and 1 female all had primary PRK to correct hyperopia with a mean spherical equivalent refraction of +7.26 ± 0.95 D. PRK retreatment was performed for residual hyperopia a mean of 9.5 ± 1.44 months after primary hyperopic PRK. The mean spherical equivalent refraction that was treated was +4.67 ± 0.81 D.

Bilateral subepithelial nodular scarring of the central cornea was noted in all patients at the 1 month postoperative examination. The scarring progressed until the 3-month postoperative examination which revealed bilateral, symmetrical round scars protruding anteriorly, measuring less than 2.0 mm and located at the center of the entrance pupil. There was no change in the size or density of the lesions during the follow-up period (mean 40.66 ± 2.46 months). Seven eyes had trace haze at the paracentral cornea over the laser-ablated area and 5 eyes had no corneal haze.

Three years after PRK retreatment, the mean postoperative spherical equivalent refraction was +4.36 ± 1.83 D in 9 eyes and the refraction was unmeasurable in 3 eyes. Two eyes (16.6%) had BCVA of 20/40 or better while 5 eyes (41.6%) lost 1 line of BCVA and 7 eyes (58.3%) lost 2 or more lines of BCVA. On corneal topography, the lesions caused irregular central steepening, distorted central corneal mires and surface regularity indices greater than 2.00 in all eyes.

Corneal haze formation after hyperopic PRK occurs at the ablated area, the paracentral cornea, and usually spontaneously resolves with time. The apical nodular scars were located in the central nonablated cornea and persisted without change during the 3-year follow-up period.

Nagy[43] reported a central bump-like opacity in 3 eyes following primary PRK for hyperopic corrections between +5.00 and +6.00 D. The incidence was 1.85% (3/162) in eyes treated with hyperopic PRK for ≥+5 D. The opacity recurred in 1 eye after PTK while another opacity could only partially be removed by PTK due to the depth of the scar. Two eyes had 20/30 BSCVA and one eye had 20/25 BSCVA. Excessive steepening may produce tear film dysfunction and central corneal drying facilitating central scarring. Trophic changes within the central unablated Bowman's layer are another possible mechanism for central scarring.

Central corneal scarring is a significant complication of primary and retreatment PRK for high hyperopic corrections. The central scar does not spontaneously resolve with time and often reduces vision.

Changes in Measured Intraocular Pressure

A decrease in measured intraocular pressure (IOP) following myopic PRK has been reported in several studies.[45-46] Studies have revealed a direct correlation between the decrease in postoperative measured IOP and the decrease in central corneal thickness[47] or the magnitude of pretreatment myopia.[48] Because the central cornea remains relatively untreated in hyperopic PRK, one would expect less change in the measured postoperative IOP compared to myopic PRK.

A recent study by Munger[49] found that despite only minimal changes in the central corneal thickness (CCT), the changes in IOP after hyperopic PRK were similar to changes after myopic PRK. During the study, 191 eyes had hyperopic PRK to correct from +1.00 to +6.50 D of sphere and less than 3.75 D of cylinder. IOP and CCT were measured preoperatively and at 1, 2, 3, 6, 12, 18, and 24 months. The mean IOP was 1.0 to 1.8 mmHg lower than the preoperative IOP (P <.001) at all postoperative examinations. A mean decrease in CCT between 17.0 and 21.0 µm was measured at all postoperative visits (P <.001). However, the changes in IOP did not correlate with changes in CCT, unlike what has been demonstrated with myopic PRK. The significant reduction in CCT was unexpected because the hyperopic PRK laser ablation does not treat the central cornea. The authors speculate that after hyperopic PRK, biomechanical effects may result in stromal thinning of the central cornea.

Wang et al[50] reported that Goldmann applanation tonometry may underestimate the IOP after hyperopic LASIK. They found a significant reduction in postoperative Goldmann applanation tonometry measurements of IOP taken from the central and peripheral cornea after hyperopic LASIK. Postoperative pneumotonometry IOP measurements taken from the central and peripheral cornea were also lower than preoperative measurements but were not statistically significant.

Acute Corneal Necrosis

Acute corneal necrosis following hyperopic PRK is a rare and severe complication reported by Mietz et al.[51] A 56-year-old white male had PRK OS to correct mild hyperopia and astigmatism (+1.75 + 0.75 x 51). The patient complained of moderate pain at the day 1 postoperative visit. The examination revealed hand motion visual acuity, marked conjunctival injection, chemosis, corneal opacities, endothelial precipitates, and a fibrinous exudate in the anterior chamber. The eye did not improve with treatment directed against bacteria, fungi, and *Acanthamoeba*. An infectious etiology was not identified. A penetrating keratoplasty (PKP) was performed on postoperative day 24. An anterior zone of corneal necrosis with a moderate amount of acute inflammatory cells was seen on light microscopy. Immunohisto-chemistry and electron microscopy detected keratocyte apoptosis at the interface between necrotic and viable corneal stroma. Seventeen months following PKP the patient achieved 20/40 visual acuity with a refraction of +0.25+2.25x60.

The effect of excimer laser on corneal tissue is poorly understood. A rabbit study has demonstrated a higher incidence of apoptosis following excimer laser ablation compared to control eyes.[52] The authors believe that their patient's corneal reaction was due to the laser ablation and not related to an infectious etiology. They speculate that similar corneal reactions may be misinterpreted as infections.

Summary

Complications following excimer laser PRK (surface ablation) for hyperopia are low. Surface ablation techniques may be the ideal procedure for wavefront-guided custom excimer laser surgery. LASIK surgeons who have limited experience with PRK will need to become familiar with these potential complications. A careful preoperative examination should be performed in all refractive surgery patients to exclude conditions that may increase the risk of postoperative complications. Hopefully, as surgeons gain experience with surface ablation, the ability to avoid, identify, and successfully manage complications will improve.

References

1. Sener B, et al. Photorefractive keratectomy for hyperopia and aphakia with a scanning spot excimer laser. 1997;13:620-623.
2. O'Brart DPS, Stephenson CG, Baldwin H, et al. Hyperopic photorefractive keratectomy with the erodible mask and axicon system: two year follow-up. *J Cataract Refract Surg.* 2000;26:524-535.
3. Stevens JD, Ficker LA. Results of Photorefractive keratectomy for hyperopia using the VISX star excimer laser system. *J Refract Surg.* 2002;18:30-36.
4. Carones F, Brancato R, Morico A, et al. Photorefractive keratectomy for hyperopia using an erodible disc and axicon lens: 2 year results. *J Refract Surg* 1998;14:504-511.
5. Dausch DGJ, Klein R, Schroder E, Niemczyk S. Photorefractive keratectomy for hyperopic and mixed astigmatism. *J Refract Surg.* 1996;12:684-692.
6. Nagy ZZ, Munkacsy G, Popper M. Photorefractive keratectomy using the Meditec MEL 70 G-scan laser for hyperopia and hyperopic astigmatism. *J Refract Surg.* 2002;18:542-550.
7. Jackson WB, Casson E, Hodge W, et al. Laser vision correction for low hyperopia. *Ophthalmology.* 1998;105:1727-1738.
8. Nagy ZZ, Krueger RR, et al. Photorefractive keratectomy for hyperopia in 800 eyes with the Meditec MEL 60 laser. *J Refract Surg.* 2001;17:525-533.
9. Durrie DS. Bandage contact lenses and surface ablation. *LASEK Congress.* March 2001.
10. Sher NA, Frantz JM, Talley A, et al. Topical diclofenac in the treatment of ocular pain after excimer photorefractive keratectomy. *Refract Corneal Surg.* 1993;9:425-436.
11. Teal P, Breslin C, Arshinoff S, Edmison D. Corneal subepithelial infiltrates following excimer laser photorefractive keratectomy. *J Cataract Refract Surg.* 1995;5:516-518.
12. Arshinoff SA, Mills MD, Haber S. Pharmacotherapy of photorefractive keratectomy. *J Cataract Refract Surg.* 1996;22:1037-1044.
13. Ku EC, Lee W, Kothari HV, Scholer DW. Effect of diclofenac sodium on the arachidonic cascade. *Am J Med.* 1986;80(suppl 4B):18-23.
14. Hecker M, Foegh ML, Ramwell PW. The eicsanoids: prostaglandins, thromboxanes, leukotrienes, and related compounds. In: Katzung BG, ed. *Basic & Clinical Pharmacology.* 6th ed. Norwalk, CT: Appleton & Lange; 1995;290-306.
15. Phillips AF, Szerenyi K, Campos M, et al. Arachidonic acid metabolites after excimer laser corneal surgery. *Arch Ophthalmol.* 1993;111:1273-1278.
16. Sher NA, Krueger RR, Teal P, et al. Role of topical corticosteroids and nonsteroidal anti-inflammatory drugs in the etiology of stromal infiltrates after excimer photorefractive keratectomy. (Letter). *J Refract Corneal Surg.* 1994;10:587-588.
17. McDonald MB, Frantz JM, Klyce SD, et al. Central photorefractive keratectomy for myopia: the blind eye study. *Arch Ophthalmol.* 1990;108:799-808.
18. Faschinger C, Faulborn J, Gauser K. Infektiose hornhauntgeschwurte-einmal mit endophthalmitis nach PRK mit einmalkontaktlinse. *Klin Monatsbi Augenheilkd.* 1995;206:96-102.
19. Lavery FL. Photorefractive keratectomy in 472 eyes. *Refract Corneal Surg.* 1993;9:11-16.
20. Waked NE, Ojeimi GK. Excimer laser photorefractive keratectomy in Lebanon. *J Refract Surg.* 1995;11(3 Suppl):S270-273.
21. Wee WR, Kim JY, Choi YS, Lee JH. Bacterial keratitis after photorefractive keratectomy in a young, healthy man. *J Cataract Refract Surg.* 1997;23:954-956.
22. Lim-Bon-Siong R, Valluri S, Gordon ME, Pepose JS. Efficacy and safety of the ProTek (vifilcon A) therapeutic soft contact lens after photorefractive keratectomy. *Am J Ophthalmol.* 1998;126:328-329.
23. Kouyoumdjian GA, Forstot SL, et al. Infectious keratitis after laser refractive surgery. *Ophthalmology.* 2001;108:1266-1268.
24. Amayem A, Ali AT, Waring GO, Ibrahim O. Bacterial keratitis after photorefractive keratectomy. *J Refract Surg.* 1996;12:642-644.
25. Förster W, Becker K, Hungermann D, Busse H. Methicillin-resistant *Staphylococcus aureus* keratitis after excimer laser photorefractive keratectomy. *J Cataract Refract Surg.* 2002;28:722-724.
26. Heidemann D, Clune M, Dunn S, Chow C. Infectious keratitis after photorefractive keratectomy in a comanaged setting. *J Cataract Refract Surg.* 2000;26:140-141.
27. Malling S. Keratitis with loss of useful vision after photorefractive keratectomy. *J Cataract Refract Surg.* 1999;25:137-139.
28. Cherry PMH. The treatment of pain following excimer laser photorefractive keratectomy: additive effect of local anesthetic drops, topical diclofenac, and bandage soft contact. *Ophthalmic Surg Lasers.* 1996;27(suppl):S477-480.
29. Cherry PMH, Tutton MK, Adhikary H, et al. The treatment of pain following photorefractive keratectomy. *J Refract Corneal Surg.* 1994;10(suppl):S222-225.
30. Acheson JF, Joseph J, Spalten DJ. Use of soft contact lenses in an eye casualty department for the primary treatment of traumatic corneal abrasions. *Br J Ophthalmol.* 1987;71:285-289.
31. Pietilä J, Mäkinen P, Pajari S, Uusitalo H. Excimer laser photorefractive keratectomy for hyperopia. *J Refract Surg.* 1997;13:504-510.
32. Danjoux JP, Kalski R, Cohen P, Lawless M, Rogers C. Excimer laser photorefractive keratectomy for hyperopia. *J Refract Surg.* 1997;13:349-355.
33. Haw W, Manche E. Prospective study of photorefractive keratectomy for hyperopia using an axicon lens and erodible mask. *J Refract Surg.* 2000;16:724-730.

34. Carones F, Gobbi PG, et al. Photorefractive keratectomy for hyperopia: long-term nonlinear and vector analysis of refractive outcome. *Ophthalmology*. 1999;106:1976-1983.
35. McDonnell PJ, Moreira H, Clapham TN, et al. Photorefractive keratectomy for astigmatism: initial clinical results. *Arch Ophthalmol*. 1991;109:1370-1373.
36. Rao SK, Mukesh BN, Bakshi H, Sitalakshmi G, Padmanabhan P. Photorefractive keratectomy: the Sankara Nethralaya experience. *Ophthalmic Surg Lasers*. 1996;27(5 Suppl):S444-453.
37. Epstein SP, Fisher EM, Sternberg GJ, et al. Recurrent ocular herpes simplex keratitis following excimer laser photorefractive keratectomy in a rabbit model. *CLAO J*. 2001;27:94-99.
38. Asbell PA. Valacyclovir for the prevention of recurrent herpes simplex virus eye disease after excimer laser photokeratectomy. *Trans Am Ophthalmol Soc*. 2000;98:285-303.
39. Fagerholm P, Ohman L, Orndahl M. Phototherapeutic keratectomy in herpes simplex keratitis. clinical results in 20 patients. *Acta Ophthalmol*. 1994;72:457-460.
40. Vrabec MP, Anderson JA, Rock ME, et al. Electron microscopic findings in a cornea with recurrence of herpes simplex keratitis after excimer laser phototherapeutic keratectomy. *CLAO J*. 1994;20:41-44.
41. Beyer CF, Hill JM, Reidy JJ, Beuerman RW. Corneal nerve disruption reactivates virus in rabbits latently infected with HSV-1. *Invest Ophthalmol Vis Sci*. 1990;31:925-932.
42. Sener B, Ozdamar A, Aras C. Apical nodular subepithelial corneal scar after retreatment in hyperopic photorefractive keratectomy. *J Cataract Refract Surg*. 2000;26:352-357.
43. Nagy ZZ, Krueger RR, Süveges I. Central bump-like opacity as a complication of high hyperopic photorefractive keratectomy. *Am J Ophthalmol*. 1999;128:636-638.
44. Schipper I, Senn P, Thomann U, Suppiger M. Intraocular pressure after excimer laser photorefractive keratectomy for myopia. *J Refract Surg*. 1995;11:366-370.
45. Mardelli PG, Piebengal LW, Whitacre MM, Siegmund KD. The effect of excimer laser photorefractive keratectomy on intraocular pressure measurements using the Goldmann applanation tonometer. *Ophthalmology*. 1997;104:945-948.
46. Faucher A, Gregoire J, Blondeau P. Accuracy of Goldmann tonometry after refractive surgery. *J Cataract Refract Surg*. 1997;23:832-838.
47. Munger R, Hodge WG, Mintsioulis G, et al. Correction of intraocular pressure for changes in central corneal thickness following photorefractive keratectomy. *Can J Ophthalmol*. 1998;33:159-165.
48. Chatterjee A, Shah S, Bessant DA, Naroo SA, Doyle SJ. Reduction in intraocular pressure after excimer laser photorefractive keratectomy—correlation with pretreatment myopia. *Ophthalmology*. 1997;104:355-359.
49. Munger R, Dohadwala AA, Hodge WG, et al. Changes in measured intraocular pressure after hyperopic photorefractive keratectomy. *J Cataract Refract Surg*. 2001;27:1254-1262.
50. Wang X, Shen J, McCulley JP, et al. Intraocular pressure measurement after hyperopic LASIK. *CLAO J*. 2002;28(3):136-139.
51. Mietz H, Severin M, Seifert P, et al. Acute corneal necrosis after excimer laser keratectomy for hyperopia. *Ophthalmology*. 1999;106:490-496.
52. Gao J, Gelber-Schwalb TA, Addeo JV, Stern ME. Apoptosis in the rabbit cornea after photorefractive keratectomy. *Cornea*. 1997;16:200-208.

Chapter Eight

Hyperopic LASIK: Techniques and Results

David R. Hardten, MD and Neelu Hira, OD

Introduction

The field of refractive surgery has grown exponentially over the last several years. This growth may be due to a combination of factors. While increased safety and precision are probably the most influential, other contributing factors may include increased number of refractive surgeons and laser centers and the expanded approval of new technology and treatment modalities. Most of the early efforts were focused on treating myopia because it is technically an easier refractive error to treat. Myopic patients are more dependent on glasses and thus they have benefited tremendously from these relatively safe and predictable procedures in enhancing their quality of life. There is now increasing interest and consumer demand in applying these same procedures and technologies to treat hyperopia.

Changing the radius of corneal curvature with LASIK remains the most common means of changing the eyes refractive error, as it accounts for two-thirds of the refractive power in the eye. Recent studies have shown predictable results in low to moderate levels of hyperopia in patients treated with hyperopic laser-assisted in situ keratomileusis (H-LASIK). As with myopia, several modalities in addition to LASIK for surgically managing hyperopia exist including hexagonal keratectomy (HK), automated lamellar keratoplasty (ALK), Holmium-YAG, laser thermal keratoplasty (LTK), corneal inlay, clear lens extraction, intraocular lens (IOL) implantation, conductive keratoplasty (CK) or hyperopic photorefractive keratectomy (HPRK).[1-11] However, each of these procedures have their own potential shortcomings, and so have been used in limited situations. H-LASIK is discussed in this chapter.

Prevalence and Anatomy

Hyperopia is a common vision problem, affecting a significant portion of the population. Approximately half of the population over the age of 50 years is hyperopic, with an increasing incidence of hyperopia from 21.1% in individuals between 43 and 54 years of age to 68.5% in those 75 years of age or older.[12] Hyperopia occurs when light entering the eye focuses behind the retina, instead of directly on it. It is caused by a cornea that is flatter, or an eye that is shorter than the emmetropic eye. Correction of hyperopia can be achieved with spectacles, contact lenses, or refractive surgery, all allowing light to focus directly on the retina.

Young patients with low to moderate hyperopia are able to correct their distance vision with the help of accommodation. These patients may not require corrective lenses to see clearly at a distance, but can experience blurred near vision, headaches, and eye strain. In patients with severe hyperopia, accommodation alone may be inadequate and thus require corrective lenses to correct both distance and near vision. Also loss of accommodation with age affects both distance and near vision. The age at which a hyperope requires correction for near or distance depends on the amount of their hyperopia.

Patient Selection

A thorough preoperative comprehensive eye examination with emphasis on the following key elements aids the surgeon in determining the appropriate refractive surgical procedure and helps select patients with good outcomes. In general, patients should be at least 18 years of age to allow for relative stability of their correction due to growth of the eye. Patients should discontinue soft contact lenses 2 weeks and rigid gas permeable (RGP) contacts 3 to 4 weeks prior to this evaluation, due to the possibility of contact lens-induced corneal warpage.

History is helpful in determining patient's goals, vocation, avocation, knowledge of the procedure, and motivation for choosing refractive surgery. A comprehensive ocular and systemic history along with complete list of medications and drug allergies should be obtained. Both aided and unaided visual acuity should be documented for future comparison. Pupil size in both bright and dim illumination should be documented. Some surgeons may choose to use a laser with a larger treatment zone in patients with large pupils to reduce the likelihood of postoperative glare and halos, although it is difficult to predict preoperatively which patients may experience problems with glare and halos after surgery. Eye dominance should be noted as some surgeons may treat the non-dominant eye first. This is also useful in patients wanting monovision correction. All patients desiring monovision after H-LASIK should try contact lenses to establish tolerance of monovision first.

Cycloplegic refraction and keratometry should be stable. For H-LASIK cycloplegic refraction is helpful to uncover latent hyperopia and avoid obvious future regression.

The anterior segment should be thoroughly evaluated for any abnormalities. Blepharitis, meibomitis, and dry eyes need to be managed prior to surgery to avoid a longer, more difficult postoperative recovery period. Screening for keratoconus, corneal dystrophies, scars, or neovascularization needs to be performed. The presence of significant lens changes should be noted. Gonioscopy should be performed on all patients with shallow angles as these patients are at higher risk of angle closure.[13] It is important to document intraocular pressures (IOP) which help to rule out ocular hypertension and glaucoma. There have been reports of underestimation of tonometric reading with Goldmann applanation tonometer in patients who have undergone H-LASIK. This appears to be due to changes in corneal curvature.[14,15] Some patients are also more vulnerable to IOP spikes, which may occur with the use of postoperative steroids.

The posterior segment should be carefully evaluated with a dilated fundus exam to rule out any optic nerve, macula, and retina problems. Any treatable pathology should be addressed prior to surgery. Pachymetry should be used to determine corneal thickness. Post-surgical ectasia is probably less common with hyperopic LASIK, but can occur in patients with very thin residual bed thickness after LASIK, or in patients with preexisting keratoconus. Computerized corneal topography helps screen for corneal warpage, irregular astigmatism, extreme keratometric values, corneal thickness, and to rule out keratoconus. Wavefront analysis is helpful in ruling out patients with aberrations of the visual system other than spherical hyperopia or astigmatism, so-called higher order aberrations. Patients with significant higher order aberrations may have better results with wavefront treatment of their hyperopia. Patients with a displaced apex on topography are more likely to have significant higher order aberrations and may have better results with a wavefront directed treatment (Figure 8-1).

Risks, benefits, and alternatives should be discussed with the patient at the initial evaluation with emphasis on presbyopia, halos, glare, dry eyes, possible retreatments, and risk of loss of best-corrected visual acuity (BCVA). Patients should be supplied appropriate reading materials to supplement their understanding of the procedure and informed consent should be obtained.

Patients at Higher Risk

Refractive surgery in patients with the following conditions may have a higher risk of postoperative complications.

Ocular

Patients with an unstable refraction will not have a stable refraction postoperatively. Patients with functional monocularity take risk in their only functional eye. Keratoconus causes unstable irregular astigmatism that progresses over time, which is not specifically addressed by the surgery. Anterior membrane

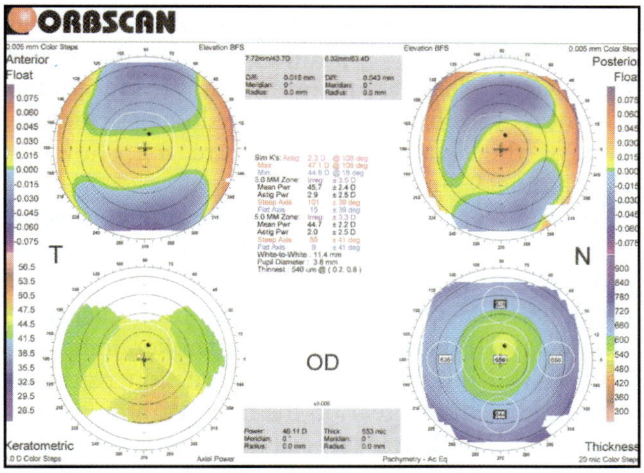

Figure 8-1. Preoperative LASIK corneal topography in a patient with a decentered apex. Centering the hyperopic ablation on this patient's cornea over the pupil may lead to irregular astigmatism postoperatively.

basement dystrophy may lead to epithelial sloughing at the time of the procedure. *Herpes simplex* keratitis may recur following the procedure. Patients with a history of *herpes zoster* may have neurotrophic corneas or uveitis, which may be problematic postoperatively. Patients with dry eyes will have dry eye symptoms postoperatively. Patients with significantly thin corneas may not have enough tissue remaining in the stromal bed to enable sufficient correction with the laser.

Systemic

Collagen vascular, autoimmune, immunodeficiency diseases, and other systemic diseases may affect wound healing postoperatively.

Medications

Patients taking isotretinoin (Accutane, Roche, Nutley, NJ) or amiodarone (Cordarone, Wyeth, Madison, NJ) may have collection of the drug in the cornea or abnormal healing responses with ocular surgery.

Other

During pregnancy or lactation, women may have hormonal changes that may affect refractive error or wound healing. Diabetes remains a relative risk factor due to unstable refraction in patients without tight blood sugar control and delayed wound healing. Patients with glaucoma, where the IOP is being measured serially, should know that IOP may be underestimated by Goldmann applanation tonometry.

Historical Perspectives

LASIK as first reported by Pallikaris et al in the 1990's has fast become the most popular surgical technique in correcting myopia and several recent studies have shown promising results in treating low to moderate levels of hyperopia.[16] LASIK is a two-step procedure; first a microkeratome is used to create a hinged corneal flap, this is followed by excimer laser ablation of the corneal stroma. At this time, FDA approval limits the application of H-LASIK to patients with 0 to 6.00 D of hyperopia with or without up to 6.00 D of astigmatism with Summit Autonomous (LADARVision, Alcon, Cleveland, Ohio) and hyperopia in the range of +0.50 D to 5.00 D with or without astigmatism up to +3.00 D with VISX (Star S2/S3).[17]

Microkeratomes

Several different microkeratomes are available for use in LASIK. The microkeratome head consists of 3 key components: a motor, an oscillating blade, and interchangeable plates. The thickness of these determine the thickness of the flap (usually 160 to 180 µm). The main differences along those microkeratomes are the method of assembly, the location of the corneal flap's hinge, and automated or manual translation across the cornea during the procedure.

Alternatives to blades containing microkeratomes include the use of high-speed water jet and laser technology, but metal blade microkeratomes still are most commonly utilized, and have the longest track record.[18,19]

Lasers

Many different excimer lasers have been successfully used to treat low to moderate levels of hyperopia. Each laser has a unique combination of the ablation zone parameters, beam profile, and beam delivery mechanism. For hyperopic correction, more laser energy is directed to the peripheral cornea in an annular zone around the central optical zone resulting in central steepening relative to corneal periphery. A treatment area of greater than 8.0 mm and an optical zone between 5.5 to 6 mm is typically utilized.

Operative Technique

The surgeon should confirm identity of patients and make sure proper parameters are entered into the computer. All instruments should be sterile and cali-

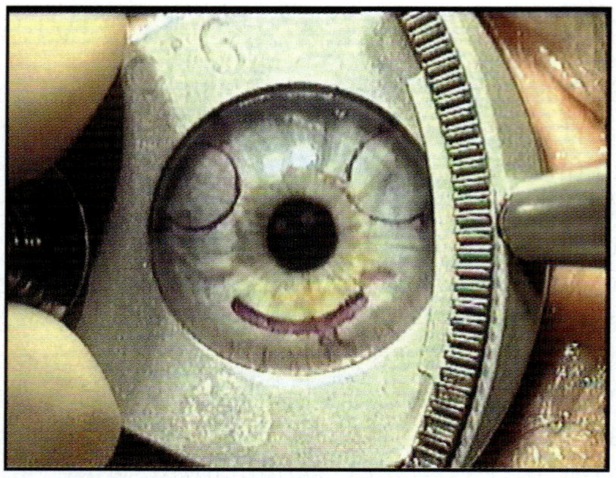

Figure 8-2. Hansatome keratome with 9.5 mm on eye.

brated. Room temperature should be accounted and adjusted for in planning the procedure. Approximately 5 to 10 minutes before the procedure, 5 mg of diazepam are given to the patient to alleviate the anxiety of undergoing the procedure and to help them sleep postoperatively.

The patient is then positioned under the microscope, with the head carefully aligned to make sure the iris is perpendicular to the laser beam. Careful centration with the eye aligned in the *x*, *y*, and *z* planes is crucial.

Topical anesthesia is then applied to the eye. The eyelids are prepared with diluted povidone-iodine solution and a lid speculum is inserted to open the eyelids. Eyelashes should be kept away from the surgical field by the use of adhesive drapes or a closed, bladed lid speculum. The contralateral eye is taped shut to prevent cross-fixation and dehydration of the cornea.

The microkeratome should be inspected for any defects in the blade or function of the moving parts. It is also vital to confirm that the excimer laser will be able to deliver treatment after the corneal flap is reflected. The cornea can be marked with ink before creating the corneal flap with the microkeratome to more easily realign the corneal flap in the event that a free flap is created.

The suction ring is placed using a bimanual technique where the shaft of the suction ring is held in the fingers of one hand and a finger from the other hand provides additional support on the ring itself. A large suction ring is used for hyperopic LASIK to make certain that the flap will be large enough to put the larger hyperopic ablation under the flap. Once adequate placement has been achieved the suction is engaged by foot control (usually done by the technician). Adequate intraocular pressure (above 65 mmHg) is then verified, with one useful method being an applanation lens (Barraquer tonometer). When adequate suction is achieved, the patient will confirm the temporary loss of visualization of the fixation light. Figure 8-2 shows a Hansatome, 9.5-mm ring on eye.

Before the pass of the microkeratome, several drops of artificial tears are placed on the cornea. This lubrication reduces the likelihood of a corneal epithelial defect occurring during the microkeratome pass. If using a two-piece microkeratome, the head is slid onto the post of the suction ring and advanced until the gear on the microkeratome head engages the track. It is important to again verify that the suction ring is still firmly attached to the globe at this point by gently lifting the suction ring upward, making sure that the suction is not lost. The surgeon then activates the microkeratome using forward and reverse foot controls, the suction is turned off after the microkeratome pass and the suction ring can then be carefully removed. In cases where the stromal bed is too small or irregular for a good result, the laser ablation should not be performed, and the flap is carefully placed back into position.

Before lifting the flap, a moist cellulose sponge is used to remove any cells, debris, or excess fluid from the top of the flap that otherwise might get onto the stromal bed. Using forceps, the flap can be lifted and directed toward the hinge.

A dry or slightly moist cellulose sponge is then used to carefully remove any excess fluid from the stromal surface. Hydration of the stromal bed needs to be adjusted evenly and consistently in all cases. It is important at this point to minimize the procedure time in order to prevent stromal dehydration and subsequent overcorrection. Uneven hydration can lead to central islands and/or irregular astigmatism. Excess pooling of fluid can often be found near the hinge after folding back the flap and any excess fluid should be removed. This is especially important in hyperopic ablations, as the ablation is larger and may require treatment close to the hinge. Use of a suction device may be helpful in these cases (Figures 8-3A through C).

The patient is then asked to fixate on the alignment target. The laser and eye tracker are activated. The surgeon should verify centration and patient fixation during the treatment. If fluid starts accumulating over the stromal surface, the laser ablation can be halted and the fluid should be removed with a cellulose sponge. The hinge should be protected if within the ablation zone.

After the ablation, the flap is then repositioned onto the bed using an irrigation cannula or an iris

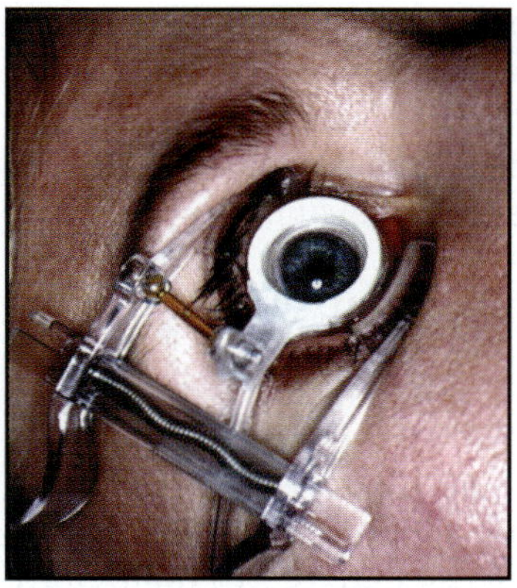

Figure 8-3A. EyeFix speculum (Minneapolis, Minn) in use on a patient.

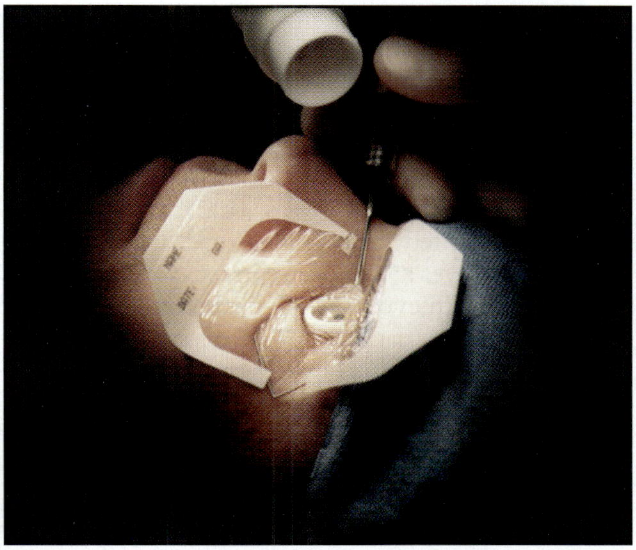

Figure 8-3B. OcuGuard handheld vacuum speculum in use on a patient.

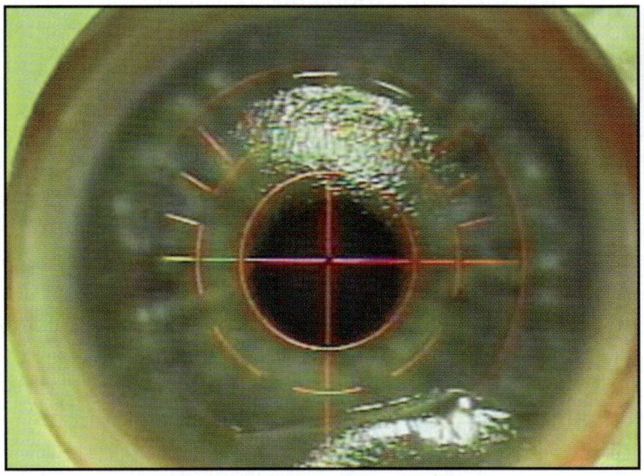

Figure 8-3C. Bleeding is controlled, and fluid is kept away from areas of ablation with the excimer laser.

sweep. Saline solution is used to remove debris from the interface. A moist cellulose sponge is then used to realign the flap. Brushing of the flap should be performed from the hinge toward the periphery of the flap.

Good adhesion of the flap is verified by stretching the flap toward the gutter. If good adhesion is present, there is minimal space in the gutter, and no movement of the flap occurs when stroking the flap with a dry sponge. A thick lubricant may be applied to the surface to prevent dehydration of the anterior flap while the interface fluid is resorbed by the endothelium. When the flap is felt to be securely in position, a drop of an antibiotic, a steroid and a lubricating agent may be applied to the cornea before removing the speculum. If bilateral LASIK will be performed, the operated eye is covered and the procedure repeated in the contralateral eye. Both eyes are then protected with transparent plastic shields until the following day.

Postoperative Care

The patient is placed on topical prophylactic antibiotics and topical steroids QID for the first week. Preservative-free lubricating drops are helpful in most patients for the first several weeks after surgery; frequent use should be encouraged.

The patient may resume most activities if the postoperative examination is normal. Instructions not to rub the eyes or have contact with contaminated environments should be reinforced in order to prevent flap displacement or infectious keratitis.

Results

The result of any refractive surgery procedure can best be discussed in terms of efficacy, predictability, safety, stability and complication rate. Using these parameters, there have been several published studies[1,2,20-35] (Table 8-1). In these studies, surgeons using various techniques—ablation diameters, optical zones, lasers, and microkeratomes—have shown H-LASIK to be a safe and predictable procedure for correcting low to moderate hyperopia. H-LASIK is less predictable and postoperative refractions are less stable in eyes with higher degrees of hyperopic and hyperopic astigmatism.[21,22,25] A 10% error in axis alignment in toric correction may result in an undercorrection of 30%.[36] Most studies have reported loss of BCVA after LASIK in high hyperopes, therefore H-LASIK in patients with greater than +5.00 D is not recommended.[21,23,24,33]

In a recent large multicenter study using LADARVision excimer laser, 88 eyes with a preoperative spherical equivalent in the range of +0.88 to +2.99 D were followed for 12 months after H-LASIK.[2] Of these eyes, 93.2% obtained a correction within ±1.00 D from target and 97.2% obtained 20/40 or better uncorrected visual acuity (UCVA). Another 29 eyes were treated in the range of +3.00 to +6.00 D, and of these eyes 85.7% were corrected within ±1.00 D and 88.5% achieved 20/40 or better uncorrected visual acuity.

In the same study, 54 eyes were treated for hyperopic astigmatism in the range of +0.50 to +2.99 sphere with -0.50 to -6.00 cylinder and 20 eyes treated in the range of +3.00 to +5.75 sphere and -0.50 to -6.99 cylinder and were followed for 12 months after H-LASIK, at which point, 92.6% and 80.0% of the eyes achieved correction with ±1.00 D respectively and 95.7% and 88.2% respectively achieved 20/40 or better uncorrected vision postoperatively. Postoperative UCVA was equal or better than preoperative best-spectacle corrected visual acuity (BSCVA) in 37% and 41% of the low and moderate sphere hyperopic eyes respectively and 35% and 47% of the low and moderate hyperopic astigmatic eyes respectively.

In another study, patients were divided into 4 groups: low hyperopia (spherical correction +1.00 to +3.00 and cylindrical correction 0 to +0.50), moderate hyperopia (spherical correction +3.25 to +6.00 and cylindrical correction 0 to +0.50), low hyperopic astigmat (spherical correction +1.00 to +3.00 and cylindrical correction +0.75 D to +2.00) and moderate hyperopic astigmat (spherical correction +3.25 to +6.00 and cylindrical correction +0.75 to +3.50).[25] They were followed for 6 months after LASIK, and 72.7%, 80.0%, 66.6%, and 44.4% of patients in each group respectively obtained 20/40 or better uncorrected visual acuity. 81.8%, 80%, 55.5%, and 77.7% were within ±1.00 D of emmetropia in each group respectively.

H-LASIK works well to correct consecutive hyperopia after myopic LASIK. A recent study treated 36 eyes for consecutive hyperopia after myopic LASIK and followed them for 3 months.[37] The pre-retreatment range was +0.63 to 2.63 D. Of these eyes, uncorrected visual acuity of 20/20 and 20/40 or better was achieved in 66.7% and 94.4% of the eyes respectively. Accuracy of the treatment was high with 55.5% within ±0.50 D and 94.4% within ±1.00 D of intended correction. H-LASIK has also been used to treat hyperopic overcorrection seen after radial keratotomy (RK). A stable refraction for at least 6 months before LASIK is mandatory. Patients who wear soft or hard contact lenses should abstain from using them for at least 2 and 4 weeks respectively. A careful evaluation of the RK incisions is necessary because the presence of epithelial inclusion cysts can predispose to subsequent epithelial ingrowth.[38]

LASIK Enhancements

Regression rates in H-LASIK are lower than in H-PRK.[33,39] The exact cause of this is yet unknown. Epithelial hyperplasia may play a role in H-LASIK. Arbelaez reported higher enhancement rates in high hyperopia and hyperopic astigmats.[22] In their study, 7% in the spherical group and 15% in the toric group required enhancements. Zadok reported a higher enhancement rate of 25%.[24] Most other studies did not include retreatment results.

The initial consideration when deciding to perform a LASIK enhancement is to determine the possible reason for failure of the prior procedure. Errors may be related to inadequate preoperative refraction, improper laser ablation, abnormal corneal hydration during the procedure, an excessive or inadequate healing response, induced corneal ectasia, or new ocular pathology. A careful analysis of anterior and posterior corneal elevations maps should be performed to rule out a decentered ablation or iatrogenic corneal ectasia.

Patient selection and appropriate timing are key for a successful LASIK enhancement. Waiting at least 3 months before considering an enhancement is recommended.[40] Patients with refractive instability should not undergo an enhancement procedure. The stability of the postoperative refraction appears to be related to the magnitude of the ablation, with higher refractive errors requiring longer time periods. A practical estimation is to use the preoperative refraction in diopters, and multiply this number by 3 to determine the number of months to wait after the initial H-LASIK procedure. In other words, waiting at least 9 months in a patient with a preoperative refraction of +3.00 D.

Regarding the decision of recutting the cornea versus lifting the flap, studies have shown the effectiveness and predictability of using different techniques.[41,42] Both procedures have advantages and disadvantages, which should be considered based on the patient's individual needs. Flap lifting is probably the preferred method in most patients, as major flap complications may be more likely to occur with recutting versus lifting the flap.[42] The flap edge can be marked at the slit lamp and lifted before the laser ablation. Unfortunately, this method requires flap manipulation and has been reported to be associated

Table 8-1

Summary of Selected Recent Hyperopic-LASIK Studies

Author (Study year)	*Laser Microkeratome*	*Follow-up (mos)*	*Number of eyes*	*Refractive Range (D) Spherical Equivalent*	*Cylinder*	*Uncorrected Visual Acuity 20/20%*	*Uncorrected Visual Acuity 20/40 (%)*	*Manifest Retraction Spherical Equivalent ±0.50 (%)*	*Manifest Retraction Spherical Equivalent ±1.00 (%)*	*Best-Corrected Visual Acuity 2 lines (%)*
Spherical Hyperopia										
Ditzen et al	MEL 60	12	20	+1.00 to +4.00		NA	95	NA	85	5
(1998)[20]	ACS		23	+4.25 to +8.00		NA	90	NA	58	4.3
Goker et al (1998)[21]	Keracor 116 ACS	18	54	+4.25 to +8.00		14.8	66.66	38.88	75.92	6.8
Argento et al	Keracor 116/117	6	138	+1.25 to +2.50		70.3^	94.1	Overall	100	0
(1998)[1]	ACS		153	+2.25 to +4.75		75.0^	100	48.30%	95.3	2
			170	+5.50 to +8.50		45.3^	87.8		71.4	0
Arbelaez et al	Keracor 117C	12	24	+1.00 to +3.00		42	95	55	91	0
(1999)[22]	ACS		20	+3.10 to +5.00		25	93	44	83	0
			16	+5.10 to +9.00		0	50	38	50	13
Esquenazi et al (1999)[23]	Keracor 117CT ACS	24	61	+1.25 to +8.50		47	82	67	74	5
Zadok et al	Nidek EC-5000	6	45	+1.00 to +3.00		42.2	95.6	NA	88.9	0
(2000)[24]	ACS		27	+3.00 to +5.00		25.9	77.8	NA	51.8	1.4
Salz et al	LADARVision	12	88	+0.88 to +2.99		54.8	97.2	78.4	93.2	4.5
(2001)[2]	B&L Hansatome		29	+3.00 to +6.00		42.3	88.5	60.7	85.7	0
Pineda-	Nidek EC-5000	6	22	+1.00 to +3.00	0 to +0.50	14	72.7	54.5	81.8	0
Fernandex et al (2001)[25]	LSK-One		10	+3.25 to +6.00	0 to +0.50	0	80	40	80	0
Davidorf et	VISX Star S2	6	16	+0.38 to +5.50		40	90	NA	NA	0
al (2001)[26]	B&L Hansatome		15	+0.63 to +4.13		40	90	NA	NA	0
			18	+1.25 to +3.50		40	90	NA	NA	0

Table 8-1

Summary of Selected Recent Hyperopic-LASIK Studies (continued)

Author/ Study year	*Laser Microkeratome*	*Follow-up (mos)*	*Number of eyes*	*Refractive Range (D) Spherical Equivalent*	*Cylinder*	*Uncorrected Visual Acuity 20/20%*	*Uncorrected Visual Acuity 20/40 (%)*	*Manifest Retraction Spherical Equivalent ±0.50 (%)*	*Manifest Retraction Spherical Equivalent ±1.00 (%)*	*Best-Corrected Visual Acuity 2 lines (%)*
				Simple and Compound Hyperopic Astigmatism and Mixed Astigmatism						
Argento et al (1997)[27]	Keracor 116/117	6	11	+1.00 to +2.50	+2.00 to +5.00	63.7^	90.1	45.5	81.9	0
	Chiron Micro-keratome (Model 600, 657, 694		53	+2.50 to +4.25	+2.00 to +5.75	60.4^	73.6	45.7	95.9	3.8
			51	-0.88 to +4.25	+0.50 to +7.25	76.5^	92.2	72	100	3.9
Chayet et al (1998)[28]	Nidek EC-5000	3	41*	+0.67±1.33!	-3.82±0.95!	44	85	78	90	0
Lindstrom et al (1999)[29]	VISX Star S2 B&L Hansatome	6	46	+0.50 to +6.00	0 to +5.00	21	79	47	63	0
Barraquer et al (1999)[30]	Schwind-Keratome	6	18	+1.50 to +3.50	0 to -5.00	NA	71	NA	100	0
	Automated		30	+3.51 to +6.00	0 to -4.50	NA	71	NA	80	0
	Linear		18	+6.01 to +10.0	0 to -4.00	NA	71	NA	77	0
	Microkeratome									
Salz et al (2001)[2]	LADARVision	12	54	+0.50 to +2.99	-0.50 to -6.00	59.6	95.7	77.8	92.6	1.9
			20	+3.00 to +5.75	-0.50 to -6.00	35.3	88.2	60	80	0
			38	-1.75 to +2.375	-1.25 to -6.00	47.2	94.4	73.7	94.7	0
Pineda-Fernandez et al (2001)[25]	Nidek EC-5000	6	18	+1.00 to +3.00	+0.75 to +2.00	0	66.6	50	55.5	5.5
	LSK-One Microkeratome		18	+3.25 to +6.00	+0.75 to +3.50	0	44.4	38.8	77.7	0
Rashad (2001)[31]	Technolas Carriazo-Barraquer Manuel micro-keratome	12	85	+1.25 to +5.00	0 to +3.00	24.7	92.9	61.2	89.4	0
Tabbara et al (2001)[32]	Keracor 117C ACS	6	80	+0.50 to +12.00	-4.25 to +3.50	44	97.5	58	84	1.25

*Includes simple myopic astigmatism eyes.
!Mean+ standard deviation only (range not reported)
^ 20/25

with a higher risk for epithelial ingrowth.[43] In a large comparative study of lift versus recut enhancements, there was no significant difference in epithelial ingrowth between cases that were lifted and cases that had repeat cuts.[41] However, a second cut can result in loose lamellar wedges of stromal tissue, and some surgeons advocate a deeper cut to avoid the previous interface.[44] A deeper cut, though, may still allow a lamellar wedge of tissue that is thicker and may cause more problems if it becomes displaced.

Complications

Regarding the safety of any refractive surgery procedure, one must consider intraoperative and postoperative complications.[45] Hyperopes tend to have flatter corneas and H-LASIK requires a larger flap. Therefore, intraoperative flap complications may be more common than in myopic eyes, especially as reported in earlier studies.[1] An incomplete flap may occur with premature cessation of the microkeratome advancement, due to interference with lids and lashes, drapes, or speculums. Epithelial defects can occur due to inadequate lubrication of the cornea before the microkeratome pass and due to toxicity of anesthetics, especially in the older hyperopic population. This can increase the risk of epithelial ingrowth and diffuse lamellar keratitis. Decentration is more of a problem with H-LASIK due to smaller effective optical zone, small flap size (which leaves little room to center the ablation), poor fixation (which is more of a problem with hyperopes as amblyopia is more common and H-LASIK takes a longer time to perform). Also hyperopes tend to have smaller eyes and palpebral apertures, which makes it difficult to apply and center suction ring.[46] Decentration can result in glare, irregular astigmatism and decrease in (BCVA). Laser equipped with eye tracking devices and external fixation targets are recommended for H-LASIK to decrease decentration. Studies by Esquenazi and Ditzen reported incidence of vertical decentration by 1 to 1.5 mm in 2% and 4.7% of the cases respectively.[20,23] All of their patients lost 2 lines of BSCVA. Punctate epithelial keratopathy is most commonly seen after H-LASIK in patients with pre-existing dry eyes or blepharitis. Over- and undercorrection may occur from problems with the preoperative refractive information, or from tissue under or over response to the laser energy. Goker et al reported undercorrection and regression >2.00 D in 13% of cases.[21] Epithelial ingrowth into the interface between the cap and stromal bed can occur, and may be more common in the older hyperope with a larger flap and treatment area. Rarely, the epithelial ingrowth progresses into the central visual axis, causing irregular astigmatism. Earlier studies by Goker and Ditzen reported the incidence of epithelial ingrowth of 31.4% and 14% respectively.[20,21] Later studies report a much lower incidence of epithelial ingrowth of 0% and 1% respectively.[25,31]

Discussion

In hyperopic LASIK the paracentral cornea is ablated to flatten the corneal periphery, thereby steepening the central cornea. Studies have shown that H-LASIK and H-PRK are similar in safety, predictability, and efficacy in low to moderate hyperopes.[47] H-PRK had problems with increased regression, haze, and decreased BCVA as the ablation zone filled due to epithelium hyperplasia. In H-PRK, regression was reported to occur up to 1 year.[39,48] In H-LASIK, there is less regression and stabilization can be achieved as early as 1 month as the epithelium and the Bowman's layers are left intact and a peripheral transition zone is utilized. With longer follow-up, additional regression may be seen. Also H-LASIK is associated with less postoperative pain and rapid visual recovery. However, there is the potential of microkeratome-induced complications.

Earlier H-LASIK studies had problems as small ablation zones resulted in glare, halos, irregular astigmatism, and more regression after treatment, and larger ablations often exceeded flap size obtained by most microkeratomes at that time. Most of the earlier studies utilized the Automated Corneal Shaper (Chiron, Miami, Fla). It created a corneal flap diameter of 8.5 mm, which was smaller than the ablation zone of 9.0 mm need for H-LASIK. To allow for larger ablation, these surgeons intentionally decentered the flap nasally by 0.5 to 1 mm. This resulted in nasal scars due to ablation of the flap hinge and the intact epithelium beyond the flap and temporal epithelial ingrowth.[20,22,23] Later studies utilized microkeratomes capable of creating larger flap diameters or superior hinges which allowed for the ablation to occur within the exposed stromal bed. This also resulted in better centration.[2,31]

The importance of the optical zone size was also realized early on, as studies by Ibrahim showed poor results due to small optical zone.[33] As smaller optical zone is more sensitive to decentration and possibly linked to higher rate of regression. Later, Argento et al noted increased post-operative refractive stability and decreased incidence of undercorrection by changing the optical zone diameter from 4.4 to 4.8 mm to 5.0 to 5.5 mm.[1] In another study, Davidorf et al used VISX Star S2, kept single repetition rate (10 Hz), and varied the ablation profile (5 x 9 mm, 5.5 x 8.5 mm, and 6 x 9 mm-inner and outer border of the annular zone of maximum ablation). Their results showed that even though postoperative UCVA was the same in all groups, there was a tendency toward undercorrection in the 5 x 9 group and overcorrection in the 6 x 9 group. With each 0.5-mm increase in the optical zone size, there was a 2.5% increase in desired correction. Thus, there was a tendency toward overcorrection with progressing large optical zone diameter (6 x 9 group versus 5 x 9 group).[26]

H-LASIK tends to induce mild astigmatism.[21,23,25] Pineda-Fernandez et al speculate that this may be due to ablation compromising the hinge of the flap resulting in less increase in corneal curvature in that area.[25] Also postoperative astigmatism may be induced due to corneal flap not being parallel to the treatment zone.

Many surgeons find that adjusting the amount of treatment using a nomogram based on their actual surgical results improves their refractive surgery outcome. Most surgeons tolerate an early overcorrection in order to obtain long term emmetropia, because H-LASIK has a greater incidence of regression than myopic LASIK.

As the techniques, lasers, microkeratomes and individual surgeon nomograms continue to improve and advances such as wavefront guided technology become widely introduced, H-LASIK will continue to evolve and the results will continue to improve, and one day will enjoy the same success as myopic LASIK.

References

1. Argento CJ, Cosentino MJ. Laser in situ keratomileusis for hyperopia. *J Cataract Refract Surg*. 1998;24:1050-8.
2. Salz JJ, Stevens CA, LADARVision LASIK hyperopia Study Group. LASIK correction of spherical hyperopia, hyperopic astigmatism, and mixed astigmatism with the LADARVision excimer laser system. *Ophthalmology*. 2002;109(9):1647-56; discussion 1657-8.
3. Grandon SC, Sanders DR, Anello RD, Jacobs D, Biscaro M. Clinical evaluation of hexagonal keratotomy for the treatment of primary hyperopia. *J Cataract Refract Surg*. 1995;21(2):140-149.
4. Kezirian GM, Gremillion CM. Automated lamellar keratoplasty for the correction of hyperopia. *J Cataract Refract Surg*. 1995;21(4):386-392.
5. Durrie DS, Schumer DJ, Cavanaugh TB. Holmium: YAG laser thermokeratoplasty for hyperopia. *J Refract Corneal Surg*. 1994;10:S277-S280.
6. Ehrlich MI, Nordan LT. Epikeratophakia for the treatment of hyperopia. *J Cataract Refract Surg*. 1989:15(6):661-6.
7. Lyle WA, Jin GJ. Clear lens extraction for the correction of high refractive error. *J Cataract Refract Surg*. 1994; 20(3):273-276.
8. Hardten DR. Phakic iris claw artisan intraocular lens for correction of high myopia and hyperopia. *Int Ophthalmol Clin*. 2000;40(3):209-221.
9. Sanders DR, Martin RG, Brown DC, et al. Posterior chamber phakic intraocular lens for hyperopia. *J Refract Surg*. 1999;15:309-315.
10. Asbell PA, Maloney RK, Davidorf J, et al. Conductive keratoplasty for the correction of hyperopia. *Trans Am Ophthalmol Soc*. 2001;99:79-84; discussion-7.
11. Williams DK. One year results of laser vision correction for low to moderate hyperopia. *Ophthalmology*. 2000;107:72-5.
12. Wang Q, Klein BE, Klein R, Moss SE. Refractive status in the Beaver Dam study. *Invest Ophthalmol Vis Sci*. 1994; 35:4344-7.
13. Paciuc M, Velasco CF, Naranjo R. Acute angle-closure glaucoma after hyperopic laser in situ keratomileusis. *J Cataract Refractive Surg*. 2002;26(4):620-3.
14. Alonso-Munoz L, Lleo-Perez A, Rahhal MS, Sanchis-Gimeno JA. Assessment of applanation tonometry after hyperopic laser in situ keratomileusis. *Cornea*. 2002; 21(2):156-60.
15. Zadok D, Raifkup F, Landao D, Frucht-Pery J. Intraocular pressure after LASIK for hyperopia. *Ophthalmology*. 2002;109(9):1659-61.
16. Pallikaris IG, Papatzanaki NE, Stathi EZ, et al. Laser in situ keratomileusis. *Lasers Surg Med*. 1990;10(5):463-8.
17. *FDA-Approved Lasers for LASIK*. www.fda.gov/cdrh/LASIK/lasers.htm; 2003.
18. Krueger RR, Parolini B, Gordon El, et al. Nonmechanical microkeratomes using laser and waterjet technology. In: Pallikaris IR, Siganos DS, eds. *LASIK*. SLACK Incorporated: Thorofare, NJ;1998, 81-105.
19. Ratkay-Traube I, Juhasz T, Horvath C, et al. Ultra-short pulse (femtosecond) laser surgery. In-vitro use in LASIK flap creation. *Ophthalmol Clin North Am*. 2001;14(2):347-55.
20. Ditzen K, Huschka H, Pieger S. Laser in situ keratomileusis for hyperopia. *J Cataract Refract Surg*. 1998;24:42-7.
21. Goker S, Er H, Kahvecioglu C. Laser in situ keratomileusis to correct hyperopia from +4.25 to +8.00 diopters. *J Refract Surg*. 1998;14:26-30.
22. Arbelaez MC, Knorz MC. Laser in situ keratomileusis for hyperopia and hyperopic astigmatism. *J Refract Surg*. 1999;15:406-14.
23. Esquenzai S, Mendoza A. Two-year follow-up of laser in situ keratomileusis for hyperopia. *J Refract Surg*. 1999;15(6):648-52.
24. Zadok D, Maskaleris G, Montes M, et al. Hyperopic laser in situ keratomileusis with the Nidek EC-5000 excimer laser. *Ophthalmology*. 2000;107:1132-7.
25. Pineda-Fernandez A, Rueda L, Huang D, Nur J, Jaramillo J. Laser in situ keratomileusis for hyperopia and hyperopic astigmatism with the Nidek EC-5000 excimer laser. *J Refract Surg*. 2001;17(6):670-5.

26. Davidorf JM, Eqhbali F, Onclinx T, Maloney RK. Effects of varying the optical zone diameter on the results of hyperopic laser in situ keratomileusis. *Ophthalmology*. 2001;108(7):1261-5.
27. Argento CJ, Cosentino MJ, Biondini A. Treatment of hyperopic astigmatism. *J Cataract Refract Surg*. 1997;23:1480-90.
28. Chayet AS, Magallanes R, Montes M, et al. Laser in situ keratomileusis for simple myopic, mixed, and simple hyperopic astigmatism. *J Refract Surg*. 1998;14(Suppl):S175-6.
29. Lindstrom RL, Hardten DR, Houtman DM, et. al. Six-month results of hyperopic and astigmatic LASIK in eyes with primary and secondary hyperopia. *Trans Am Ophthalmol Soc*. 1999; 97:241-255; discussion 255-260.
30. Barraquer C, Gutierrez AM. Results of laser in situ keratomileusis in hyperopic compound astigmatism. *J Cataract Refract Surg*. 1999;25:1198-204.
31. Rashad KM. Laser in situ keratomileusis for the correction of hyperopia from +1.25 to +5.00 diopters with the Technolas Keracor 117C laser. *J Refract Surg*. 2001; 17(2):113-22.
32. Tabbara KF, El-Sheikh HF, Islam SM. Laser in situ keratomileusis for the correction of hyperopia from +0.50 to +11.50 diopters with the Keracor 117C laser. *J Refract Surg*. 2001;17(2):123-8.
33. Ibrahim O. Laser in situ keratomileusis for hyperopia and hyperopic astigmatism. *J Refract Surg*. 1998; 14(Suppl):S179-82.
34. Suarez E, Torres F, Duplessie M. LASIK for the correction of hyperopia and hyperopia with astigmatism (review). *Int Ophthalmol Clin*. 1996;36:65-72.
35. Reviglio VE, Luna JD, Rodriguez ML, et al. Laser in situ keratomileusis using the LaserSight 200 laser: results of 950 consecutive cases. *J Cataract Refract Surg*. 1999;25:1062-8.
36. Stevens JD. Astigmatic excimer laser treatment: theoretical effects of axis misalignment. *Eur J Implant Ref Surg*. 1994;6:310-318.
37. Rojas MC, Haw WW, Manche EE. Laser in situ keratomileusis enhancement for consecutive hyperopia after myopic overcorrection. *J Cataract Refract Surg*. 2002; 28(1):37-43.
38. Linebarger EJ, Hardten DR, Lindstrom RL. Laser-assisted in situ keratomileusis for correction of secondary hyperopia after radial keratotomy. *Int Ophthalmol Clin*. 2000; 40(3):125-132.
39. Vinciguerra P, Epstein D, Radice P, Azzolini, M. Long-term results of photorefractive keratectomy for hyperopia and hyperopic astigmatism. *J Refract Surg*. 1998; 14:(Supplement)S183-S185.
40. Durrie DS, Vande Garde TL. LASIK Enhancements. *Int Ophthalmol Clin*. 2000;40(3):103-10.
41. Davis EA, Hardten DR, Lindstrom M, Samuelson TW, Lindstrom RL. LASIK enhancements: a comparison of lifting to recutting the flap. *Ophthalmology*. 2002; 109(12):2308-13; discussion 2313-4.
42. Domniz Y, Comaish IF, Lawless MA, et al. Recutting the cornea versus lifting the flap: comparison of two enhancement techniques following laser in situ keratomileusis. *J Refract Surg*. 2001;17(5):505-10.
43. Probst LE, Machat JJ. Enhancement techniques and results. In: Machat JJ, Slade SG, Probst LE, eds. *The Art of LASIK*. 2nd ed. Thorofare, NJ: SLACK Incorporated; 1999;225-238.
44. Pallikaris IG, Papadaki T, Siganos DS. Complex LASIK enhancements. In: Probst LE, ed. *Complex Cases with LASIK: Advanced Techniques and Complication Management*. Thorofare, NJ: SLACK Incorporated; 2000:355-365.
45. Hardten DR, Lindstrom RL. Management of LASIK Complications. *Operative Techniques in Cataract and Refractive Surgery*. 1998;1(D):32-39.
46. O'Brart DP. The status of hyperopic laser-assisted in situ keratomileusis. *Current Opinion in Ophthalmology*. 1999; 10(4):247-52.
47. el-Agha MS, Johnson EW, Bowman RW, et al. Excimer laser treatment of spherical hyperopia: PRK or LASIK? *Trans AM Ophthalmol Soc*. 2000;98:59-66; discussion-66-9.
48. Carones F, Brancato R, Morico A, Vigo L, Venturi E, Gobbi PG. Photorefractive keratectomy for hyperopia using an erodible disc and Axicon lens: 2-year results. *Refract Corneal Surg*. 1998;14:504-511.

Chapter Nine

HYPEROPIC LASIK: COMPLICATIONS AND MANAGEMENT

Louis E. Probst, MD

INTRODUCTION

The safety profile of LASIK has dramatically improved over the last 8 years. The LASIK technology has improved with better microkeratomes and scanning excimer lasers that allow for bigger and smoother ablation zones. Surgeon experience has also increased dramatically. These factors have reduced the number of intraoperative contraindications for LASIK. The postoperative complications have also been reduced by the increased awareness of the contraindications for LASIK. LASIK is an elective procedure; therefore, the complication rate must be low in order for it to be an accepted refractive procedure. Most LASIK complications can be corrected so that no long-term problems persist. However, there are some uncommon complications that can have permanent visual consequences. There are a few LASIK complications that are unique for hyperopic corrections. LASIK complications can be conveniently divided into intraoperative, early postoperative, and late postoperative complications.

INTRAOPERATIVE LASIK COMPLICATIONS

Intraoperative LASIK complications are often preventable with the appropriate safeguards of the surgical system. If the equipment is defective or setup incorrectly, a complication is almost assured. Therefore, the key to minimizing LASIK complications is prevention. Proper training and high degree of focus is essential for both the surgeon and the surgical technicians to minimized operative errors.

A recent retrospective study evaluated the intraoperative flap complications in 84,771 cases of LASIK with the automated corneal shaper (ACS) or the Hansatome.[1] The rate of all flap complications was 0.302%, failures to achieve intraocular pressure in 0.034%, partial flaps in 0.099%, buttonholes in 0.07%, thin or irregular flaps 0.087%, free flaps in 0.012% of eyes. There were 134 right eye complications and 122 left eye complications. No patient developed an intraoperative flap complication in both eyes. Flap complications have been found to be more common with the ACS as compared to the Hansatome,[2] as success with the ACS is more surgeon experience dependent.

PREVENTION OF INTRAOPERATIVE COMPLICATIONS

Prior to the LASIK procedure, all the equipment should be checked as any failure of the equipment could result in a flap complication. This is often

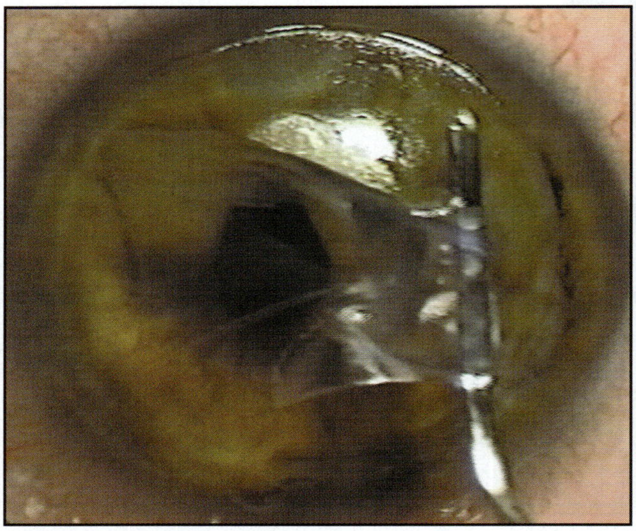

Figure 9-1. Intraoperative view of a buttonhole flap with the cannula protruding through the center of the buttonhole.

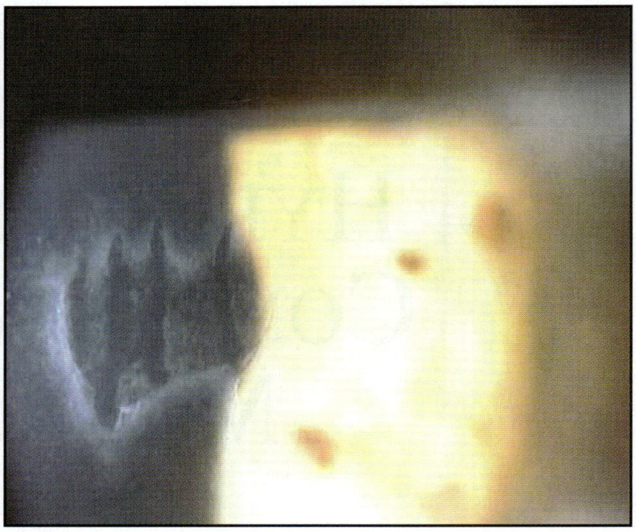

Figure 9-2. One month after a buttonhole with an irregular haze pattern surrounding buttonhole.

referred to as the "preflight checklist." The microkeratome blade should be checked before every LASIK procedure. The microkeratome blades supplied by the manufacture can be defective. Nicks or irregularities of the cutting edge will produce a linear ridge through the flap or a split flap.[3] It is difficult to check the microkeratome blade once it is loaded in the microkeratome, as the edge is not well reflected by the light of the microscope. Once the blade is loaded in the microkeratome, it should be checked to make sure it is mobile. It is possible to hear the sound of the microkeratome motor running and have no blade movement if the blade is loaded into the head incorrectly. If a microkeratome pass is made with an immobile blade, a thin irregular flap will result. A test run should then be performed of the microkeratome to ensure that it is running smoothly in the microkeratome track. The resistance level on the Hansatome box gauge should be less than 20. If the gauge is running in the 20 to 30 range, a drop of proparacaine on the blade and the gears usually causes the resistance to drop into the below 20 range. If the resistance is in the 20 to 30 range, the microkeratome should be reassembled as there is excessive blade resistance. Low levels of suctions have been experienced due to suction tubing that was not properly inserted into the suction unit. Therefore, it is important to always check the suction at the beginning of each day to make sure the suction unit is functioning properly. Finally, it is important to confirm the intraocular pressure (IOP) has risen to an adequate level prior to performing the keratectomy. The pressure should be well above 90 mmHg when checked with the 90 mm Barraquer tonometer.

Buttonhole and Irregular Flaps

Buttonhole flaps occur when the keratectomy has been performed without adequate suction. The microkeratome procedures a meniscus-shaped flap that is thinner in the center so any additional thinning due to the low suction results in a break in the center of the flap, creating a buttonhole flap. Although an increased risk of button-hole flaps have been suggested with steep corneal keratometry readings (>50.00 D), this has not been the experience of this author or published in the literature.[4]

Clinical

The buttonhole flap is evident immediately after the microkeratome has completed the reverse pass. The central aspect of the cornea will appear irregular with a 2 to 3 mm diameter irregular circle in the center representing the buttonhole. If the flap is lifted, it will be thin and difficult to manipulate (Figure 9-1). The defect through the center of the flap will be obvious (Figure 9-1). The stromal bed has a clear area in the center about 2 to 3 mm in size that is slightly elevated representing the uncut area of cornea where the epithelium is still present. After 1 month, haze will form around the edges of the buttonhole (Figure 9-2).

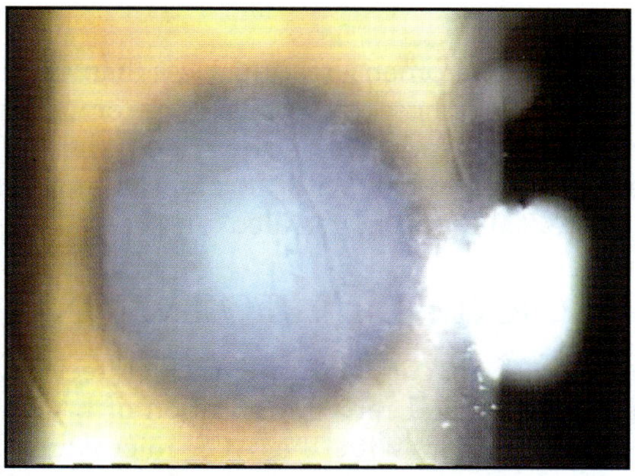

Figure 9-3. Central corneal haze and irregular striae after a thin flap.

Management

Performing the laser ablation will result in an irregular astigmatism with central corneal haze. If the buttonhole is identified immediately, the flap should not be lifted. Gentle interface irrigation will allow the flap to be refloated into position. If the flap has been lifted, the flap should be replaced, and then refloated into position. This can be difficult as the flap is thin and very unstable. The eye is allowed to heal for at least 3 months. LASIK can be performed again using a deeper plate. Topical steroids are tapered during the healing phase to reduce the risk of haze formation. Although immediate transepithelial photorefractive keratectomy (PRK) has been reported following flap complications,[5] this technique is not recommended by the majority of refractive surgeons.

Prevention

Buttonhole flaps can be prevented with techniques and precautions discussed above. The keratectomy should never been performed without excellent suction and a perfect blade.

Thin Flaps

The average flap thickness for each microkeratome is variable. The Hansatome generally cuts about 40 µm thinner than the depth indicated on the depth plate. There is also considerable standard deviation in the average cut thickness, which is generally about 25 µm.[6,7] Therefore the flap thickness can vary considerably, often between 100 and 200 µm. The Nidek (Japan) MK-2000 microkeratome also cuts about 20 µm thinner than the depth plate number.[8] Because of this variation, the LASIK surgeon has little room for error if the flap is thin.

Clinical

Thin flaps can be immediately identified after the keratectomy as they tend to role along the distal cut edge. Flaps of 100 µm or more do not demonstrate this pattern. Very thin flaps can be associated with complete buttonhole flaps or partial buttonhole flaps when the central flap is only composed of epithelium. If the suction level was poor or the blade was not moving during the keratectomy, the flap and the stromal bed will be irregular. This is best seen with the reflections of the microscope illumination lights. Striae are also more prominent with thin LASIK flaps. The superficial corneal stromal is less hydrated than the deeper stromal so the stromal bed of a thin flap will appear less moist and more reflective. Once a very thin flap has healed, a hazy area with irregular striae will form in the center of the cornea (Figure 9-3).

Management

When a thin flap is achieved the surgeon must evaluate the flap and the stromal bed. If the stromal bed is smooth and the flap itself is smooth, LASIK can still be performed with an excellent outcome. If the stromal bed is not smooth or there are perforations or buttonholes of the flap, then performing the laser ablation will result in irregular astigmatism with central corneal haze.

In the case of an irregular flap with an irregular stromal bed, the flap should then be replaced and the cornea allowed to heal for 3 months. LASIK can be performed again using a deeper plate. Topical steroids are tapered during the healing phase to reduce the risk of haze formation.

Prevention

Thin flaps are prevented with the safeguards listed above. The keratectomy should never been performed without excellent suction and a perfect blade.

Free Cap

A free cap occurs when the microkeratome does not stop to create a hinge, but rather continues across the cornea severing the flap from the bed, thereby creating a free cap. Free caps usually occur for 2 reasons. In eyes with very flat preoperative keratectomies, a free cap can occur on some microkeratomes such as the ACS when the K's are less than 41.00 D. A free cap can also occur if there is a very

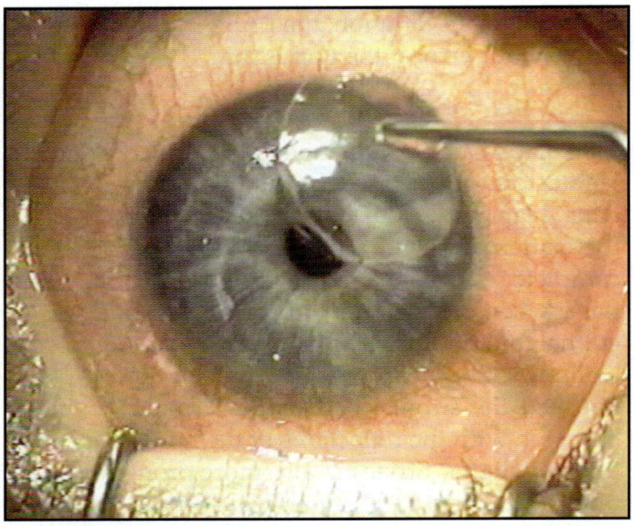

Figure 9-4. This free cap maintains some rigidity as it has a normal thickness.

thin flap due to inadequate pressure. This flap would tend to be smaller in diameter, more central in the cornea, with an irregular edge.

Clinical

Free caps are circular and completely separated from the stromal bed. If the free cap is thin, the edges may be irregular and the free cap will fold onto itself when manipulated. If the free cap is of normal thickness, it will maintain rigidity when lifted (Figure 9-4).

Management

If the suction level was low and the stromal bed is irregular, the flap should be replaced and allowed to heal without performing the excimer laser ablation. If the free cap occurred because of low preoperative keratometry reading, the stromal bed may be smooth and the free cap of normal thickness. In this case, the ablation can be continued with an excellent outcome. The free cap should be carefully placed epithelial side down on a drop of balanced salt solution (BSS) in the anti-desiccation chamber while the ablation is being performed. The anti-desiccation chamber should be then covered with a sterile container to ensure that it is not inadvertently knocked off the surgical tray. Once the ablation is performed the free cap can be replaced and aligned using the alignment marks that were placed prior to the keratectomy. It is important to ensure that the epithelial side of the free cap is up and that the epithelial marks are well aligned otherwise astigmatism will be induced postoperatively because of incorrect flap orientation.

Prevention

In eyes with keratometry readings less than 42.00 D, it is advisable to use the Hansatome or a larger microkeratome head (9.5) on the Nidek MK-2000. I have performed LASIK with the Hansatome on K's less than 37.00 D and not created a free cap.

Corneal Perforation

Perforation of the cornea during the keratectomy is the most feared and rare complication of LASIK. It was first reported with the ACS microkeratome when the depth plate was not properly screwed into the microkeratome head. Without the depth plate to restrict the cut depth, the blade would cut straight into the cornea causing penetration into the anterior chamber with extrusion of the intraocular contents due to the elevated IOP. When the Hansatome was introduced with a fixed depth plate, this problem was thought to be eliminated. However this problem was more recently reported during the early introduction of the Nidek MK-2000 microkeratome. Once again, it was the incorrect assembly of the microkeratome that allowed this complication to occur. Nidek has since required that a plastic wedge is placed in the hinge of the MK-2000 that prevents corneal perforation even if the head is not properly assembled.

Clinical

This complication is obvious during the advancement of the microkeratome as there is a sudden release of jet of fluid as the cornea is penetrated following by a loss of suction with beeping from the suction pump. The suction should be disengaged immediately. Removal of the microkeratome reveals the penetration, which could be associated with extruded iris and/or lens material.

Management

Corneal perforation is managed by preserving as much intraocular tissue as possible, suturing the corneal incision to restore the anterior chamber, and immediate referral for further evaluation/surgery that may be required. An emergency surgical kit that includes a needle driver and sutures should available in every laser center.

Prevention

Careful microkeratome assembly is critical for successful LASIK. LASIK staff should be well trained for correct assembly as well as the pitfalls of incorrect assembly. The surgeon should always check the microkeratome to insure that it has been properly assembled.

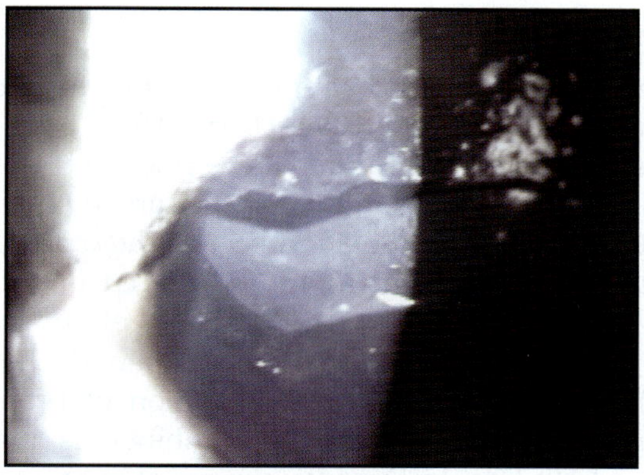

Figure 9-5. Loose flap of epithelium after LASIK.

Laser-Related Complications

Laser-related complications are perhaps the most frustrating LASIK complications as they are usually completely preventable. The most embarrassing complication is incorrect laser programming. Often this task is left to a technician who may read a number incorrectly or simply have a typing error. The most insidious programming problems occur with prescription transposition errors. On rare occasions, the excimer laser will actually fail in the middle of a procedure.

Clinical

There is little to warn of incorrect laser programming during the procedure. The result will become obvious postoperatively when the patient does not achieve a good UCVA. If there was a transposition error, or an astigmatism axis error the resultant astigmatism may be magnified in a new axis.

Management

Errors in laser programming can be corrected by an enhancement procedure; however, the best strategy is prevention with multiple checks. If laser failure occurs, the flap should be replaced and the patient is taken from the surgical room. The percentage of the correction performed should be recorded in case all data is lost from the laser. The laser company should be called to determine the cause of the failure. Often, with company guidance, steps can be taken that return the laser to full functioning. Most excimer lasers have the procedure in memory so the patient can be brought into the room and the procedure continued from the previous point with no detrimental effect on the outcome. Patient reassurance during this phase is critical to maintain confidence.

Prevention

It is essential to check and double-check all programming prior to performing LASIK. One technician can read the programming to the other technician verifies the information to ensure that they both have confirmed the numbers. It is very easy to make transposition errors when converting from plus to minus cylinder; therefore, the refraction calculations should also be checked. It is helpful to compare the axis and sign of the refractive astigmatism with the astigmatism on the topography to make sure that they are similar. Any discrepancy—particularly those 90 degrees apart—may indicate a transposition error.

Intraoperative Epithelial Defects and One-Drop LASIK

Intraoperative epithelial defects (IED) during LASIK can results in a number of highly undesirable complications including prolonged visual recovery, postoperative pain, diffuse lamellar keratitis (DLK), and epithelial ingrowth. Therefore, the LASIK surgeon must strive to avoid this complication in every way possible. A recent study evaluated the risk factors for IED defects during LASIK.[9] IED occurred in 9.7% of 247 eyes. IED significantly increased with older age, preoperative corneal thickness, and maintenance of suction ring vacuum during the reverse pass of the microkeratome. Less preoperative drops resulted in less IED. In patients undergoing bilateral LASIK, the incidence of IED was much higher in the second eye if the first eye developed an IED.

Clinical

IED are noted immediately after the keratectomy as irregular areas along the epithelial surface of the cornea. A flap of epithelium can sometimes be seen hanging over the corneal flap (Figure 9-5). The displaced epithelium is usually edematous and grey in appearance. IED can be <1 mm or as large as the entire corneal flap. The flap is usually intact and healthy beneath the defect. IED usually occur along the superior edge of the flap where the epithelium is less adherent.

Management

If an epithelial defect occurs during the treatment of the first eye, the surgeon should continue with the laser treatment, replace the LASIK flap, and place a bandage contact lens over the eye, if the defect is greater than 3 mm is size. If the defect is extremely

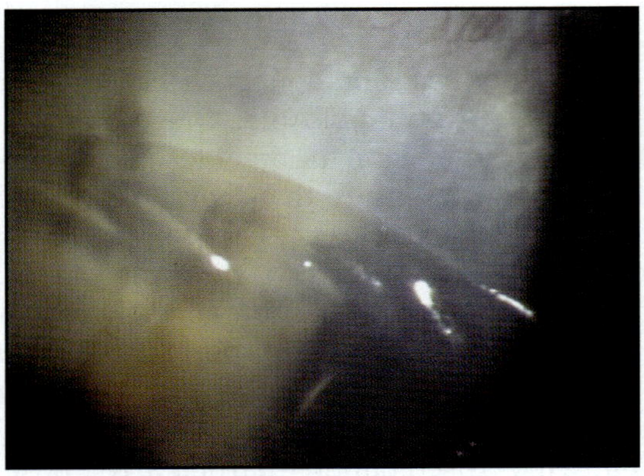

Figure 9-6. Loose superior epithelium immediately after LASIK.

large, it may be elected not to proceed with the treatment of the second eye until the first eye has healed.

The patient must be observed daily for evidence of infection and a prophylactic antibiotic should be used postoperatively at least until the epithelial defect has healed. For small epithelial defects, reassurance that the foreign body sensation will resolve, lubrication, topical NSAIDs to reduce the foreign body sensation, and a topical steroid to control potential interface inflammation may be all that is required. Small epithelial defects will generally heal with 1 to 3 days. For larger epithelial defects, a bandage contact lens should be carefully inserted with care not to disturb the flap. A bandage contact lens with a base curve of 8.4 mm generally fits well. Topical NSAIDs have been associated with sterile corneal infiltrates therefore they should only be used for 3 to 4 days.[10,11] Topical steroids should be used every at least every few hours as the risk of interface keratitis is higher with larger defects. Oral agents such as sedatives or narcotic agents are rarely required and are used only in selective cases as it is far better to have the patient aware of any continued discomfort so that the center can be notified. Pressure patching is contraindicated as patient eye movement against the firmly applied eyelid may create excessive shearing forces and displacement of the flap. After lubricating drops to hydrate the contact lens (CTL) and topical anesthetic have been instilled into the eye, the bandage CTL can be removed. The ideal technique for CTL removal is to have the patient look up while at the slit-lamp biomicroscope; in this manner the inferior aspect of the CTL is visible and may slide down. Using fine non-toothed forceps, the inferior aspect of the CTL is firmly grasped and the CTL pulled down and away from the eye.

Prevention

One technique that is extremely effective for reducing epithelial defects is "One-Drop LASIK".[12] No preoperative drops are put in the eye prior to LASIK to minimize the toxic keratopathy that greatly increases the risk of epithelial defects. The patient is brought into the laser room and placed under the laser. One drop of topical anesthetic is placed in the eye and then a Murocel (Bausch & Lomb, Rochester, NY) sponge soaked in a combination of proparacaine, NSAIDs, steroid, and antibiotic is placed under both lids. In this way we are able to achieve appropriate anesthesia, anti-inflammatory, and antibiotic effect in the eye while reducing the time of exposure so there is limited opportunity for the development of a toxic keratopathy.

Patients that have pre-identified weakness with the epithelium including anterior basement membrane dystrophy or loose epithelium or skin conditions such as acne rosacea are prone to epithelial defects. These patients will be better treated with a nasal hinge flap as the rotary movement of the Hansatome will cause more epithelial friction with a greater incidence of epithelial defects. I currently use a nasal hinge flap in approximately 90% of my standard myopic LASIK cases and a superior hinge flap for hyperopes, wide zone ablations, mixed astigmatism, and large pupils.

Loose Epithelium

Loose epithelium may be noted prior to the LASIK procedure or more commonly after the keratectomy. This occurs more commonly in patients over the age of 40 years and in those with a history suggesting loose epithelium such as recurrent corneal erosions, previous eye trauma, or obvious anterior basement membrane dystrophy.

Clinical

Loose epithelium can present in different manners depending on the level of severity. Mildly loose epithelium will present with a rippled appearance along the cornea surface, and most will commonly sign along the superior flap edge after the keratectomy (Figure 9-6). Severe loose epithelium can result in large sheets of detached epithelium after the keratectomy with epithelial defects. There is usually some attached epithelium along the inferior flap edge.

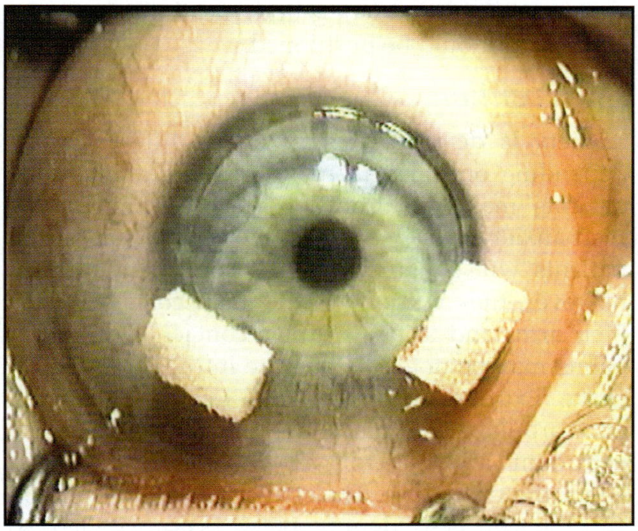

Figure 9-7. Sponges are used to control corneal bleeding during LASIK.

Management

Loose epithelium identified after the keratectomy can generally be replaced with gentle pressure along the surface of the flap. Surprisingly, this epithelium will remain in the new replaced position as long as the rest of the epithelium is intact and attached. Large flaps of detached or displaced epithelium are best removed while carefully preserving the remaining attached epithelium. A bandage contact lens should then be placed on the eye and left in place for 1 to 3 days to allow the epithelium to attach to the basement membrane of the cornea. Careful removal of the contact lens should reveal healthy attached epithelium.

Prevention

Loose epithelium identified preoperatively should alert the LASIK surgeon to a higher risk of epithelial loss and defects during the LASIK procedure. While the "one-drop LASIK" technique and a careful surgical technique can prevent these complications, PRK or LASEK should be considered for low spherical corrections to avoid the risk altogether. If LASIK is still the preferred procedure, a nasal hinged microkeratome will minimize the risk of loose epithelium and epithelial defects.

Neovascular Bleeding During LASIK

When LASIK was first performed using nasal hinge flaps with the ACS microkeratome, corneal bleeding was not common. The 8.5-mm flap rarely intersected the corneal vessels and if it did, only the superior vessels were involved, which was not a problem to control.

Clinical

With the advent of larger flaps particularly with those created by the Hansatome, it is not uncommon to have corneal neovascular bleeding during the LASIK procedure. Hyperopes tend to have smaller eyes with a greater incidence of neovascular bleeding. Generally, neovascular bleeding occurs immediately after the keratectomy along the superior flap edge. It may be self limited, lasting for less than a minute or persist for several minutes depending on the size of the vessels cut and the coagulation status of the patient. There are occasions when bleeding occurs 360 degrees around the cornea and can cause difficulties both during the ablation and after the procedure because of bleeding underneath the flap.

Management

Once the flap is cut and it is obvious that there is neovascular bleeding, the suction ring can be left in place and downward pressure from the suction ring can tamponad some of the bleeding vessels. The flap is lifted and the bleeding vessels can be dried with a dry Murocel spear.

If there is continued bleeding that could extend into the ablation area, dry rectangles of instrument wipe cut in 2 x 4-mm segments are placed on the area of bleeding (Figure 9-7). These are available from Hurricane Medical (Bradenton, Fla) (Probst LASIK sponge) or can be prepared beforehand by the surgical technician by simply taking an instrument wipe and cutting it into those segments. This allows the ablation to be performed without further interruption. The sponges can be removed and the flap replaced with copious irrigation to make sure there is no further bleeding underneath the flap. The same sponges which have been soaked in Iopidine (Alcon, Fort Worth, Tex) (apraclonidine HCl) are placed over the areas of bleeding. Iopidine is used as it is an alpha 2 agonist with a vasoconstrictive effect without the pupillary dilation that occurs with phenylephrine. The sponges are left in place for approximately 1 minute while the flap is adhering to the stromal bed.

Prevention

There are several maneuvers that can be used to prevent bleeding during the LASIK procedure. When the 9.5-mm suction ring is first placed on the eye, neovascular vessels extending into the exposed cornea will be cut. In this case, the ring can be switched to the 8.5-mm ring so that the neovascular bleeding can be minimized. I do not use 8.5-mm ring routinely as this ring more commonly decenters, which does not occur to same degree with the 9.5-mm ring. Pretreatment with Alphagan (Allergan, Irvine, Calif) (brimonidine tartrate) has been suggested to reduce the incidence of intraoperative bleeding; however, this potential benefit must be balanced with the increased with of postoperative slipped flaps.

The Anxious Patient

There is a reasonably high incidence of general anxiety disorder in the population in general, which is of course magnified by the normal fears associated with the LASIK procedure. There are also patients who are claustrophobic who may be fearful if they have had past experience with an MRI. Younger patients are more anxiety prone than the older patients. They have difficulty controlling their anxiety as well as being extremely sensitive around their eyes, which seems to be a trait particularly common to young males.

Clinical

Anxiety is displayed in countless ways by patients; however, the best measure of identifying the problem is noting increased tension in the surgical suite. As soon as this is noted, the surgeon must make a careful analysis of the source of the problem and address it before further complications arise.

Management

If a patient appears to be anxious, they should be isolated from the other patients so that the anxiety is not propagated throughout the center.

Anxious patients should be evaluated and treated as quickly as possible rather than have them wait while their anxieties build. Preoperative sedation should be used generously whenever someone appears to be anxious. The anxiety prior to LASIK is related to a feeling of helplessness and a loss of control. Patients need to understand that there is not immediate need to do LASIK. Patients should also understand that they can have only one eye treated. Some patients appreciate being able to check their vision with their first eye before continuing with their second eye. Sometimes it is helpful to have the husband, wife, parent, or friend hold the patient's hand during the procedure. If there is any sense of anxiety when the patient is underneath the laser, the procedure should be postponed.

Prevention

Anxiety is demonstrated in many different ways depending on the personality of the patient. Some patients make identification easy by announcing their anxiety as they arrive at the center. Introverted patients will sit quietly in the consultation room; however, they will often leave their coats on, cross their arms and legs, avoid eye contact, and sweaty palms may be noted during the introductory handshake. Extroverted patients will talk in loud tones, pace around the room, make multiple trips to the bathroom, and talk to everyone they can to find about the procedure. The challenge for the surgeon and the staff is to identify every anxious patient so they can be appropriately addressed prior to LASIK.

Deep-Set Eyes

Deep-set eyes are more difficult to treat as the palpebral opening is crowded by the prominent orbital bones.

Clinical

Patients with deep-set eyes can be identified preoperatively by their small palpebral fissures, prominent superior orbital rim, and prominent cheek bones. This problem is far more common in men due to a prominent supra-orbital rim but can occur in both sexes. A highly myopic spectacle correction can make the problem appear worse due to the minification effect of the spectacles. Patients with small heads and faces and Asian patients do not generally have deep set eyes; however, the small palpebral opening introduces similar challenges. Hyperopic patients tend to have small orbits that limit access to the globe for LASIK.

Management

These patients are best avoided until the LASIK surgeon becomes proficient in LASIK. Different techniques can help provide more exposure. Downward pressure on the speculum will often result in slight proptosis. An adjustable wire eyelid speculum usually offers the most exposure with the least interference with the suction ring. Once the speculum has been maximally expanded, a short wait will allow further expansion of a few millimeters. A lateral canthotomy and retrobulbar injection can be performed to increase exposure; however, these aggressive techniques are not well received by the patients. A very effective but technically more difficult tech-

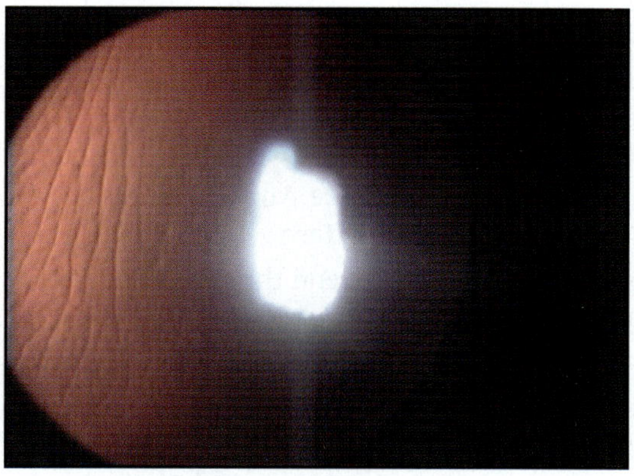

Figure 9-8. Peripheral striae are demonstrated by retroillumination.

nique to perform LASIK in very small orbits is to use the suction ring alone to separate the eyelids without a speculum. Peri-orbital skin can get caught in the microkeratome when LASIK is done without a speculum so caution is required with this technique.

Prevention

If adequate exposure cannot be obtained and the prescription is small, PRK or LASEK may be safer refractive options in properly informed patients.

Exophthalmic Eyes

Large orbits or exophthalmic eyes are ideal first cases to perform as exposure is maximal. However, there is often considerable orbital fat that allows for a certain amount of spring or ballottement to these eyes when applying the suction ring. This excessive movement can make fixation with the suction ring and the microkeratome pass slightly more difficult as the globe is not stationary. Redundant conjunctiva is often found in exophthalmic eyes that can occlude the suction ring holes without elevation of the true intraocular pressure, giving "pseudo-suction," which is a normal suction pressure reading on the base unit while the intraocular pressure remains low.

Management

It is important that the surgeon does not become overconfident and careless because of the excellent exposure. Downward pressure on the speculum can render the eye less mobile in the orbit. Redundant folds of conjunctiva should be pushed away for the limbal region to avoid "pseudo-suction." Careful attention to checking the intraocular pressure will avoid thin flaps caused by "pseudo-suction."

Prevention

In cases when the interaction of the microkeratome and the eye is difficult or the suction level is inadequate, the surgeon should always remember that PRK or LASEK may be safer refractive options in properly informed patients.

Early Postoperative Complications

Flap Striae

Striae of the LASIK flap occur when it is folded onto itself. Striae generally have 3 sources including misalignment of the corneal flap after flap replacement, movement of the corneal flap during the first postoperative day, and the "tenting effect" of the corneal flap over the ablated stromal bed. Obviously, a displaced flap or dislodged flap will also be associated with striae.

Clinical

Normally the striae are oriented horizontally with a nasal hinge and vertically with the superior hinge. Displaced flaps will often have oblique striae. Retroillumination of the fixation light and aiming beam through the dilated pupil provides accurate localization of the flap striae and will help identify striae in cases of unexplained reduction of BCVA (Figure 9-8). Fluorescein staining of the corneal will also assist is identifying subtle striae. If the striae have occurred due to flap movement or displacement after LASIK, the flap may be noted to have shifted 1 to 2 mm leaving an area of exposed stromal bed. It is helpful to grade striae to assist with the description of their severity and to plan treatment (Table 9-1, Figures 9-9 to 9-11).

Management

Most flap striae occur within the first hour after LASIK. Flap striae become more difficult to remove as the length of the postoperative course increases therefore identification of the striae on the first postoperative day is imperative. The indications for the treatment of striae include flap striae that extend through the visual axis, striae causing a decrease in BCVA or diplopia, or striae inducing regular or irregular astigmatism. There have been several techniques described for the removal of flap striae. These include the stretch and smooth technique,[13] flap hydration with hypotonic saline epithelial debridement,[14] flap applanation, phototherapeutic keratectomy,[15] and flap suturing.[16]

Table 9-1

Probst Classification of Flap Striae

Grade 1	Grade 2	Grade 3
♦ Fine parallel lines in lines ♦ Difficult to identify ♦ Identification obvious ♦ Not in visual axis ♦ No reduction in UCVA or BCVA *No treatment required*	♦ Fine parallel lines in flap ♦ Identification obvious ♦ Extent through visual axis ♦ BCVA reduced to 20/25 to 20/40 ♦ Less than one diopter of induced astigmatism ♦ Patient may complain of diplopia *Treatment may be required due to the reduction in the BCVA or the induced astigmatism*	♦ Large parallel or "basket weave" pattern ♦ Extend through visual axis ♦ BCVA worse than 20/40 ♦ One or more diopters of induced astigmatism ♦ Patient may complain of blur, diplopia, and glare *Treatment required to restore BCVA and reduce astigmatism, diplopia, and glare*

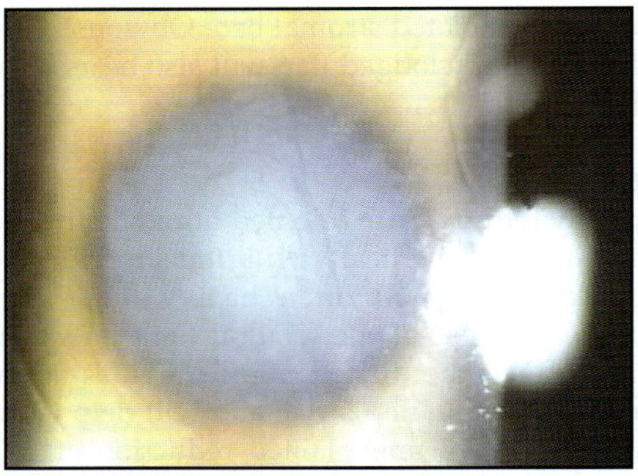

Figure 9-9. Grade 1 mild vertical striae may not affect the visual performance.

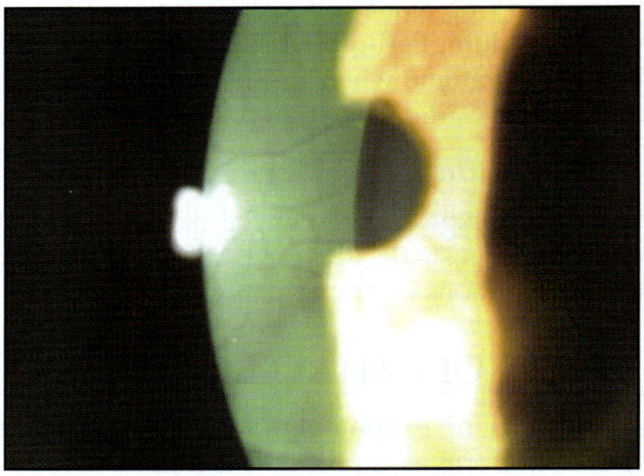

Figure 9-10. Grade 2 striae in a "basket weave" configuration will reduce the BCVA.

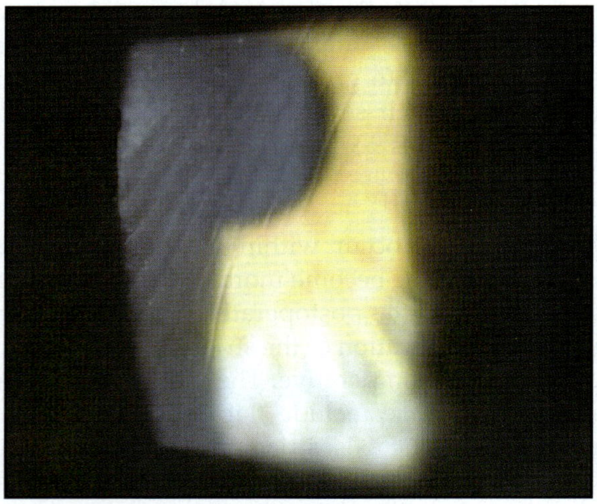

Figure 9-11. Grade 3 severe vertical striae may occur with a displaced flap.

The stretch and smooth technique is the most recognized. The flap edge is first marked at the slit lamp to allow for easy lifting of the flap once the patient is under the microscope. No flap alignment markings are necessary as the flap will be re-aligned in a more correct position when replaced. The flap is then reflected back onto the conjunctiva. The stromal surface of the flap is hydrated with BSS solution for 30 to 60 seconds. Some surgeons have suggested the using a hypotonic irrigation fluid of 80% BSS and 20% sterile water mixture to induce flap hydration to assist is flap removal. The flap is replaced in the stromal bed and floated into position with interface irrigation. The flap is left for 5 minutes to attach to the stromal bed and dry the epithelial surface. The side of blunt forceps is used to stretch flap perpendicular to the striae for 5 to 10 minutes or until epithelial defects start to occur. At the end of the procedure striae will still be visible after stretching but will be gone in 24 hours. This technique is effective in 90% of striae; however, it can be repeated in 2 to 4 weeks if necessary.

Prevention

Intraoperative attention to the repositioning of the flap with minimal manipulation once it has been replaced into the correct position. Postoperatively, patients are instructed to avoid rubbing or squeezing the eye. Patients wear eye protection 24 hours a day for the first week to prevent any eye trauma while the flaps are healing.

Dislodged Flap

A dislodged flap (flap subluxation or dehiscence) occurs when the flap is completely separated from the stromal bed. This most commonly occurs during the first 24 hours postoperatively as the flap is still adhering to the stromal bed. Rarely, late dislocation of the flap can occur with cornea trauma.[17,18] With proper LASIK technique and postoperative care, the incidence flap movement should be less than 1/1000 although an incidence of over 1% has been reported.[19]

Clinical

With nasal flaps, the dislodged flap is found rolled onto the nasal conjunctiva. If the flap has been dislodged for a few hours, it is usually very edematous. The patients are acutely aware of this problem as their vision is extremely blurred (<20/200) and the eye can be painful. With superior hinged flaps, the dislodged flap is usually found 4 to 5 mm onto the nasal conjunctival. Epithelium can be seen growing over the area of exposed stromal bed (Figure 9-12). The flap will have obvious striae and folds; however, they may be disguised by the flap edema.

Management

Patients with a dislodged flap should be treated as urgently as possible. Prior to treatment, lubrication and an eye patch can improve the discomfort. Once at the surgical center, the flap is unrolled and smoothed out. The stromal side of the flap and the stromal bed must be thoroughly cleaned of all debris and mucous. The epithelium growing over the area of the exposed stroma should also be removed. The flap is then replaced and allowed to adhere to the stromal bed for at least 5 minutes because of the edematous state. The flap striae should then be treated as described above. Finally, a bandage contact should be placed on the eye to safeguard a repeat

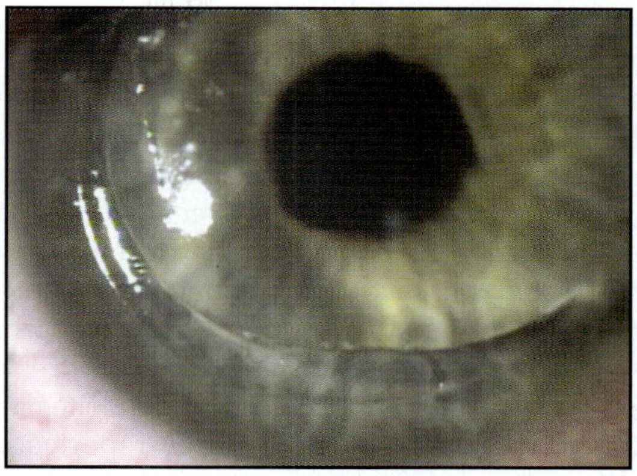

Figure 9-12. Superiorly dislodged flap with exposed stromal bed inferiorly.

dislodgement of the flap. When managed properly, the outcome should not be compromised by flap dislodgement.[19]

Prevention

For the first postoperative day, patients are advised to go home and have a 4-hour sleep. This is the critical step to allow their eyes to heal without disturbance immediately after the procedure. For the first postoperative week, patients should be warned not to touch or rub their eyes. Patients should be sent home wearing sunglasses or clear eye shields and instructed to wear these whenever possible. The shields should be worn at night. Patients can participate in any activity that does not involve touching, rubbing, irritating, or squeezing their eyes.

Infection

Infections rarely occur after LASIK; however, a recent review of the world literature found that 41 cases have been reported to date.[20] The causative organisms vary from gram positive bacteria to atypical mycobacteria, fungal, and viral pathogens. The infection is usually acquired intraoperatively, but may also be caused by postoperative contamination. While infections are generally unilateral, a bilateral infection after bilateral LASIK has now been reported.[21]

Clinical

The majority of the bacterial keratitis patients present within 72 hours of the surgery with an acute onset of symptoms.[20] Bacterial infection should be suspected whenever a localized infiltrate is identified either on the surface of the flap or at the flap interface. The infective infiltrate is generally a single and localized, about 1 to 2 mm in size, and white/gray in color with hazy with indistinct margins. If located on the surface of the cornea, it may be slightly elevated and associated with an epithelial defect. If allowed to progress without treatment, it will slowly increase in size like an early cornea ulcer. Inflammation of the cornea with surrounding interface keratitis, conjunctival injection, and an anterior chamber reaction may all occur if the infection persists. Reactivation of *herpes simplex*[22] and *zoster*[23] viral infections that present with corneal dendrites in the postoperative period have also been reported after LASIK. Fungal infections after LASIK have a delayed onset and have been related to topical prolonged steroid use after LASIK.[24]

Management

Any suspected corneal infection should be treated immediately. For suspected bacterial infections, hourly topical fluoroquinolones are the obvious first course of treatment. Topical steroids should be discontinued or reduced. Patients should be followed daily. If the infiltrate is larger than 1 mm, increasing in size, or associated with ocular inflammation, a full evaluation by a corneal specialist is recommended. Cultures with microbiological evaluation and fortified antibiotics may be required. If the infiltrate is under the flap, the flap will need to be lifted, cultures taken of the infiltrate from the stromal bed, the infiltrate should be removed, the interface irrigated, and antibiotics place in the interface before the flap is replaced. The keratitis can result is some corneal scarring. A BCVA of 20/40 or better can be obtained in the majority of the patients.[20]

Corneal epithelial dendrites that occur in any postoperative LASIK patient, particularly those with a past history of *h. simplex* keratitis or *h. zoster*, should be treated immediately with the appropriate topical and oral antiviral therapy.

Prevention

Prevention of epithelial defects during and after LASIK should greatly reduce or eliminate the risk of a superficial bacterial corneal infection. Infection at the flap interface is avoided by preventing contamination of the instruments used to treat the interface. Microkeratomes heads are sterilized for each patient. New sterile blades are used for each patient. Instruments should also be sterilized. Disposable instruments such as microkeratomes or cannulas ensure the sterility of that step of the procedure. Sterile BSS is used for interface irrigation. While LASIK is not currently a true "sterile" procedure, all efforts that move in this direction should further reduce the risk of infection.

If a patient had a past history of *h. simplex* or *h. zoster* infection, a prophylactic course of oral antiviral is recommended 1 week prior and 1 week after the LASIK procedure. Doses of acyclovir from 200 to 800 mg 5 times per day have been recommended by various LASIK experts. I have personally treated at least 20 patients with a past history of herpetic keratitis with this regimen and never experienced viral reactivation.

Diffuse Lamellar Keratitis (Sands of Sahara)

DLK is referred to by several names, including Sands of Sahara, Sands, non-specific diffuse interface keratitis, and LASIK interface keratitis (LIK). DLK and Sands are the most common terms. The cause of DLK has remained somewhat of an enigma. Holland et al have demonstrated the risk of DLK from the bacterial cell wall endotoxins that build up in the wet autoclave reservoirs.[25] Epithelial defects have been associated with focal DLK.[26] DLK has been reported months after LASIK associated with ocular inflammation,[27] ocular trauma,[28] and without an obvious etiology.[29] Other causes that have been proposed but remain unproven include cleaning solutions,[30] talc from gloves, meibomian gland secretions, microkeratome oil, rust on instruments, blade debris, iodine skin cleaners, and carboxymethylcellulose lubrication drops.[31] DLK is a postoperative interface inflammation that occurs in the 24 to 72 hour postoperative period. Late activation of DLK without an identified cause has also been reported.[29] The incidence is thought to be 1:200 to 1:500 cases, but may occur in sequential patients (outbreaks) at a specific location.

Clinical

DLK presents with varying severity, and with patient symptoms ranging from asymptomatic to mild pain, photophobia, and decrease in vision (usually a hyperopic shift). The presentation of DLK can be graded according to the severity of the presentation (Table 9-2, Figures 9-13 through 9-20).[32] The clinical appearance typically begins in the periphery and is confined to the flap interface without extension into the surrounding stroma. Untreated, this may lead to central inflammation affecting visual acuity secondary to induced hyperopia or irregular astigmatism. It may present with multiple foci, which are diffusely distributed and are often more concentrated around interface debris. Early, subtle DLK may be difficult to differentiate from postoperative superficial punctate keratitis (SPK) or mild interface debris. SPK is always on the corneal surface and will stain with fluorescein. DLK is at the level of the interface and does not stain with fluorescein. There is no anterior chamber reaction in DLK except in the most advanced cases.

Management

Early identification and intervention are the key steps for successful management of DLK. When grades 1 or 2 DLK are identified, the patient should immediately be started on topical steroid every 1 to 2 hours and an antibiotic QID for prophylaxis against infection.[33] If grade 3 DLK is identified or grade 2 DLK has not resolved after several days of treatment, the flap should be lifted and the interface irrigated. All these measures aim to prevent the progression to grade 4 DLK with central accumulation of cells, central corneal haze and striae, decreased BCVA, and a hyperopic shift. Grade 4 DLK also requires urgent flap irrigation along with flap stretching, and frequent topical steroids after. While PTK has been suggested as another treatment for DLK,[34] this can cause iatrogenic hyperopia.

Prevention

Because epithelial defects have been associated with DLK, the LASIK surgeon should strive to avoid epithelial defects whenever possible. Autoclaves reservoirs of wet autoclaves should be drained and cleaned at the end of each day. Instruments should also be cleaned and dried at the end of each day. These maneuvers aim to eliminate the wet environment that could allow the proliferation of gram negative bacteria that produce the bacterial cell wall endotoxins proposed to be an etiological agent of DLK. Dry autoclaves may offer a safer method of sterilization if DLK becomes recurrent. Disposable instruments offer another method of avoiding a toxic contaminant to the LASIK process. Topical steroids should be used for all patients for a few days after LASIK to suppress any subclinical inflammation.

Late Postoperative LASIK Complications

Epithelial Ingrowth

Carr and coworkers[35] reviewed the risk factors and the incidence of epithelial ingrowth following 1246 consecutive cases of LASIK. Epithelial ingrowth underneath the flap following LASIK was identified in 14.7% of cases. While most of these cases had small amounts of self-limited insignificant ingrowth, 1.7% of all the LASIK cases required flap revision for the removal of significant ingrowth. In another study of 3,786 eyes, significant epithelial ingrowth occurred in 0.9% of primary LASIK cases and 1.7% of enhancement cases.[36]

Preoperatively, any factor that contributes to an epithelial defect will increase the risk of epithelial ingrowth. This includes anterior basement membrane dystrophy and a history of recurrent erosions. Helena and colleagues found that ingrowth was associated with some cases of postoperative inflammation.[37] Carr and coworkers[35] found that postoperative epithelial defects, repeat LASIK rather than primary LASIK, postoperative flap slippage within 24 hours, and microperforation at the time of simultaneous Arc-T were significant risk factors for epithelial ingrowth after LASIK. Prior surgeon experience was found to be significantly protective against epithelial ingrowth. All of these factors are likely related to a disturbance of the epithelial layer during LASIK. Once the epithelium is stimulated to replicate and migrate to heal an epithelial defect, the incidence of epithelial ingrowth will increase.

Clinical

Most commonly, the patient is asymptomatic and the ingrowth is identified on a scheduled postoperative visit as a faint gray line extending less than 2 mm in from the flap edge. The ingrowth can be so discrete that it may be passed over with a quick inspection of the cornea. Epithelial ingrowth can be associated with a mild foreign body sensation that generally indicates an epithelial irregularity along the flap edge associated with the ingrowth. The visual acuity will be unaffected or drop one line of BCVA[37] except in the most severe cases when progression occurs into the visual axis.

The ingrowth is best identified with the direct focal tangential illumination of the slit-lamp biomicroscope. It is generally white to gray in color and can be seen to be located beneath the corneal flap with tangential slit-beam illumination. White to gray areas of stromal haze can occur in areas of previous ingrowth or surrounding an active area of ingrowth. Irregular fluorescein staining and pooling is often identified at the flap edge associated with the ingrowth. Surface irregularities associated with the epithelial ingrowth can be identified with corneal topography.[37] Retroillumination through the dilated pupil can also be useful to delineate the margins of large sheets of ingrowth that have extended near the

Table 9-2

Grading of Diffuse Lamellar Keratitis

1. Grade 1 DLK

   Clinical Presentation

   - Focal, white to gray, granular material in the LASIK flap interface 1 to 7 days after LASIK
   - No other ocular inflammation/ anterior chamber reaction
   - Normal visual acuity

   Treatment

   - Intensive topical steroids every hour with follow-up every 2 to 3 days to ensure complete resolution

   Prognosis

   - Excellent after topical steroids and one week for stabilization

2. Grade 2 DLK

   Clinical Presentation

   - Diffuse, white to gray, granular material under the LASIK flap interface 1 to 7 days after LASIK
   - No other ocular inflammation/anterior chamber reaction
   - Normal visual acuity

   Treatment

   - Interface irrigation has an immediate curative effect
   - Intensive hourly topical steroids after irrigation
   - Follow-up daily to ensure resolution

   Prognosis

   - Excellent after interface irrigation, topical steroids and one to two weeks of stabilization

3. Grade 3 DLK

   Clinical Presentation

   - Diffuse, confluent, white to gray, granular material under the LASIK flap interface 1 to 7 days after LASIK
   - Slight conjunctival injection
   - No anterior chamber reaction
   - Reduced visual acuity

   Treatment

   - Interface irrigation has an immediate curative effect
   - Intensive hourly topical steroids after irrigation
   - Follow-up daily to ensure resolution
   - Repeat irrigation in 1 to 2 days if the inflammation does not resolve
   - Topical steroid and antibiotics can been placed on the stromal bed to directly address the area of inflammation

   Prognosis

   - Excellent after interface irrigation, topical steroids, and several weeks of stabilization

4. Grade 4 DLK

   Clinical Presentation

   - Diffuse, confluent, white to gray, granular material under the LASIK flap interface 1 to 7 days after LASIK
   - Inflammation localized to a 2 to 4 mm area of intense central inflammation
   - Central interface striae in area of inflammation
   - Slight conjunctival injection

Table 9-2

Grading of Diffuse Lamellar Keratitis (continued)

- No anterior chamber reaction
- Markedly reduced visual acuity

Treatment

- Interface irrigation has an immediate effect
- Wipe the stromal bed with Murocel sponges
- Topical steroid and antibiotics can been placed on the stromal bed to directly address the area of inflammation
- Intensive hourly topical steroids after irrigation
- Follow-up daily to ensure resolution
- Repeat irrigation in 1 to 2 days if the inflammation does not resolve

Prognosis

- Reduced BCVA and irregular astigmatism with residual hyperopia will persist after the resolution of the inflammation due to the residual interface haze and stromal thinning
- Persistent interface striae may also reduce the final BCVA

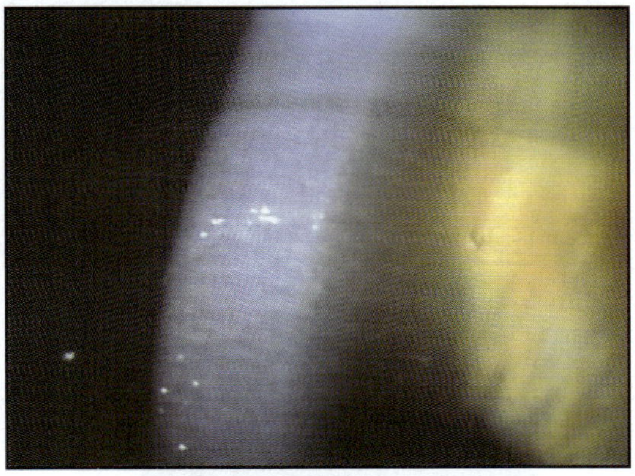

Figure 9-13. Grade 1 DLK underneath a superior epithelial defect one day after LASIK.

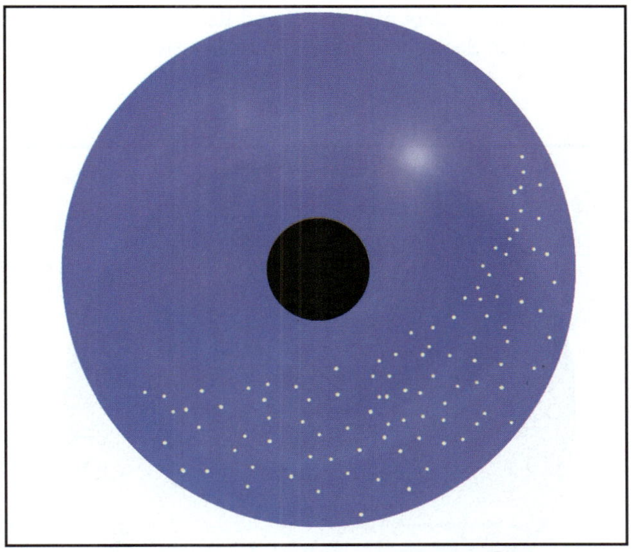

Figure 9-14. Grade 1 DLK illustration. (Reprinted from *J Cataract Refract Surgery,* 26, Linebarger EJ, Hardten DR, Lindstrom RL, Diffuse lamellar keratitis: Diagnosis and management, 1072-1077, Copyright 2000, with permission from the American Society of Cataract and Refractive Surgery and the European Society of Cataract and Refractive Surgeons.)

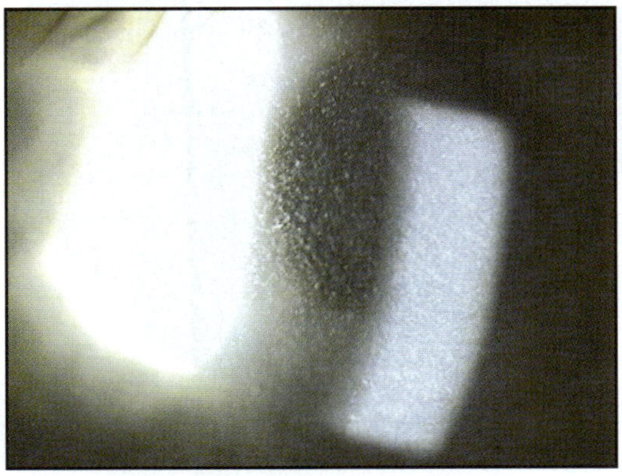

Figure 9-15. Grade 2 DLK three days after LASIK.

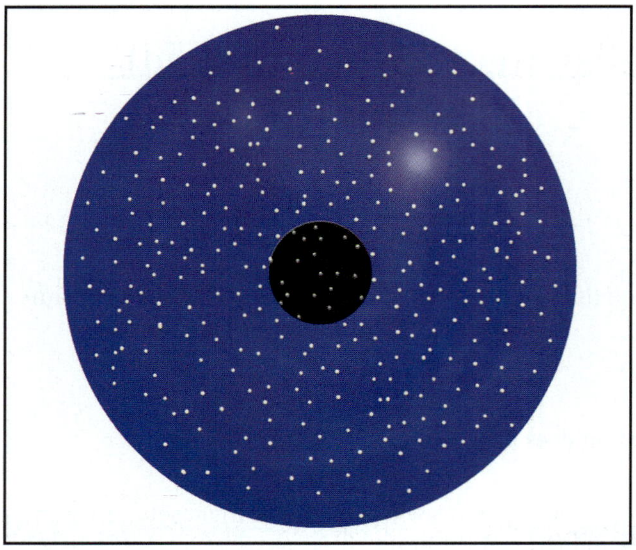

Figure 9-16. Grade 2 DLK illustration. (Reprinted from *J Cataract Refract Surgery,* 26, Linebarger EJ, Hardten DR, Lindstrom RL, Diffuse lamellar keratitis: Diagnosis and management, 1072-1077, Copyright 2000, with permission from the American Society of Cataract and Refractive Surgery and the European Society of Cataract and Refractive Surgeons.)

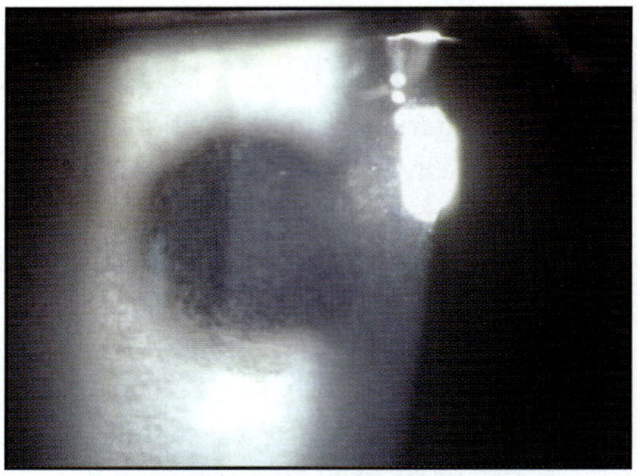

Figure 9-17. Grade 3 DLK with obvious inflammatory diffuse material in the flap interface.

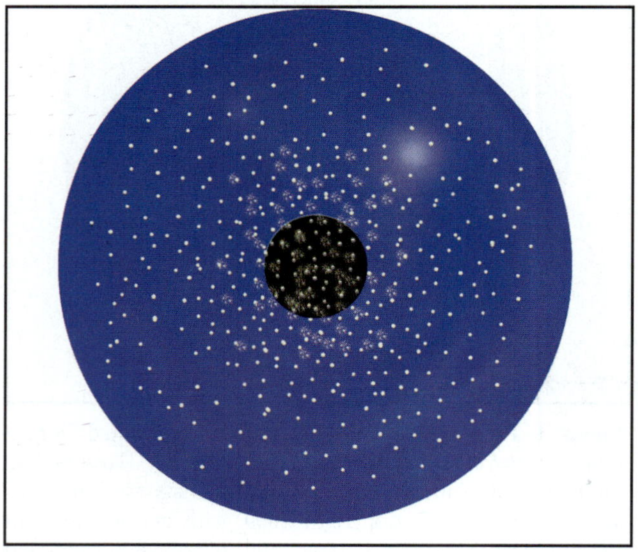

Figure 9-18. Grade 3 DLK illustration. (Reprinted from *J Cataract Refract Surgery,* 26, Linebarger EJ, Hardten DR, Lindstrom RL, Diffuse lamellar keratitis: Diagnosis and management, 1072-1077, Copyright 2000, with permission from the American Society of Cataract and Refractive Surgery and the European Society of Cataract and Refractive Surgeons.)

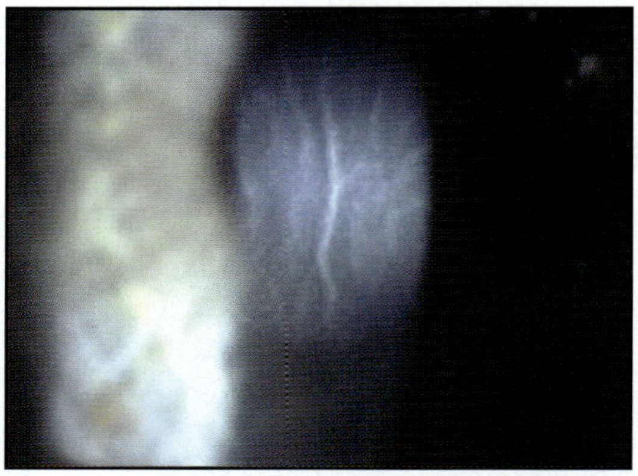

Figure 9-19. Grade 4 DLK with central flap haze and striae.

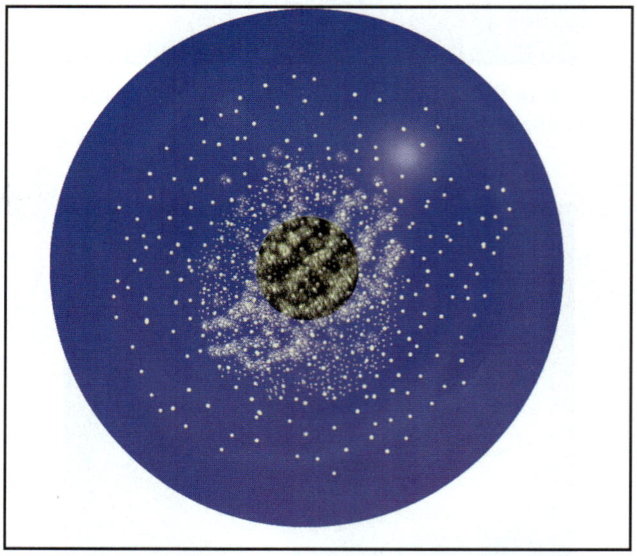

Figure 9-20. Grade 4 DLK illustration (Reprinted from *J Cataract Refract Surgery,* 26, Linebarger EJ, Hardten DR, Lindstrom RL, Diffuse lamellar keratitis: Diagnosis and management, 1072-1077, Copyright 2000, with permission from the American Society of Cataract and Refractive Surgery and the European Society of Cataract and Refractive Surgeons.)

Table 9-3

Probst/Machat Epithelial Ingrowth Classification

- Grade 1. Thin ingrowth, 1 to 2 cells thick, limited to within 2 mm of flap edge, transparent, difficult to detect, well delineated white line along advancing edge, no associated flap changes, non-progressive (Figure 9-21).

  No treatment required.
- Grade 2. Thicker ingrowth, discreet cells evident within nest, at least 2 mm from flap edge, individual cells translucent, easily seen on slit-lamp, no demarcation line along nest, corneal flap edge rolled or gray, no flap edge melting or erosion, usually progressive (Figure 9-22).

  Requires non-urgent treatment within 2 to 3 weeks.
- Grade 3. Pronounced ingrowth, several cells thick, greater than 2 mm from flap edge, ingrowth areas opaque, obvious on slit-lamp, white geographic areas of necrotic epithelial cells with no demarcation line, corneal flap margins rolled with thickened whitish-gray appearance. Progression results in large areas of flap melting from collagenase release from the necrotic epithelium. Confluent haze develops peripheral to the flap edge as flap pulls away leaving exposed stromal bed in contact with surface epithelium (Figure 9-23).

  Urgent treatment required with close follow-up, as recurrences are more common due to the altered flap edges.

visual axis. Epithelial ingrowth usually occurs on the superior and inferior regions of the nasal based flap made with the Chiron Vision ACS (Miami, Fla), although any region of the flap may be affected. The Hansatome tends to be associated with inferior epithelial ingrowth.

Epithelial ingrowth following LASIK can occur in a number of different patterns that can be divided into a classification system of grades that assist with identification and treatment (Table 9-3). Grade 1 is the most common pattern with a fine white line 2 mm inside the flap edge, which is seen in up to 10% of patients (Figure 9-21). This type of ingrowth generally demonstrates very slow progression that arrests without treatment in a few weeks. Grade 2 and grade 3 ingrowth are more aggressive forms that tend to be progressive and often require treatment. The affected area should have slit-lamp measurements of the extension of the ingrowth from the flap edge. It can occur in patterns epithelial pearls or nests, strands, and sheets (Figures 9-22 and 9-23). Grade 4 ingrowth is the most aggressive pattern of ingrowth. It is characterized by strands of epithelial cells streaming underneath the flap toward the visual axis often as early as the first 3 weeks following LASIK. This can be associated with flap edge melting (Figure 9-24). This pattern of epithelial ingrowth obviously requires urgent treatment to prevent further progression.

Management

Indications for treatment of epithelial ingrowth following LASIK include greater than 2 mm of ingrowth from the flap edge, documented progression, associated flap melting, or a disturbance of BCVA which can be attributed to the ingrowth.

Epithelial ingrowth removal has been described by several different methods. Generally the flap is lifted and the epithelial ingrowth is removed from the stromal bed and the stromal side of the flap (Figure 9-25). Because the ingrowth is generally transparent, great care must be used to remove all the ingrowth. Ingrowth that has been present for a short time (<4 weeks) generally slides of the stromal with gentle pressure from a Murocel spear. When the ingrowth has been present for longer, it tends to be more adherent so a dull surgical blade can be used to scrape the ingrowth off the stromal bed. The flap can then be replaced and the interface is generously irrigated to remove any additional epithelial cells. Generally, these two steps are all that is required for complete epithelial removal without recurrence.

Surgeons have suggested that alcohol can be applied to the stromal area of ingrowth to ensure that all the epithelial cells are destroyed.[38] Because alcohol can be toxic to the stromal, this technique should be used sparingly. Phototherapeutic keratectomy of approximately 10 μm has been used by some surgeons to successfully clean the bed after epithelial

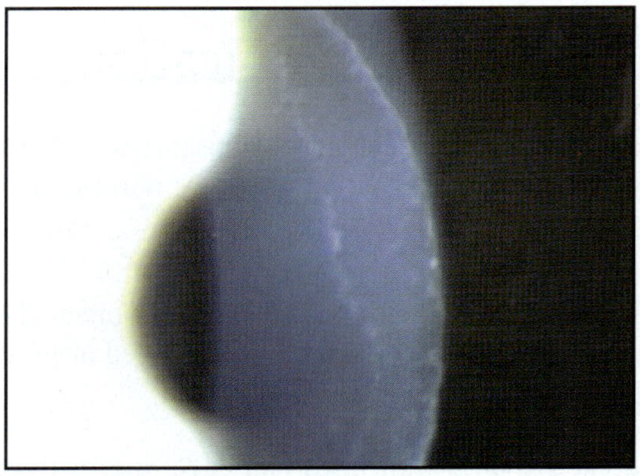

Figure 9-21. Grade 1 epithelial ingrowth with a faint white border inside the flap edge.

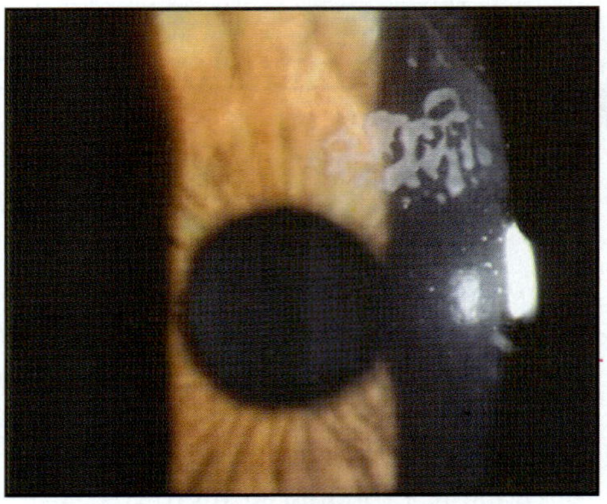

Figure 9-22. Grade 2 epithelial ingrowth with a superior "grape-like" cluster of epithelium under the flap.

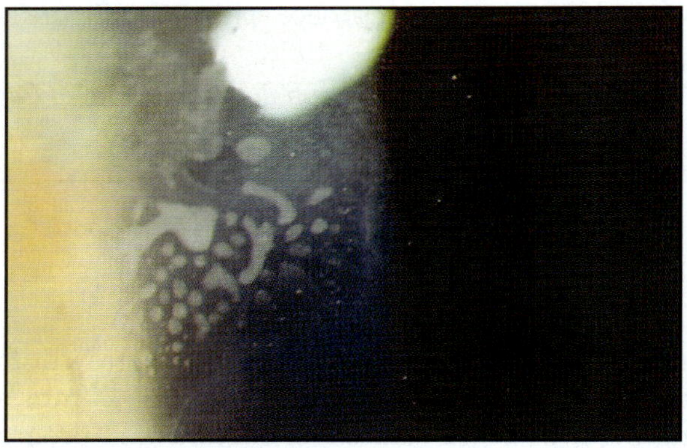

Figure 9-23. Grade 3 epithelial ingrowth with diffuse clusters of epithelial cells extending more than 2 mm from the flap edge.

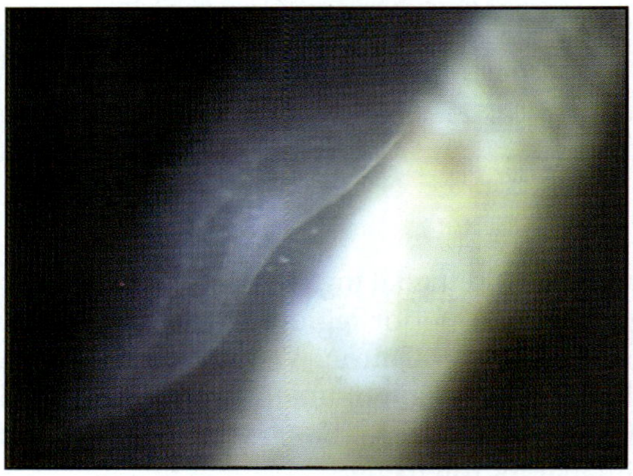

Figure 9-24. Grade 4 epithelial ingrowth is often associated with a flap edge melt.

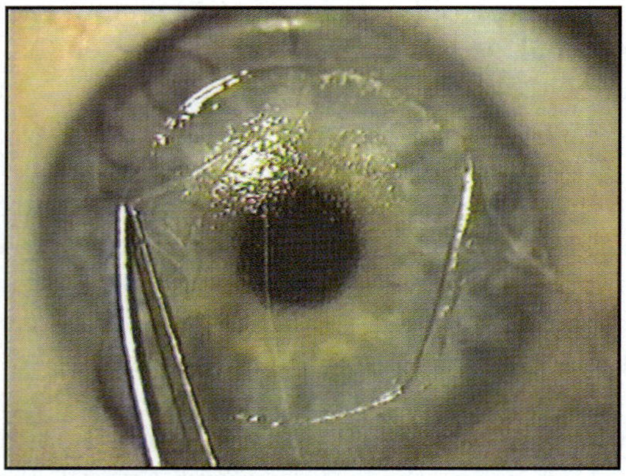

Figure 9-25. The translucent sheet of epithelial ingrowth can be peeled off the stromal bed with forceps.

ingrowth removal.[39] As they may induce a refractive effect, this technique is best reserved for recurrent cases of ingrowth. Suturing of the flap to the stromal bed has also been reported as successful for recurrent cases of epithelial ingrowth.[40] Epithelial flap removal or corneal transplant may rarely be required.[39]

Prevention

Preoperatively, anterior basement membrane dystrophy, a history of recurrent corneal erosions, advanced age, or a history of ingrowth in the other eye would all increase the risk of epithelial ingrowth following LASIK. When one or more of these factors are identified preoperatively, the refractive surgeon must carefully consider whether another refractive option such as PRK would be safer with less potential postoperative complications.

Errors in Refractive Outcome

The variability in the corneal healing after LASIK has made LASIK enhancements inevitable. With modern hyperopic LASIK techniques and excimer lasers the enhancement rate can be generally estimated as 10% per diopter of spherical correction and 10% per diopter of astigmatic correction. Regression is particularly common with correction over 3.0 D of hyperopia.

Clinical

Hyperopic LASIK undercorrections are noted immediately as the patient's postoperative UCVA on day 1 will be poor. Regression of the refractive effect usually occurs over the next several months, but rarely can occur years after the primary LASIK. In either case, the patient will be unable to function without glasses or contacts if the undercorrection and regression is significant and bilateral. Patient may also complain of night glare.

Management

Patients with residual refractive errors should be prescribed temporary glasses by the end of the first week of surgery or fit with disposable CTL after 1 to 2 weeks. Patient symptoms dramatically reduce once some form of temporary correction is obtained pending additional surgical treatment. Refractive stability should be achieved prior to performing any LASIK enhancement. Generally it could be estimated that approximately 1 month is required for each diopter of LASIK correction in order to achieve refractive stability. In practice however most LASIK enhancements are not performed earlier than the 3- to 4-month time period, and most large enhancements can be performed at the 6- to 7-month postoperative LASIK period and achieve excellent results.

The Orbscan will underestimate the thickness of the cornea for LASIK enhancement; therefore, accurate pachymetry of the cornea is best obtained with ultrasound measurements. As in primary LASIK, at least 250 µm of posterior stroma or a total corneal thickness of 410 µm should be preserved following a LASIK enhancement in order to ensure that the risk of long term corneal ectasia is minimized. If posterior corneal ectasia on the Orbscan is greater than 50 µm, this indicates that the cornea may be showing some early signs of ectasia and instability as a result of the original LASIK procedure, which may be contributing to the refractive regression. Irregular topographic patterns are also a contraindication to LASIK enhancement. The pupil size should be measured to allow for appropriate settings of the ablation zone size.

It is important to evaluate older patients with late "regression" for potential cataract formation because a LASIK enhancement will only temporarily solve their problem, as once the nuclear sclerosis progresses further they will require a cataract procedure. With eyes less than 410 µm of thickness, the Holmium LTK procedure offers an alternative method of correcting spherical iatrogenic hyperopia for up to 3.00 D.

Lifting the original corneal flap is the preferred technique for enhancement as recutting over the original flap can occasionally result in a free wedge of tissue that is difficult to manage.[41] This technique is still effective if a smaller 8.5-mm flap was used as the steepening effective of the hyperopic enhancement is within the treatment optical zone with the blend zone providing no refractive effect.

Prevention

All patients should have a cycloplegic refraction to ensure that accommodation does not occur during the preoperative refraction. Tight control of the operating room environment will improve the consistency of the results. Humidity should be kept in the 30% to 40% range and the temperature between 65 to 75°F. Low room humidity and high temperatures have been associated with over-corrections. The LASIK nomogram should be set to target slight myopia so that the effect of regression is minimized.

Postoperative Keratectasia Following LASIK

Corneal ectasia following LASIK has been recognized as an uncommon complication of LASIK. In a study of 2873 eyes, 19 eyes (0.66%) developed post-LASIK ectasia.[42] None of the eyes with ectasia had less than 8.00 D of preoperative myopia or a residual corneal bed thickness greater than 325 µm.

Clinical

Corneal ectasia usually presents from 1 to 12 months after the original LASIK procedure.[43-45] The patients often had large LASIK corrections of over 8.00 D. Most cases involve a final corneal thickness of less than 400 µm associated with the ectasia with less than 250 µm of presumed posterior corneal stroma however exceptions to this rule have been reported.[46,47] Ectasia is usually associated with regression of the refractive effect, loss of UCVA and BCVA, and irregular astigmatism. Topography demonstrates irregular astigmatism often with inferior steepening of the cornea. The Orbscan will demonstrate posterior corneal ectasia on the posterior float map with a deep orange to red color in the central area of the cornea with maximum thinning in the same area of the pachymetry map (Figure 9-26). Furthermore, this ectasia may be contributing to the regressive effect of the cornea.

Management

Any signs of corneal ectasia on the anterior corneal or posterior cornea should preclude any further LASIK as this could exacerbate the ectasia. Patients are best treated with hard CTL if these can be comfortably fit. Unfortunately, some of these patients must go on the corneal transplantation in order to restore functional vision.

Prevention

Patients with keratoconus or other corneal thinning disorders identified on topography should not have LASIK as LASIK will hasten the onset of keratectasia.[48-50] At least 250 μm of posterior stroma should be preserved following a LASIK in order to ensure that the risk of long term corneal ectasia is minimized. If we assume that the original corneal flap was approximately 160 μm, this means that the minimum corneal thickness that should be preserved after a LASIK enhancement would be approximately 410 μm.[51]

The LASIK surgeon should carefully calculate the ablation depth per diopter of their excimer laser to determine how many diopters of correction can still be performed while preserving the adequate amount of corneal thickness. Generally most excimer lasers used at a 6-mm optical zone will remove approximately 13 μm per diopter and but as the optical zone or the blend zone are increased this depth can increase to at least 15 D per micron and sometimes up to 20 μm per diopter.[51]

Night Vision Disturbances: Halos and Glare

Night vision problems after LASIK have been reported extensively in the media; however, the incidence of significant night vision symptoms is not common. A study of 236 eyes treated with the Bausch & Lomb 217C laser for mild to moderate myopia found that while mild to moderate glare was reported by 10% more patients at the 6 months follow-up, there was no significant increase in marked or severe glare or halos.[52] There were no significant changes in night driving symptoms at any level after LASIK. Hyperopic LASIK tends to be performed on older patients with smaller pupil sizes however it also produces a smaller effective optical zone so the incidence of night vision problems is similar.

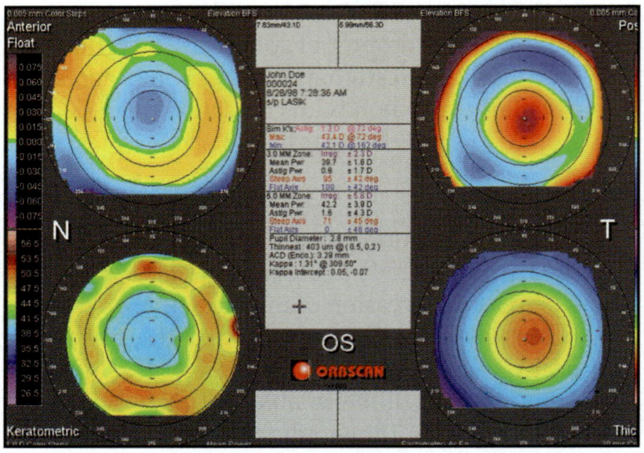

Figure 9-26. Postoperative LASIK Orbscan demonstrating posterior ectasia on the posterior float map.

Clinical

There are two potential night vision problems that occur after LASIK. Halos are the concentric blur circles that surround a point source of light, such as a car headlight, when viewed at night. Halos occur when the optical zone size of the laser treatment are smaller than the mesopic pupil size. Glare is the distortion radiating from light sources at night. Glare occurs because of the optical aberrations of the optical system that are magnified when the pupil dilates at night. Topography can clearly identify the small effective optical zones associated with halos (Figure 9-27).

Management

Patients that do experience night glare postoperatively should be seen immediately as the loss of ability to night drive can be a very stressful event. Patients are reassured that these symptoms generally abate over 3 to 6 months. Over the recovery phase, the treatment of dry eyes and any residual refractive error or monovision often improve the symptoms. For those patients who still have difficulties, night driving glasses, turning on the car dome light when driving, and rarely 1/8% pilocarpine drops just before night driving allow the patients to manage during the recovery phase. Alphagan has recently been found to reduce pupillary dilation at night with far less side effects than the pilocarpine.[53] For those rare patients with persistent night glare, custom/wavefront LASIK should offer a refined method of enlarging the treatment zones in the next 12 months.

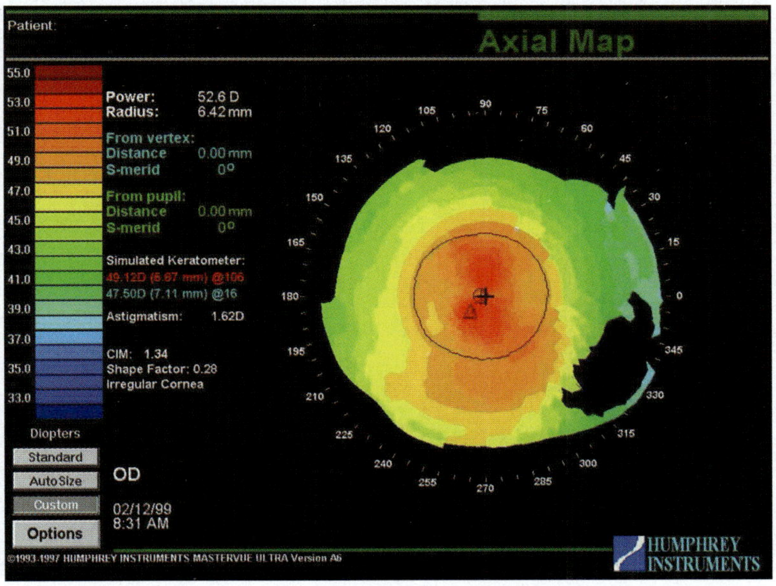

Figure 9-27. Topography after hyperopic LASIK demonstrates relatively small optical effective optical zone.

Prevention

Pupillometry should be performed in all LASIK patients preoperatively to identify those with pupils larger than 6 mm in dim light. While the risks for night glare are multi-factorial, the current most accepted treatment is to adjust the blend zone of the treatment correction to cover the measured pupil size.

De-Centration

De-centration of excimer laser is much less common now that the excimer lasers have eye trackers that allow the center of the laser ablation to be locked onto the center of the pupil. The incidence of decentrations of 0.5 mm or more has been found to occur in 20.8% of eyes after PRK.[54]

Clinical

The patient may be noted to have an undercorrection or induced astigmatism. The patient may complain of diplopia[55] and halos at night. De-centration may produce both a reduction of BCVA secondary to irregular astigmatism and a reduction of uncorrected visual acuity from the associated undercorrection, because the maximally treated area is not aligned. The diagnosis of de-centration is made topographically (Figure 9-28). Nasal de-centration is more common with the use of miotics and temporal decentrations with attempts to avoid hitting the nasally hinged flap. Dilatation makes all centration more difficult. When an eye tracker is used most of these difficulties above can be avoided; however, decentrations can still occur when the visual axis of the eye is several millimeters off the center of the pupil. This situation most commonly occurs with a large-angle kappa.

Management

Various techniques with variable success have been described for the treatment of decentrations including masking techniques to expand the ablation zone, transepithelial ablation opposite to the de-centered ablation,[55,56] or simply correction of the residual refraction with an expanded zone. Custom wavefront LASIK offers the promise of précising, treating the de-centered ablation to re-center the ablation and expand the optical zones to improve the night vision problems. Although there is limited experience with this technique at the present time, it offers so much more potential over the previous methods that any patient with a de-centered ablation at this time should consider waiting for a custom LASIK enhancement.

While patients are waiting for custom LASIK, there are several temporizing measures that can improve the patients functioning. Spectacle correction will correct any induced astigmatism; however, contact lenses will provide better improvement in the quality of the vision. The best improvement will be with an RGP CTL. Alphagan drops can be helpful to minimize pupillary dilation at night, which should reduce night vision symptoms.

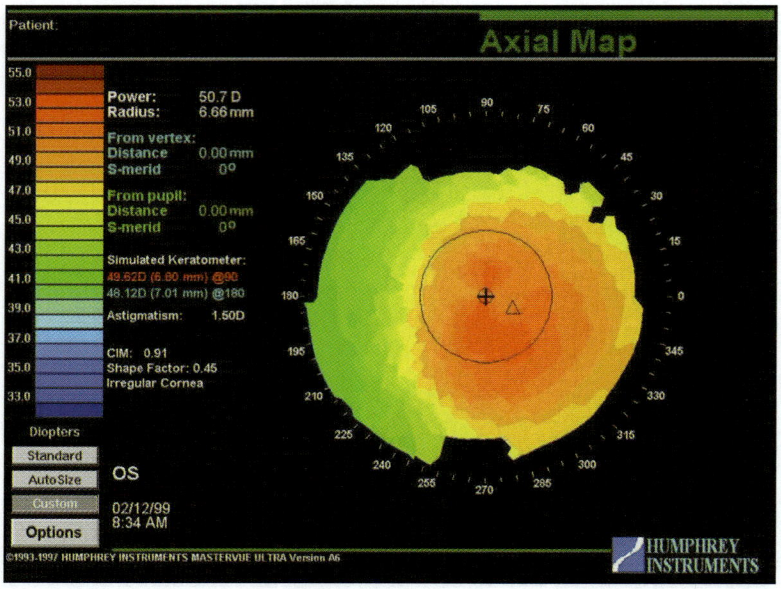

Figure 9-28. De-centered and small zone ablation after hyperopic LASIK with often be associated with night glare.

Prevention

De-centrations are avoided by appropriate centration of the laser ablation. Generally the laser ablation should be centered on the center of the pupil unless the patient's fixation, as measured preoperatively or through the operating microscope, is noted to be off the center of the pupil. Most surgeons advise that the laser ablation should then be placed between one-half and one-third the distance from the center of the pupil to the visual axis.

IRREGULAR ASTIGMATISM

Irregular astigmatism refers to irregularities in the cornea surface identified on corneal topography that do not follow the regular "bow tie" pattern of astigmatism.

Clinical

Irregular astigmatism can occur alone; however, it is usually associated with other LASIK complications such as flap complication, advanced DLK, or or a de-centered ablation. When irregular astigmatism occurs alone it is often attributed to an asymmetrical healing response of the cornea after LASIK.

Patients will complain of reduced UCVA, blurred vision, diplopia, and glare at night. Irregular astigmatism is often associated with a reduced BCVA. Topography will demonstrate the areas of asymmetrical elevation or depression of the cornea within the visual axis (Figure 9-29).

If the cause of the lost BCVA after LASIK is unclear, several additional tests can identify the cause. Hard CTL over-refraction will identify subtle corneal pathology. If the hard CTL over-refraction corrects the vision to 20/20, the problem is usually corneal irregularity. If the BCVA remains reduced, the pathology may involve the lens or the retina. Potential acuity meter (PAM) testing will identify retinal pathology. If the PAM testing is normal, the retinal function is normal, the problem is usually cornea or lens related. If the PAM BCVA is reduced, the problem is retinal. Using these two tests, the loss of BCVA related to cornea irregularity can be identified.

Management

Irregular astigmatism associated with other LASIK complications can often be improved or eliminated if the other complication is addressed. Persistent irregular astigmatism or irregular astigmatism that occurs alone is difficult to treat with current laser systems. Although techniques many have been described using broad beam lasers,[57] they are not recommended. Custom wavefront LASIK offers great promise for the treatment of patients with irregular astigmatism. While there has been little experience in this area to date, treatments should be available utilizing this method in the near future.

While patients are waiting for custom LASIK, CTLs offer the best method for the correction of irregular astigmatism. Soft CTLs will provide up to a 50% improvement in the vision while hard CTLs can

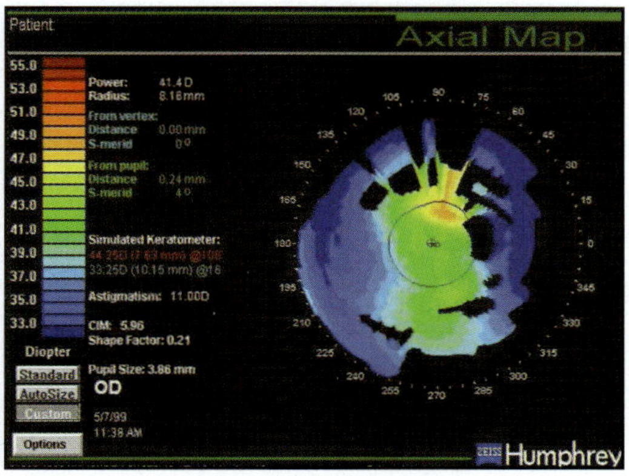

Figure 9-29. Irregular astigmatism on topography 1 year after grade-4 DLK.

offer full improvement if the patient is agreeable to their use.

Prevention

If irregular astigmatism is identified prior to the primary LASIK procedure, it is usually considered a contraindication for standard LASIK as the standard laser ablation pattern cannot correct the irregular pattern so it will persist after treatment. Irregular astigmatism associated with a history of prior hard CTL use may resolve after the contacts have been out for several weeks to months. Irregular astigmatism also occurs with forme fruste keratoconus.

Prior to using the excimer laser, the quality of the laser beam should be tested to ensure that there are no irregularities of the beam. The LASIK technique should be performed in a manner that allows even application of the laser treatment to avoid irregular astigmatism.

Post-LASIK Dry Eyes

The dry eye after LASIK is due to the creation of a temporary neurotrophic cornea by severing the corneal nerves during the creation of the LASIK flap.[58,59] The cause of the dry eye decreased corneal sensation with decrease feedback to the lacrimal gland with reduced tear production.[60] Confocal microscopy has demonstrated that the number of stromal nerve fiber bundles decreases by 90% immediately after LASIK.[61] During the first year after LASIK, the nerve fiber bundles gradually return, although by year 1 their number remains less than half of that before LASIK. Nasal hinge flaps have been shown by Eric Donnenfeld, MD, to sever less of these nerves because it preserves the nasal nerves and hence dry eyes are less of a risk because the neurotrophic cornea is less severe.[62]

Clinical

The post-LASIK dry eye presents immediately after the procedure. The patient experiences the "burning" sensation of the classic dry eye and the vision is often reduced if a dry eye keratopathy affects the central cornea. The symptoms are resolved temporarily with topical lubrication but may return less than 1 hour after application. Generally the symptoms resolve over the first postoperative month but can rarely persist for up to 1 year. Post-LASIK patients are often very frustrated by the dry eye problem as they have usually not experienced this prior to LASIK. After hyperopic LASIK, the dry eye can be caused by both the neutrotrophic cornea and the reduced tear film of the steeper central cornea. This can cause a central superficial punctate keratitis that can dramatically effect both the UCVA and BCVA (Figure 9-30).

Management

The post-LASIK dry eye should be assessed with the same approach used with the classic dry eye patient. Decreased tear secretion could occur due to the post-LASIK neurotrophic cornea but also exacerbated by a pre-existing lacrimal gland disease. Large palpebral fissures and meibomian gland dysfunction can increase the evaporative loss of tears. LASIK patients with dry eyes should be evaluated for all these conditions as this can all for the most effective treatment as well as patient education.

After the LASIK procedure frequent lubrication is suggested up to every hour even in normal patients to ensure good healing of the cornea. Punctal plugs are put in the lower punctum if symptoms persist. If the dry eye problems persist after 1 month, silicone plugs should be inserted in the upper punctum. Lubrication should be continued at least 4 to 6 times day with non-preserved viscous artificial tears. Rarely ointment can be used at prior to bed each night. Topical steroid may be useful for treating the inflammatory component of the dry eye as well as any associated eye allergy. Loteprednol etabonate 0.5% is particularly useful as it is not associated with increased risk of cataract or elevated IOP. In rare instances bandage contact lenses may be required. Environmental controls for dry eyes including a bedroom humidifier and protective sunglasses may also be useful for patients that have chronic dry eye problems. It is important to continue to see the dry eye patient to continue to provide reassurance to encourage them that the corneal signs and symptoms are resolving slowly.

Prevention

During the preoperative process it is important to identify patients with dry eyes. If the patient gives a history of dry eyes or obviously has evidence of dry eyes including a small-tear meniscus or superficial punctate keratitis it is helpful to get their epithelium healed with lubricating drops prior to the procedure. Dry eyes should be particularly suspected in patients that are already using topical lubrication prior to LASIK or that have skin conditions such as acne rosacea. Another group of patients that should particularly be suspected for dry eyes are premenopausal women, because they tend to have the most dry-eye complaints after the LASIK procedure. Schirmer testing is useful in all patients suspected of dry eyes. Punctal plugs should be used quite liberally in order to minimize the postoperative dry eye. The author prefers to use silicone punctal plugs because they are effective for 1 to 12 months after the procedure. Collagen plugs are only effective for 1 to 2 weeks so frequently need replacement.

During the LASIK procedure it is best to use a nasal hinge flap for dry eye patients in order to avoid as much as possible the neurotrophic keratopathy.[62] During the LASIK procedure, every effort should be made to preserve the epithelium as epithelial defects will prolong healing and exacerbate the post-LASIK dry eye symptoms. Other procedures could also be considered such as PRK or LASEK, which may preserve more of the corneal sensation and hence be less prone to creating a neurotrophic keratopathy. These two procedures involve surface ablation of the cornea and therefore should not be performed for corrections greater than -6.00 D as they would have a greater incidence of corneal haze.

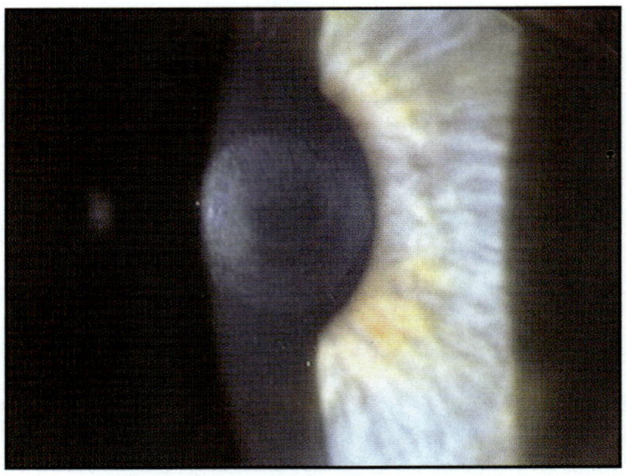

Figure 9-30. Central superficial punctate keratitis after a large hyperopic LASIK correction associated with a reduction in the UCVA and the BCVA.

Vitreoretinal Complications After LASIK

There has been a theoretical risk of increased risk of retinal detachment after LASIK due to the alteration of anterior retina from the suction ring. While the myopic population is already at an increased risk of detachment, no direct cause effect relationship has been identified.[63] A recent retrospective reviews of a large numbers of LASIK cases (38,823) found that the rate of retinal detachment was 0.08%.[64] Other complications noted to occur at a low frequency after LASIK include lattice degeneration (0.3%), posterior vitreous detachment (0.1%), macular hemorrhage (0.1%), retinal tear without retinal detachment (0.1%),[64] and choroidal neovascularization (0.1%).[66] Although the incidence of vitreo-retinal pathologic conditions in myopic eyes after LASIK is low, it is necessary to screen LASIK candidates. Preoperatively and postoperatively, lattice degeneration and other retina lesions should have long-term follow-up.[63-65]

References

1. Jacobs JM, Taravella MJ. Incidence of intraoperative flap complications in laser in situ keratomileusis. *J Cataract Refract Surg.* 2002 Jan;28(1):23-8.
2. Knorz MC. Flap and interface complications in LASIK. *Curr Opin Ophthalmol.* 2002 Aug;13(4):242-5.
3. Ellies P, Binisti P, Dighiero P, Saragoussi JJ, Bourges JL, Renard G. Blade defect responsible for a severe laser-assisted in situ keratomileusis complication. *Arch Ophthalmol.* 2002 Nov;120(11):1592-3.
4. Leung AT, Rao SK, Cheng AC, Yu EW, Fan DS, Lam DS. Pathogenesis and management of laser in situ keratomileusis flap buttonhole. *J Cataract Refract Surg.* 2000 Mar;26(3):358-62.
5. Jain VK, Abell TG, Bond WI, Stevens G Jr. Immediate transepithelial photorefractive keratectomy for treatment of laser in situ keratomileusis flap complications. *J Refract Surg.* 2002 Mar-Apr;18(2):109-12.
6. Shemesh G, Dotan G, Lipshitz I. Predictability of corneal flap thickness in laser in situ keratomileusis using three different microkeratomes *J Refract Surg.* 2002 May-Jun;18(3 Suppl):S347-51
7. Gokmen F, Jester JV, Petroll WM, McCulley JP, Cavanagh HD. In vivo confocal microscopy through-focusing to measure corneal flap thickness after laser in situ keratomileusis. *J Cataract Refract Surg.* 2002 Jun;28(6):962-70.
8. Arbelaez MC. Nidek MK 2000 microkeratome clinical evaluation. *J Refract Surg.* 2002 May-Jun;18(3 Suppl):S357-60.

9. Tekwani NH, Huang D. Risk factors for intraoperative epithelial defect in laser in-situ keratomileusis. *Am J Ophthalmol.* 2002 Sep;134(3):311-6.
10. Teal P, Breslin C, Arshinoff S, Edmison D. Corneal subepithelial infiltrates following excimer laser photorefractive keratectomy *J Cataract Refract Surg.* 1995 Sep;21(5):516-8.
11. Probst LE, Machat JJ. Corneal subepithelial infiltrates following photorefractive keratectomy. *J Cataract Refract Surg.* 1996 Apr;22(3):281.
12. Probst LE. One drop LASIK. *LASIK II Course.* San Diego, Calif: ASCRS; 2001.
13. Probst LE, Machat JJ. Removal of flap striae following laser in situ keratomileusis. *J Cataract Refract Surg.* 1998 Feb; 24(2): 153-155.
14. Kuo IC, Ou R, Hwang DG. Flap haze after epithelial debridement and flap hydration for treatment of post-laser in situ keratomileusis striae. *Cornea.* 2001 Apr;20(3):339-41.
15. Carpel EF, Carlson KH, Shannon S. Folds and striae in laser in situ keratomileusis flaps. *J Refract Surg.* 1999 Nov-Dec;15(6):687-90.
16. Lam DS, Leung AT, Wu JT, et al. Management of severe flap wrinkling or dislodgment after laser in situ keratomileusis. *J Cataract Refract Surg.* 1999 Nov;25(11):1441-7.
17. Aldave AJ, Hollander DA, Abbott RL. Late-onset traumatic flap dislocation and diffuse lamellar inflammation after laser in situ keratomileusis. *Cornea.* 2002 Aug; 21(6):604-7.
18. Sakurai E, Okuda M, Nozaki M, Ogura Y. Late-onset laser in situ keratomileusis (LASIK) flap dehiscence during retinal detachment surgery *Am J Ophthalmol.* 2002 Aug;134(2):265-6.
19. Recep OF, Cagil N, Hasiripi H. Outcome of flap subluxation after laser in situ keratomileusis: results of 6 month follow-up. *J Cataract Refract Surg.* 2000 Aug;26(8):1158-62.
20. Pushker N, Dada T, Sony P, Ray M, Agarwal T, Vajpayee RB. Microbial keratitis after laser in situ keratomileusis. *J Refract Surg.* 2002 May-Jun;18(3):280-6.
21. Suresh PS, Rootman DS. Bilateral infectious keratitis after a laser in situ keratomileusis enhancement procedure.*J Cataract Refract Surg.* 2002 Apr;28(4):720-1.
22. Perry HD, Doshi SJ, Donnenfeld ED, Levinson DH, Cameron CD. *Herpes simplex* reactivation following laser in situ keratomileusis and subsequent corneal perforation. *CLAO J.* 2002 Apr;28(2):69-71.
23. Jarade EF, Tabbara KF. Presumed reactivation of herpes zoster ophthalmicus following laser in situ keratomileusis. *J Refract Surg.* 2002 Jan-Feb;18(1):79-80.
24. Peng Q, Holzer MP, Kaufer PH, Apple DJ, Solomon KD. Interface fungal infection after laser in situ keratomileusis presenting as diffuse lamellar keratitis. A clinicopathological report. *J Cataract Refract Surg.* 2002 Aug;28(8):1400.
25. Holland SP, Mathias RG, Morck DW, Chiu J, Slade SG Diffuse lamellar keratitis related to endotoxins released from sterilizer reservoir biofilms *Ophthalmology.* 2000 Jul;107(7):1227-33; discussion 1233-4.
26. Haw WW, Manche EE. Late onset diffuse lamellar keratitis associated with an epithelial defect in six eyes. *J Refract Surg.* 2000 Nov-Dec;16(6):744-8.
27. Keszei VA. Diffuse lamellar keratitis associated with iritis 10 months after laser in situ keratomileusis. *J Cataract Refract Surg.* 2001 Jul;27(7):1126-7.
28. Weisenthal RW. Diffuse lamellar keratitis induced by trauma 6 months after laser in situ keratomileusis. *J Refract Surg.* 2000 Nov-Dec;16(6):749-51.
29. Probst LE, Foley L. Late-onset interface keratitis after uneventful laser in situ keratomileusis. *J Cataract Refract Surg.* 2001 Jul;27(7):1124-5.
30. Nakano EM, Nakano K, Oliveira MC, Portellinha W, Simonelli R, Alvarenga LS. Cleaning solutions as a cause of diffuse lamellar keratitis. *J Refract Surg.* 2002 May-Jun;18(3 Suppl):S361-3.
31. Samuel MA, Kaufman SC, Ahee JA, Wee C, Bogorad D. Diffuse lamellar keratitis associated with carboxymethylcellulose sodium 1% after laser in situ keratomileusis. *J Cataract Refract Surg.* 2002 Aug;28(8):1409-11.
32. Linebarger EJ, Hardten DR, Lindstrom RL. Diffuse lamellar keratitis: identification and management. *Int Ophthalmol Clin.* 2000 Summer;40(3):77-86.
33. Linebarger EJ, Hardten DR, Lindstrom RL. Diffuse lamellar keratitis: diagnosis and management. *J Cataract Refract Surg.* 2000 Jul;26(7):1072-7.
34. Leu G, Hersh PS. Phototherapeutic keratectomy for the treatment of diffuse lamellar keratitis. *J Cataract Refract Surg.* 2002 Aug;28(8):1471-4.
35. Carr JD, Nardone R Jr, Sulting RD, Thompson KP, Waring GO III. Risk factors for epithelial ingrowth after LASIK. *Invest Ophthalmol Vis Sci.* 1997;38(4):S232.
36. Wang MY, Maloney RK. Epithelial ingrowth after laser in situ keratomileusis. *Am J Ophthalmol.* 2000 Jun;129(6):746-51.
37. Helena MC, Meisler D, Wilson SE. Epithelial growth within the lamellar interface after in situ keratomileusis (LASIK). *Cornea.* 1997;16(3):300-305.
38. Haw WW, Manche EE. Treatment of progressive or recurrent epithelial ingrowth with ethanol following laser in situ keratomileusis. *J Refract Surg.* 2001 Jan-Feb;17(1):63-8.
39. Domniz Y, Comaish IF, Lawless MA, Sutton GL, Eckshtein R, Collins MB, Rogers CM. Epithelial ingrowth: causes, prevention, and treatment in 5 cases. *J Cataract Refract Surg.* 2001 Nov;27(11):1803-11.
40. Rowsey J. Suture laser-assisted in situ keratomileusis flaps after epithelial ingrowth removal. *Arch Ophthalmol.* 2002 Nov;120(11):1601.
41. Domniz Y, Comaish IF, Lawless MA, Rogers CM, Sutton GL. Recutting the cornea versus lifting the flap: comparison of two enhancement techniques following laser in situ keratomileusis. *J Refract Surg.* 2001 Sep-Oct;17(5):505-10.
42. Pallikaris IG, Kymionis GD, Astyrakakis NI. Corneal ectasia induced by laser in situ keratomileusis. *J Cataract Refract Surg.* 2001 Nov;27(11):1796-802.

43. Seiler T, Koufala K, Richter G. Iatrogenic keratectasia after laser in situ keratomileusis. *J Refract Surg.* 1998 May-Jun;14(3):312-7.
44. Geggel HS, Talley AR. Delayed onset keratectasia following laser in situ keratomileusis. *J Cataract Refract Surg.* 1999 Apr;25(4):582-6.
45. Argento C, Cosentino MJ, Tytiun A, Rapetti G, Zarate J. Corneal ectasia after laser in situ keratomileusis. *J Cataract Refract Surg.* 2001 Sep;27(9):1440-8.
46. Ou RJ, Shaw EL, Glasgow BJ. Keratectasia after laser in situ keratomileusis (LASIK): evaluation of the calculated residual stromal bed thickness. *Am J Ophthalmol.* 2002 Nov;134(5):771-3.
47. Spadea L, Palmieri G, Mosca L, Fasciani R, Balestrazzi E. Iatrogenic keratectasia following laser in situ keratomileusis. *J Refract Surg.* 2002 Jul-Aug;18(4):475-80.
48. Rao SN, Raviv T, Majmudar PA, Epstein RJ. Role of Orbscan II in screening keratoconus suspects before refractive corneal surgery. *Ophthalmology.* 2002 Sep;109(9):1642-6.
49. Schmitt-Bernard CF, Lesage C, Arnaud B. Keratectasia induced by laser in situ keratomileusis in keratoconus. *J Refract Surg.* 2000 May-Jun;16(3):368-70.
50. Holland SP, Srivannaboon S, Reinstein DZ. Avoiding serious corneal complications of laser assisted in situ keratomileusis and photorefractive keratectomy. *Ophthalmology.* 2000 Apr;107(4):640-52.
51. Probst LE, Machat JJ. Mathematics of laser in situ keratomileusis for high myopia. *J Cataract Refract Surg.* 1998 Feb;24(2):190-5.
52. Balazsi G, Mullie M, Lasswell L, Lee PA, Duh YJ. Laser in situ keratomileusis with a scanning excimer laser for the correction of low to moderate myopia with and without astigmatism. *J Cataract Refract Surg.* 2001 Dec;27(12):1942-51.
53. McDonald JE 2nd, El-Moatassem Kotb AM, Decker BB. Effect of brimonidine tartrate ophthalmic solution 0.2% on pupil size in normal eyes under different luminance conditions. *J Cataract Refract Surg.* 2001 Apr;27(4):560-4.
54. Azar DT, Yeh PC. Corneal topographic evaluation of decentration in photorefractive keratectomy: treatment displacement vs intraoperative drift. *Am J Ophthalmol.* 1997 Sep;124(3):312-20.
55. Yap EY, Kowal L. Diplopia as a complication of laser in situ keratomileusis surgery. *Clin Experiment Ophthalmol.* 2001 Aug;29(4):268-71.
56. Alkara N, Genth U, Seiler T. Diametral ablation—a technique to manage decentered photorefractive keratectomy for myopia. *J Refract Surg.* 1999 Jul-Aug;15(4):436-40.
57. Buzard KA, Fundingsland BR. Treatment of irregular astigmatism with a broad beam excimer laser. *J Refract Surg.* 1997 Nov-Dec;13(7):624-36.
58. Toda I, Asano-Kato N, Komai-Hori Y, Tsubota K. Dry eye after laser in situ keratomileusis. *Am J Ophthalmol.* 2001 Jul;132(1):1-7.
59. Wilson SE, Ambrosio R. Laser in situ keratomileusis-induced neurotrophic epitheliopathy. *Am J Ophthalmol.* 2001 Sep;132(3):405-6.
60. Ang RT, Dartt DA, Tsubota K. Dry eye after refractive surgery. *Curr Opin Ophthalmol.* 2001 Aug;12(4):318-22.
61. Lee BH, McLaren JW, Erie JC, Hodge DO, Bourne WM. Reinnervation in the cornea after LASIK. *Invest Ophthalmol Vis Sci.* 2002 Dec;43(12):3660-4.
62. Doshi S, Donnenfeld E, Solomon K, Perry H, Ehrenhaus M. LASIK patients have less post-op dry eye with nasal-hinge flap, US study suggests. *Eurotimes.* October 2001.
63. Lin J, Xie X, Du X, Yang Y, Yao K. Incidence of vitreoretinal pathologic conditions in myopic eyes after laser in situ keratomileusis. *Chung Hua Yen Ko Tsa Chih.* 2002 Sep;38(9):546-9.
64. Arevalo JF, Ramirez E, Suarez E, Cortez R, Ramirez G, Yepez JB. Retinal detachment in myopic eyes after laser in situ keratomileusis. *J Refract Surg.* 2002 Nov-Dec;18(6):708-14.
65. Ruiz-Moreno JM, Perez-Santonja JJ, Alio JL. Choroidal neovascularization in myopic eyes after laser-assisted in situ keratomileusis. *Retina.* 2001;21(2):115-20.

Chapter Ten

Wavefront-Based Treatment of Hyperopia

W. Bruce Jackson, MD, FRCSC

Introduction

Although hyperopic correction has been performed for more than a century,[1] recent surgical advancements have yielded the most promising data to date. Historically, hyperopia has been treated with a variety of procedures, including hexagonal keratotomy (HK), thermokeratoplasty (TK), keratophakia and keratomileusis, intracorneal lenses, clear lens extraction, and excimer laser surgery.

Excimer laser procedures, such as hyperopic photorefractive keratectomy (PRK) and laser-assisted in-situ keratomileusis (LASIK) have shown the most success for hyperopic correction.

The treatment of hyperopia has lagged considerably behind myopia with the earliest treatments being performed by Dausch[2] in 1991 on the Aesculap-Meditec (Germany) MEL60 utilizing a scanning slit and rotating mask. The ablation profile for the correction of hyperopia had been suggested by L'Esperance et al[3] and aims to create a smoothly transitioned annular ablation in the stroma at the periphery of a defined optical zone that effectively steepens the central visual axis while flattening the periphery. Early results using a 4-mm diameter optical zone which tapered to 7 mm for corrections under 5.00 D were more stable and predictable than those above 5.00 D but the major problems were regression, decentration, slow recovery, and loss of best spectacle-corrected visual acuity (BSCVA).[2] It soon became clear that the best results were obtained with low hyperopia up to 4.00 D with optical zones 5 to 7 mm with total ablation area extending to 8.5 to 9.5 mm.[4-6]

Similar work was done with the early VISX laser prototypes. In 1991, Sher et al[7,8] described a technique that used the Taunton Technologies LV 2000 device, an early prototype excimer laser that was acquired by VISX Inc. For the technique, a peripheral steepening using the laser was performed after the central cornea was treated to remove scars. This method, known as the "unity cut," reduced the amount of hyperopic shift seen after the central cornea was treated.

Different techniques were used by each laser manufacturer to develop this ablation profile. The Summit Apex Plus Laser (Alcon, Summit Autonomous, Fort Worth, Tex) used an axicon lens system to treat the area between 6.5 and 9.5 mm.[9,10] An erodible disc, which absorbs laser energy to produce a smooth transition zone, is also used. Other laser systems utilize smaller spots or a scanning slit to produce a circular pattern with an optical zone between 5 and 6 mm with an ablation zone out to 9 mm.[11,12]

PRK and LASIK for Hyperopia

In 1993, Dausch et al[2] reported their hyperopic PRK data for the correction of 15 low hyperopic eyes (with preoperative refractions of +2.00 to +7.50 D) to +0.53 D postoperatively and 8 highly hyperopic eyes (with preoperative refractions of +11.00 to +16.00 D) to +2.50 D postoperatively. Regression between 1 and 9 months was reported as +0.70 D for the low group and +3.0 D for the high group. Later in 1995, Dausch[13] reported similar data on 81 hyperopic eyes.

Since then, numerous studies have been reported in the literature on hyperopic PRK. Because the epithelium is removed beyond 9 mm, re-epithelialization takes an average of 4 days, range 3 to 10,[13,14] and stability of refraction and vision takes 6 to 12 months. Patients are frequently overcorrect by 1.00 D initially with drift to plano at 3 to 6 months.[12,14,15] Uncorrected visual acuity (UCVA) at 1 year varies from 46% to 70%, 20/20 or better, depending upon the refractive mean spherical equivalent. A 1-line loss of BSCVA is seen in upwards of 30% of eyes in part due to the loss in image magnification but is rarely appreciated by the patient.[14] With higher corrections, the results are not as encouraging, with more regression, loss of contrast acuity and BSCVA, and daytime visual problems.[15]

Overall, hyperopic patients are extremely pleased with the results of their surgery with many achieving a multi-focal cornea and are able to read much better than expected.[13] Complications unique to hyperopic PRK include an iron-ring,[16] central nodule formation with scarring[17,18] and relatively more loss of BSCVA than seen with myopic corrections, and acute corneal necrosis.[19] Because of the older age of the hyperopic population (50 years versus 39 for myopia) and knowing that steepening the curve of the central cornea can lead to decreased tear film break-up time,[20] it is not unexpected that these patients may experience symptoms and signs of dry eye. Decentration may occur more frequently because of the small optical zone and longer treatments but the use of an eye tracker will help decrease the incidence of this complication as well as the induced regular and irregular astigmatism, which may limit BSCVA. Lubrication is essential to prevent the corneal erosions and scarring.

In 1998, my colleagues and I[14] published results of our study that supported the safety and effectiveness of laser vision correction for treating low hyperopia. Thirty-eight patients received treatment with the VISX (Santa Clara, Calif) Star Excimer Laser System. Mean follow-up was 13.9 months, with 65 eyes with hyperopia from +1.00 D to +4.00 D. A total of 80% of eyes were within ±0.5 D and 98% of eyes were within ±1.0 D of intended manifest spherical equivalent (SE) at 1 year. At one year, 72% of eyes had UCVA of 20/25 or better and 70% had achieved preoperative BSCVA, with no eye seeing worse than 20/25. Results remained constant at 18 months. There was a tendency toward regression between months 1 and 6 with stabilization of SE between months 6 and 12. Thereafter, up to 18 months, there was some regression with a mean of +0.31 D, but the number of patients was small. There was one mild decentration and very slight decreases in mean intraocular pressure (IOP) and central corneal thickness. One patient had grade 1.00 haze develop in both eyes at 12 and 18 months; all other patients experienced trace or no haze.

In 2002, Stevens et al[12] published a study on the safety, efficacy, and predictability of PRK for hyperopic astigmatism of +1.75 to +5.00 D manifest refractive sphere and up to -2.50 D manifest refractive astigmatism using the VISX Star excimer laser system, with version 2.5 software.

Stevens concluded that PRK for hyperopia using the VISX Star excimer laser system was effective in the treatment of hyperopic astigmatism. Although no patient lost 2 or more lines of high-contrast BSCVA 1 year after treatment, there was a significant decrease in Pelli-Robson contrast acuity.

In the study, treatment was performed on 32 eyes of 21 patients. Manifest and cycloplegic refraction together with Pelli-Robson contrast sensitivity assessment was performed prior to surgery and 1, 3, 6, 12, and 24 months after treatment. Eighty-four percent of the surgical procedures were reviewed 1 year postop. Corneal epithelial healing was complete between day 4 and 10. Twelve months after treatment, 93% achieved 20/40 or better UCVA and 19 eyes (70%) achieved 20/20. The mean spherical equivalent refraction was reduced from +2.90 at baseline to +0.10 D at 1 year and +0.40 D at 2 years; 65% of eyes had a refraction within ±0.50 D. Four patients had further treatment by LASIK for undercorrection in 3 eyes and overcorrection in 1 eye.

Also in 2002, Nagy et al[11] conducted a study to compare the results of traditional laser photoablation and wavefront-supported customized ablation (WASCA) in hyperopic PRK (H-PRK). They concluded that WASCA-guided H-PRK treatment was safe and predictable. The results were slightly superior to traditional PRK for hyperopia in terms of UCVA and BSCVA, although additional studies with longer follow up and larger samples are needed. Wavefront-guided PRK for hyperopia has been reported to result in less halo and nighttime glare when compared to patients treated with traditional PRK. Also Nagy noted that with wavefront guided PRK, patients had not lost contrast sensitivity after 6-month follow-up as seen with traditional PRK.[11,12]

In the prospective study, two treatment groups, each comprising of 40 eyes of 20 patients, were compared. Wavefront aberrations were examined using a Shack-Hartmann aberrometer. H-PRK was performed with the Asclepion-Meditec (Germany) MEL 70 flying-spot excimer laser. Preoperative refraction was similar in the two groups. In the traditional H-PRK group (Group 1) preoperative refraction was +3.10 ± 0.85 D, and in the WASCA-guided group (Group 2) it was +2.90 ± 0.80 D. The follow-up time was 6 months.

In Group 1, mean postoperative refraction was +0.14 ± 0.24 D, and in Group 2, -0.10 ± 0.25 D. Mean UCVA was 0.92 ± 0.16 in Group 1 and 0.95 ± 0.18 in Group 2. Mean BSCVA was 0.96 ± 0.04 in Group 1 and 1.06 ± 0.13 in Group 2. In Group 1, 67.5%, and in Group 2, 85% were within ±0.50 D of target refraction. Regarding change of BSCVA in Group 1, 5%, and in Group 2, 20% gained 1 Snellen line; in Group 1, 10%, and in Group 2, 12.5% lost 2 Snellen lines. In Group 2, the root mean square (RMS) value for the higher order aberration increased from the initial 0.134 to 0.257 μm at 6 months after surgery.

Wavefront guided treatments still increased the RMS value for higher order aberrations postoperatively despite the improvement in UCVA, which raises the possibility that a decrease in higher order aberrations is not a prerequisite for improvement in subjective visual acuity following wavefront guided PRK treatments.[22,23] Panagopoulou[22] has demonstrated that the higher order aberrations increase less at 3 months with PRK (1.3 versus 1.8 times) compared to LASIK using WASCA.

LASIK, the procedure that combines a lamellar corneal flap and ablating the underlying cornea with the excimer laser, also has been effectively used for the correction of hyperopia since the late 1990s.

Results for hyperopic LASIK[23-26] are very similar to those for hyperopic PRK but refractive stability occurs sooner with less regression, and there is less discomfort and follow-up.[27] It is for these reasons that hyperopic LASIK is the current preferred procedure. A review of the literature by Nagy[11] led him to conclude that the refractive results, efficacy, and predictability depend more on the type of excimer laser beam delivery system than on the refractive procedure used (PRK or LASIK).

The treatment of spherical hyperopia does better in both low and high hyperopia groups compared to eyes with a high hyperopic astigmatic component.[11] Alessio[28] reported good results with flying-spot technology in eyes with irregular hyperopic astigmatism in the case of topography driven PRK treatments. We have noted peripheral segmental haze to be more prominent with astigmatic treatments than with spherical where haze is annular sparing the corneal center and is minimal. Surgically induced astigmatism was no more frequent with hyperopic than with myopic treatments.[29]

As with any refractive procedure, the patient must be selected carefully and, if in the presbyopic range, realize they will still need glasses for reading. Hyperopia treated with PRK should be no more than 4.00 to 6.00 D, and the patient must be counseled that visual recovery may take up to a year. Re-treatments can be performed but may result in central corneal erosions and scar formation associated with a steep cornea and poor ocular tear film.[18]

In 1998, Ditzen et al[30] reported their results for hyperopic LASIK. They concluded that LASIK for hyperopia resulted in less regression, minimal haze and better predictability and stability than surface PRK. They also noted that preoperative corneal radius appeared to be an important factor in eyes with high hyperopia.

More recently, numerous studies have been published on hyperopic LASIK. In 2002, Cobo-Soriano et al[31] analyzed the influence of preoperative corneal curvature, postoperative keratometric power, and the amount of correction on the outcomes of hyperopic LASIK. They reported that the degree of hyperopia corrected negatively influenced the outcome of hyperopic LASIK. Preoperative keratometry did not significantly influence the postoperative results and postoperative keratometry >48.00 D did not result in significant worsening of visual results when the attempted correction was less than +4.00 D.

Also in 2002, a study by Salz et al[23] supported the safety and effectiveness of the LASIK correction of spherical hyperopia, hyperopic astigmatism, and mixed astigmatism.

Lian et al[24] conducted a study, published in 2002, in which LASIK was used to treat hyperopia from +1.00 to +6.00 D with good predictability and safety. They reported that primary and secondary hyperopia required different nomograms.

In a study published in 2002, Ditzen et al[25] concluded that LASIK appeared to be safe and effective for hyperopia and hyperopia with astigmatism for corrections up to +6.00 D. They noted that large flap diameters are necessary to avoid epithelial ingrowth.

Dr. Richard J. Duffey[32] recently reported that LASIK outcomes were better for hyperopia and hyperopic astigmatism with the VISX Star S3 Smooth Scan excimer laser with infrared video tracking (ActiveTrack). The study included the first 50 consecutive hyperopic and/or hyperopic astigmatic eyes treated January through April 2001 with the VISX Star S3 Smooth Scan excimer laser with ActiveTrack enabled.

This population had a mean hyperopic SE refraction of +2.23 D (range +0.75 to +5.62 D). The mean cylinder was +0.81 D.

All patients were treated with a 5 x 9 mm optical zone at 10 Hz. For comparison, a similar group of consecutively treated hyperopic patients, with or without astigmatism and operated upon without the tracking system in late 2000, was reviewed.

In the ActiveTrack eyes at 1 month, the mean SE manifest refraction was -0.07 ± 0.32 D. At three months, this had changed to +0.04 ± 0.15 D. At 3 months, 98% of eyes had an achieved correction of ±0.50 D from the intended refractive goal. Also at 3 months, the postop UCVA was 20/20 or better in 46% of eyes, 20/25 or better in 68% of eyes, 20/30 or better in 88% of eyes, and 20/40 or better in 100% of eyes followed. At 3 months, 2% of eyes lost 1 line of BSCVA, 94% had no change, and 4% had gained 1 line. In the untracked eyes, at 3 months the mean SE refraction was +0.28 ± 0.45 D.

Aberrometry and the VISX WaveScan System

Wavefront-guided refractive surgical treatments are based on data taken directly from patients' eyes, rather than on manifest refraction.

The VISX WaveScan device generates an objective mathematical calculation of refraction across a 6 mm pupil. In addition to regular sphere, cylinder and axis, it produces an acuity map that provides all the lower and higher order aberrations, as well as a different map that looks only at the higher order aberrations. Quantitative data on RMS errors can also be obtained. The user can also look at point-spread function, Zernicke coefficients, Hartmann-Shack images, and difference maps.

In addition, the WaveScan device serves as a confirmation tool for sphere, cylinder and axis, or manifest refractions. In the postoperative setting, the WaveScan device can be used to identify and describe specific higher order aberrations that may be consistent with a patient's subjective complaint.

The VISX WaveScan system is an ophthalmic diagnostic instrument that uses a Hartmann-Shack wavefront sensor to measure the refractive error and wavefront aberrations of the human eye.[33] It is the central device in the VISX WavePrint system, which includes variable spot scanning (VSS) excimer laser energy delivery and the PreVue lens.

The Hartmann-Schack aberrometer uses thousands of lenslets (small lenses) arranged in a hexagonal array to measure the wavefront emerging across the pupil, and arranges it as a Hartmann Schack spot pattern. The aberrometer is independent of subjective patient analysis and provides an objective basis for wavefront measurement.[34]

The PreVue Lens is a diagnostic tool involving a plastic lens that is ablated with a wavefront-driven shape. It was utilized in the VISX wavefront clinical trials and proved to be a powerful tool for resolving discrepancies between wavefront and manifest preoperative refractions, addressing eyes with significant irregularities, as well as assisting the refractive surgeon with initial conversion to wavefront-driven ablations.[35]

To capture the data required to create a target ablation shape, the WaveScan device focuses a measurement beam onto the patient's retina and reflects a wavefront back through the patient's eye. As the wavefront exits, it is distorted by the optics of the eye. This wavefront is collected and analyzed by the WaveScan device, which generates two maps.[36]

One map depicts all aberrations in the exiting wavefront, including simple sphere and cylinder. The other map isolates the higher order aberrations, which constitute a much smaller proportion of the error.[37] From this information, the WaveScan VSS software calculates the "best-fit treatment table" for an individualized ablation within 0.25 μm.

The WaveScan system also can be used in combination with topography to help evaluate and understand aberrations in the optical system in order to decide how to best apply refractive surgery technology.

Results to Date

Recently, my colleagues and I have been conducting a study of wavefront-guided LASIK treatment with the VISX Wavescan.

The results to date of the first hyperopic treatment using WaveScan-guided LASIK utilizing the VISX Waveprint System showed the safety and accuracy

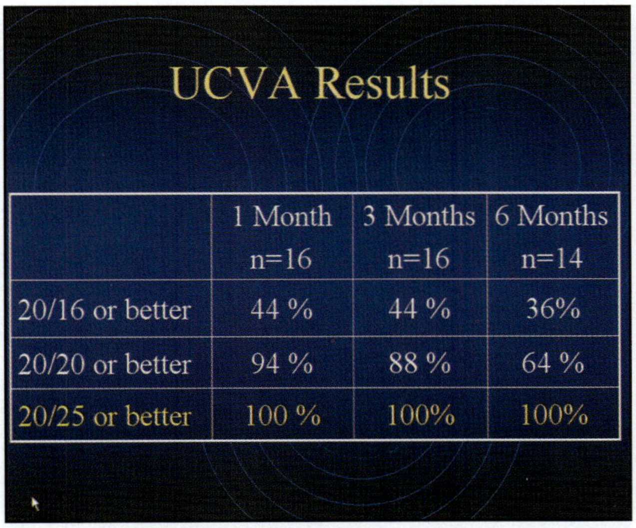

Figure 10-1. UCVA results from the VISX wavefront-driven hyperopia clinical trial with 100% of eyes achieving 20/25 or better vision at all follow-up intervals.

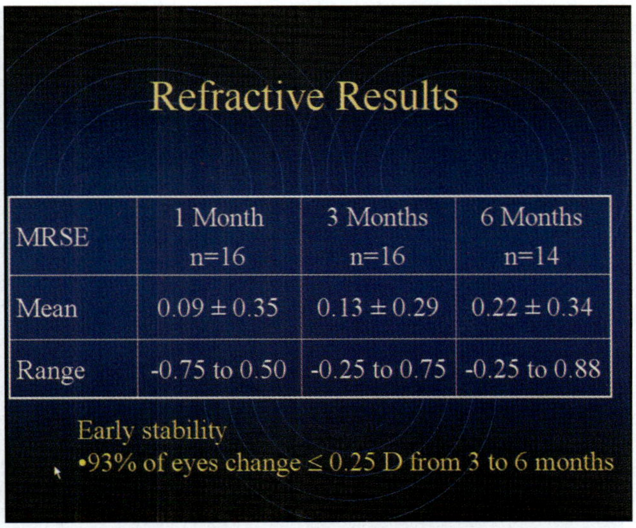

Figure 10-2. Manifest refraction spherical equivalent results over time.

of the treatment and also demonstrated excellent unaided visual acuity.

In addition, the patient group reported excellent satisfaction and the results for the new hyperopic ablation profile appeared stable at the early time-points out to 3 months. Enrollment and follow-up are continuing. While the data for the study is in the early stages and more research and follow-up are needed, the results thus far have been exciting.

The prospective, non-randomized study included 16 eyes of eight hyperopic patients (with astigmatism up to 3.00 D). Mean patient age was 50.9 (±6.5 years). The study included 3 men and 5 women. They all had bilateral LASIK treatment with a PreVue lens treatment verification using the VSS on the VISX Star S3 Active Track.

Before treating the patient with the WavePrint correction, a plastic PreVue lens was ablated to verify that the correction was an excellent option for the patient. The lens was placed in front of the patient, and if the vision could be improved to 20/20 +3 letters, the patient's cornea itself was then treated.

The Amadeus microkeratome was used in all cases. All eyes were targeted for emmetropia and there were no nomogram adjustments. Follow-up was at 1 day, 1 week and 1 month, 3 months, and 6 months.

The optical zone in the cases was blended to 9-mm total ablation area. The ablation target was created with the WaveScan Wavefront map, including up to sixth order aberrations. The variable spot scanning pulses fit to the Wavefront contour.

A treatment file was created with the WaveScan for the procedure. The file was then loaded into the VISX Star system on the floppy disk and Prevue verification was done.

For the 16 eyes of the 8 subjects the preoperative refractive error included sphere +1.66 ± 0.76 (-0.25 to +3.00 D). Cylinder was 0.64 ± 0.78 (0.0 to 2.50 D). The manifest refraction spherical equivalent (MRSE) was +1.98 ± 0.66 D (+0.63 to 3.00 D)

Preliminary Results

At 1 month for UCVA, 44% of the eyes were 20/16 or better, 94% were 20/20 or better, and 100% were 20/25 or better. At 3 months, 44% were 20/16 or better, 88% were 20/20 or better, and 100% were 20/25 or better. At 6 months, 30% were 20/16 or better, 64% were 20/20 or better; and 100% were 20/25 or better (Figure 10-1).

At 1 month, the mean SE was 0.09 ± 0.35. At 3 months, the mean SE was 0.13 ± 0.29, and at 6 months it was 0.22 ± 0.34. Early stability data showed that 93% of eyes changed 0.25 D or less from 3 to 6 months (Figure 10-2).

At 6 months postoperative, 93% were within ±0.50 D (Figure 10-3).

At 6 months for BSCVA, 79% of the eyes achieved 20/16 or better and 100% 20/20 or better. No eye lost greater than 2 lines of BSCVA (Figure 10-4). The maximum loss of BSCVA was 8 letters (2 eyes.)

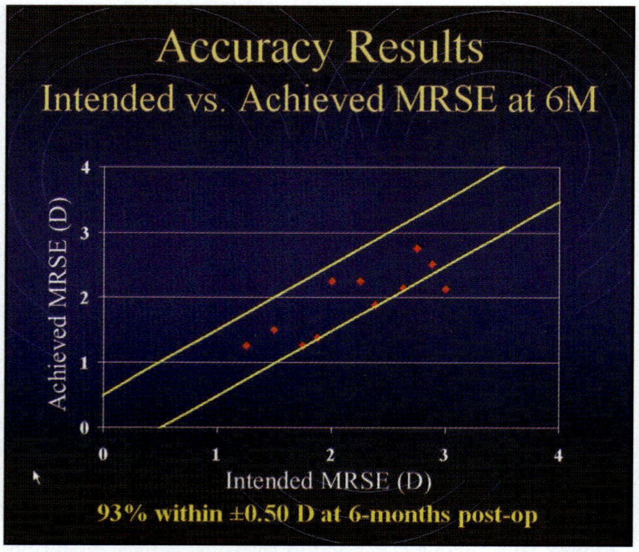

Figure 10-3. Scatterplot of manifest refraction spherical equivalent at 6 months follow-up.

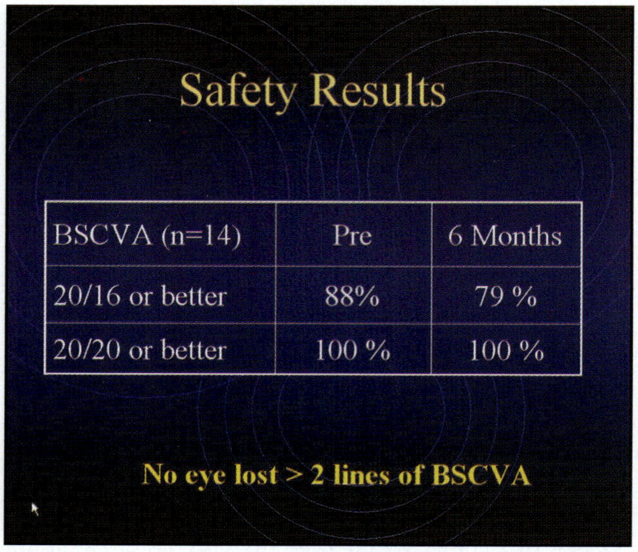

Figure 10-4. BCVA safety results.

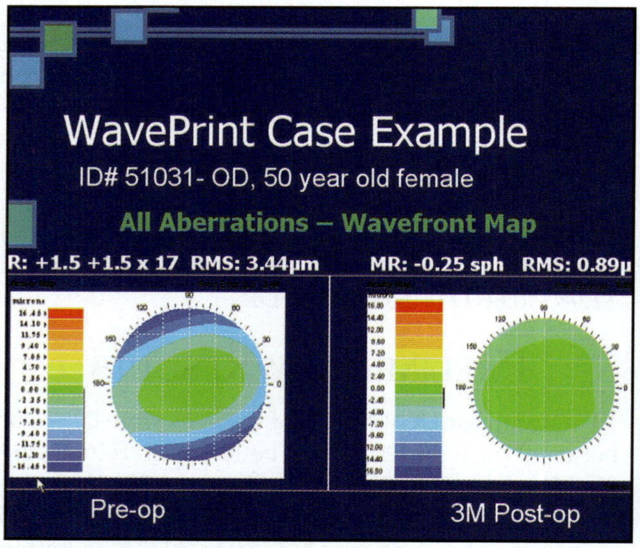

Figure 10-5. Case study from the VISX wavefront-driven hyperopia clinical trial: comparing pre- and postoperative aberration maps.

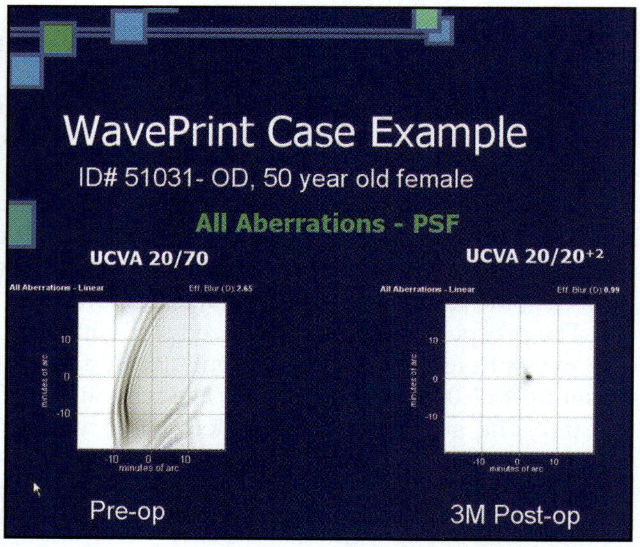

Figure 10-6. Case study from the VISX wavefront-driven hyperopia clinical trial: comparing pre- and postoperative pointspread function maps.

Case Study

A 50-year-old female underwent wavefront-guided LASIK (right eye). Her preoperative manifest refraction (MR) was +1.5 + 1.5 x 17. Postoperatively her MR was -0.25 sph with a very flat, ideal wavescan. There was also an accompanying drop in the RMS value (Figure 10-5).

An analysis of all the aberrations by point-spread function showed that her UCVA was 20/70 preoperatively, and it was 20/20 +2 postoperatively. There was a definite improvement in the point-spread function (Figure 10-6).

For higher order aberrations, there was a preoperative spherical aberration with a slight trefoil. There was marked improvement in the point-spread function for the higher order aberrations postoperatively (Figure 10-7). BSCVA also greatly improved. She was 20/20 preoperatively and 20/20+2 postoperatively (Figure 10-8).

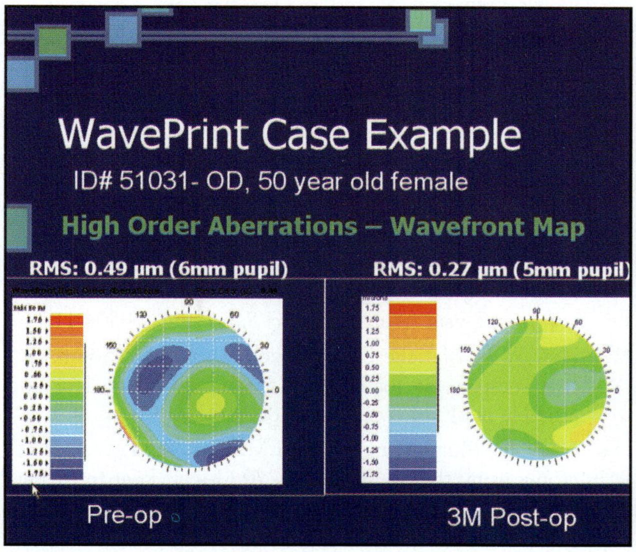

Figure 10-7. Case study from the VISX wavefront-driven hyperopia clinical trial: comparing pre- and postoperative higher order only aberration maps.

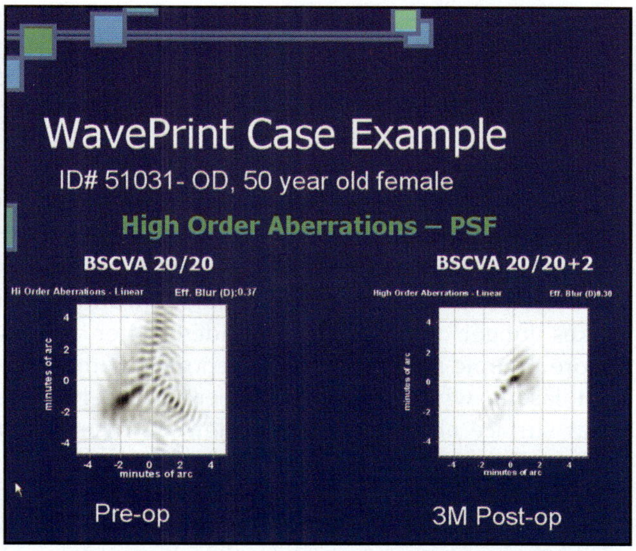

Figure 10-8. Case study from the VISX wavefront-driven hyperopia clinical trial: comparing pre- and postoperative higher order only pointspread function maps.

Comparison to Hyperopic PRK

We had performed regular hyperopic PRK on a group with a similar initial refraction as those patients who received hyperopic wavefront LASIK. The preliminary results of the hyperopic wavefront LASIK study show patients are fairing better with the Wavefront procedure compared to hyperopic PRK.

The PRK patients had an overcorrection and the UCVA was poor until approximately 6 months. However, this group was pleased because they were overcorrected and did not mind their myopia as they could read quite well during the first 3 to 6 months.

The PRK study population was made up of 26 eyes or 23 subjects. Mean patient age was 56.3 (±4 years). The study included 4 men and 19 women. For the patients, the preop sphere varied up to 3.00 D, the cylinder up to 1.50 D. The mean spherical equivalent was 2.12 ± 0.63 D.

At one month for UCVA, no patients were 20/16 or better (compared with 44% of the eyes were 20/16 or better in the Wavefront study). Only 9% were 20/20 or better, compared with 94% in the wavefront study.

For the hyperopic PRK patients, there was a -0.64 mean change in spherical equivalent from 1 week to 6 months. At 6 months 83% were ±0.50 D (compared to 93% in the wavefront group).

For BSCVA at 1 month, no eyes achieved 20/16 or better and 30% 20/20 or better, compared to 88% and 100% respectively in the Wavefront study. However, at 3 months 61% were 20/20, and 83% were 20/20 at 6 months. Two eyes lost 2 lines of BSCVA at 6 months. No eye lost greater than 2 lines of BSCVA.

Compared to the PRK, the wavefront-guided patients have a quick return and excellent vision within the first few days. LASIK shows less regression of effect than PRK. Wavefront-guided patients will be monitored for 6 to 12 months to check for regression. The nomogram will be adjusted if necessary to ensure they are plano at the 6-month mark.

Complications

In our small study of wavefront-based LASIK treatment to date, there were no serious complications. In addition, we have not observed any different complications compared to regular LASIK. Compared to PRK, the wavefront-based LASIK treatment patients had excellent vision on day one and maintained that vision.

At first, a small amount of regression of effect was observed; however, a revised nomogram from VISX corrected it.

In both PRK and LASIK (regular and wavefront) for hyperopia, it is essential that patients in the hyperopic group lubricate their eyes to avoid symptoms of dry eye and fluctuating vision.

Future

Wavefront-based LASIK treatment clearly will be the best way to treat hyperopic correction. However, surgeons will need to ensure that the keratomes provide a full 9.0-mm ablation bed.

The early results by Nagy et al[21] on wavefront hyperopic PRK, referred to earlier in this chapter, also are very promising. In the future, investigators will need to determine if surface ablation, although it takes longer to stabilize, provides better results. More myopic results are being reported with different lasers, which supports the early observations that surface ablation results in fewer higher order aberrations.

However, over time hyperopia could increase and this would lead to some loss of visual acuity. Therefore, what is gained in the short term with wavefront treatments might possibly be lost a little over time if the patient's hyperopia increases.

In addition, many hyperopes are presbyopic and as such they desire both distance and near vision. Monovision can work but the ideal would be to create a multifocal cornea allowing good distance vision and intermediate near vision without altering contrast acuity. Currently in our ongoing presbyopic study in hyperopes, called The Treatment of Presbyopia in Hyperopes Using the VISX Multifocal Ablation Pattern, most patients over 45 are opting to have both distance and near vision corrected. This study is underway and we await the results.

In general our future studies with hyperopic wavefront-based LASIK treatment will include more patients and have an expanded range of treatment. At present these treatments take longer and are limited to about 100 seconds.

VISX is in the process of increasing the Hz rate of the machine and that will allow for higher corrections.

References

1. Sher, NA. Hyperopic refractive surgery. *Curr Opin Ophthalmology*. 2001 Aug; 12(4):304-8.
2. Dausch D, Klein R, Schroder E. Excimer laser photorefractive keratectomy for hyperopia. *J Refract Corneal Surg*. 1993;9:20-28.
3. L'Esperance FA Jr., Warner JW, Telfair WB, et al. Excimer laser instrumentation and technique for human corneal surgery. *Arch Ophthalmology*. 1989;107:131-139.
4. Anschutz T. Laser correction of hyperopia and presbyopia. *Int Ophthalmol Clin*. 1994;34:107-37.
5. Dausch D, Smecka Z, Klein R, et al. Excimer laser photorefractive keratectomy for hyperopia. *J Cataract Refract Surg*. 1997;23:169-76.
6. Jackson WB, Mintsioulis G, Agapitos PJ, et al. Excimer laser photorefractive keratectomy for low hyperopia: safety and efficacy. *J Cataract Refract Surg*. 1997;23:480-7.
7. Sher NA, Bowers RA, Zabel RW, et al. The clinical use of the 193 nm excimer laser in the treatment of corneal scars. *Arch Ophthalmol*. 1991;109: 491-498.
8. Sher NA, ed. *Surgery For Hyperopia and Presbyopia*. 1st ed. Philadelphia, Pa: Williams and Wilkins; 1997;16.
9. Carones F, Brancato R, Morico A, et al. Photorefractive keratectomy for hyperopia using an erodible disc and axicon lens: 2-year results. *J Refract Surg*. 1998;14:504-11.
10. Haw WW, Manche EE. Prospective study of photorefractive keratectomy for hyperopia using an axicon lens and erodible mask. *J Refract Surg*. 2000;16:724-30.
11. Nagy ZZ, Munkacsy G, Popper M. Photorefractive keratectomy using the Meditec MEL 70 G-scan laser for hyperopia and hyperopic astigmatism. *J Refract Surg*. 2002;18:542-50.
12. Stevens JD, Ficker LA. Results of photorefractive keratectomy for hyperopia using the VISX star excimer laser system. *J Refract Surg*. 2002;18:30-6.
13. Dausch D, Landesz M. The Aesculap-Meditec excimer laser: results from Germany. In Salz JJ, ed. *Corneal Laser Surgery*. St. Louis: Mosby; 1995.
14. Jackson WB, Casson E, Hodge WG, et al. Laser vision correction for low hyperopia. An 18-month assessment of safety and efficacy. *Ophthalmology*. 1998;105:1727-38; discussion 37-8.
15. Nagy ZZ, Krueger RR, Hamberg-Nystrom H, et al. Photorefractive keratectomy for hyperopia in 800 eyes with the Meditec MEL 60 laser. *J Refract Surg*. 2001;17:525-33.
16. Bilgihan K, Akata F, Gurelik G, et al. Corneal iron ring after hyperopic photorefractive keratectomy. *J Cataract Refract Surg*. 1999;25:685-7.
17. Nagy ZZ, Krueger RR, Suveges I. Central bump-like opacity as a complication of high hyperopic photorefractive keratectomy. *Am J Ophthalmol*. 1999;128:636-8.
18. Sener B, Ozdamar A, Aras C. Apical nodular subepithelial corneal scar after retreatment in hyperopic photorefractive keratectomy. *J Cataract Refract Surg*. 2000;26:352-7.
19. Mietz H, Severin M, Seifert P, et al. Acute corneal necrosis after excimer laser keratectomy for hyperopia. *Ophthalmology*. 1999;106:490-6.
20. Golding TR, Bruce AS, Mainstone JC. Relationship between tear-meniscus parameters and tear-film breakup. *Cornea*. 1997;16:649-61.
21. Nagy ZZ, Palagyi-Deak I, Kovacs A, et al. First results with wavefront-guided photorefractive keratectomy for hyperopia. *J Refract Surg*. 2002 Sep-Oct;18(5):S620-3.
22. Panagopoulou SI, Pallikaris IG. Wavefront customized ablations with the WASCA Asclepion workstation. *J Refract Surg*. 2001;17:S608-12.
23. Salz JJ, Stevens CA. LASIK correction of spherical hyperopia, hyperopic astigmatism, and mixed astigmatism with the LADARVision excimer laser system. *Ophthalmology*. 2002;109:1647-56; discussion 57-8.

24. Lian J, Ye W, Zhou D, et al. Laser in situ keratomileusis for correction of hyperopia and hyperopic astigmatism with the Technolas 117C. *J Refract Surg*. 2002;18:435-8.
25. Ditzen K, Fiedler J, Pieger S. Laser in situ keratomileusis for hyperopia and hyperopic astigmatism using the Meditec MEL 70 spot scanner. *J Refract Surg*. 2002;18:430-4.
26. Pineda-Fernandez A, Rueda L, Huang D, et al. Laser in situ keratomileusis for hyperopia and hyperopic astigmatism with the Nidek EC-5000 Excimer laser. *J Refract Surg*. 2001;17:670-5.
27. el-Agha MS, Johnston EW, Bowman RW, et al. Excimer laser treatment of spherical hyperopia: PRK or LASIK? *Trans Am Ophthalmol Soc*. 2000;98:59-66; discussion -9.
28. Alessio G, Boscia F, La Tegola MG, et al. Topography-driven photorefractive keratectomy: results of corneal interactive programmed topographic ablation software. *Ophthalmology*. 2000;107:1578-87.
29. Yi DH, Petroll M, Bowman RW, et al. Surgically induced astigmatism after hyperopic and myopic photorefractive keratectomy. *J Cataract Refract Surg*. 2001;27:396-403.
30. Ditzen K, Huschka H, Pieger S. Laser in situ keratomileusis for hyperopia. *J Cataract Refract Surg*. 1998 Jan; 24(1):42-7.
31. Cobo-Soriano R, Llovet F, Gonzalez-Lopez F, et al. Factors that influence outcomes of hyperopic laser in situ keratomileusis. *J Cataract Refract Surg*. 2002 Sep;28(9):1530-8.
32. Duffey, R. LASIK outcomes better for hyperopia, hyperopic astigmatism. *Ophthalmology Times*. Feb. 1, 2002.
33. Kraff, C. Results of six-month wavefront-guided ablation studies for the correction of myopia using the VISX WaveScan system and STAR S3 ActiveTrak Excimer Laser system. *J Cataract Refract Surg*; submitted.
34. Hardten, DH. Using the WaveScan aberrometer, the PreVue lens and variable spot scanning. *Ophthalmology Times*. 2001, August 15.
35. O'Brien T, Kraff C. PreVue the future: Subjective verification is a powerful tool for difficult cases. *VISXInk newsletter*. Spring, 2003.
36. Harner, C. *New VISX technology*. Presented at annual meeting of American Society of Refractive and Cataract Surgeons; 2001.
37. Marcos M. Refractive surgery and optical aberrations. *Optics and Photonics News*. 2001;12(1):22-25.

Chapter Eleven

Excimer Laser Treatment of Hyperopic Astigmatism

Danish Khan, MB, BS; Amy Scally, OD; and Dimitri T. Azar, MD

Introduction

Early surgical attempts at hyperopic correction included hexagonal keratotomy (HK), automated lamellar keratoplasty (ALK), epikeratophakia, and keratophakia.[1-5] These procedures have had limited success. They were either very difficult to perform or were unstable and unpredictable and caused irregular astigmatism.[1-7]

With the introduction of the excimer laser it became possible to carve a positive lenticule out of the cornea to correct hyperopia and hyperopic astigmatism. Current conventional excimer laser ablations are based on a subtraction-shaped model, in which the profiles of the ablation are etched on the stromal surface in photorefractive keratectomy (PRK) or in laser-assisted in-situ keratomileusis (LASIK).[8-10] Most studies show that LASIK surgery used to treat myopia and compound myopic astigmatism has greater predictability than that for hyperopia and hyperopic astigmatism.[8-11]

This chapter focuses on the theoretical models of excimer laser correction of hyperopic astigmatism and the surgical results of various treatment algorithms for the correction of hyperopic astigmatism. The theoretical models are based on paraxial and arc-based assumptions.[8,9] These models assume the initial corneal surface to be spherical (pure spherical treatments) or toroidal (pure cylindrical or spherocylindrical treatments) and the final surface to be spherical over the chosen optical zone.[8-10] Furthermore, the laser systems perform as though they had to etch, from the flat surface having the same refractive index for the cornea, a lenticule whose power would correspond to the spherocylindrical error to correct.

Several studies have reported the surgical results of various excimer laser treatment approaches. PRK has been used successfully for hyperopic errors (including hyperopic astigmatism), but is complicated by regression, induced astigmatism, and corneal haze, thereby limiting its usefulness for the correction of mild hyperopic errors. Because LASIK overcomes many disadvantages of surface ablation (PRK), it has become the procedure of choice for the treatment of low to moderate hyperopic errors.[12]

Methods of Correction

Excimer laser treatment of hyperopic astigmatism involves steepening of the central cornea along the flatter meridian. Earlier laser systems accomplished this by applying a mask (Aesculap-Meditec, Germany) (Figure 11-1) or an erodable mask (Summit Apex Plus Laser, Alcon, Fort Worth, Tex) over the cornea. The Summit system also incorporates the Axicon lens to deliver additional energy between 6.5 and 9.5 mm. The Summit erodable mask

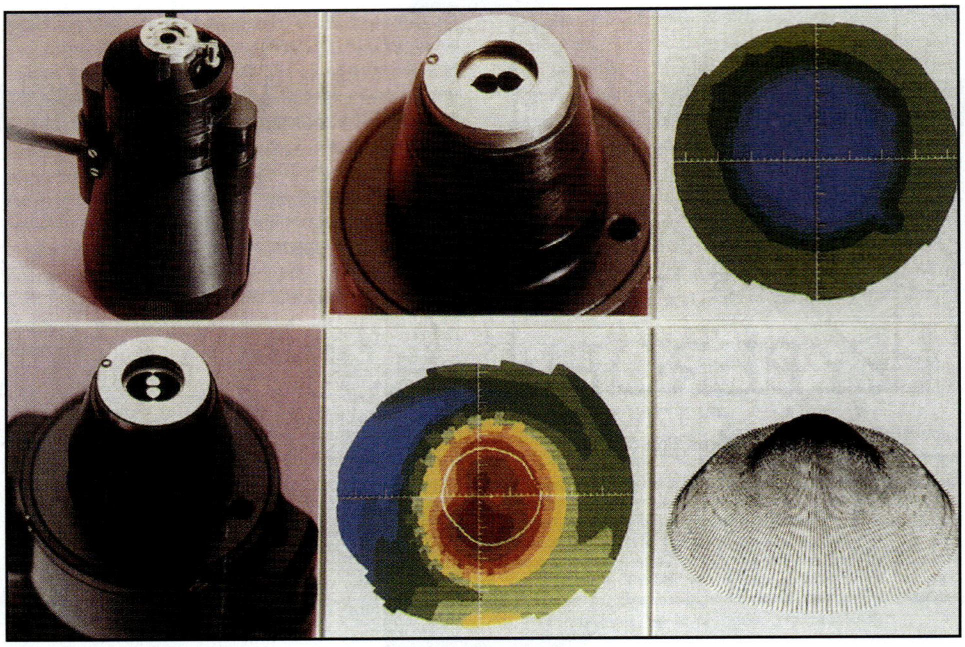

Figure 11-1. (Top left) Iris mask handpiece (Aesculap-Meditec laser) for correction of myopia and therapeutic applications. (Top center) Rotating mask for myopic corrections. (Top right) Corneal topography after correction of myopia. (Bottom left) Rotating mask for hyperopia and hyperopic astigmatism. (Bottom center), corneal topography after a hyperopic correction. (Bottom right) Computer-aided design of a hyperopic correction. (Reprinted with permission from Hardten DR. 193-nm excimer laser treatment of hyperopia. In: Azar DT, ed. *Refractive Surgery*. Stamford, CT: Appleton & Lange; 1997:481-489.)

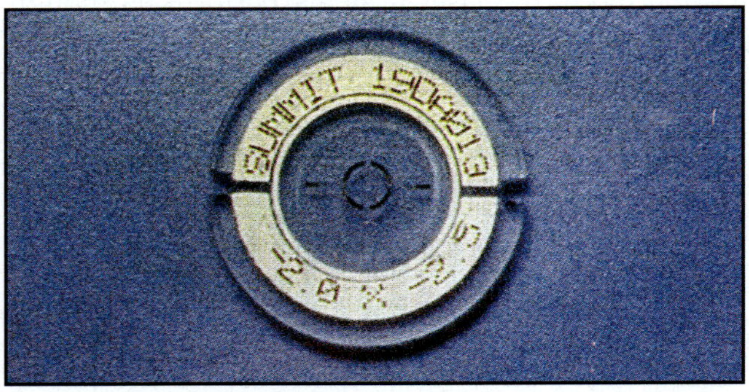

Figure 11-2. Mask system of Summit. Summit astigmatic laser disc. (Reprinted with permission from Slade SG, Doane JF. Treatment of astigmatism. In: Buratto L, Brint SF, eds. *LASIK Principles and Techniques*. Thorofare, NJ: SLACK Incorporated; 1998:250.)

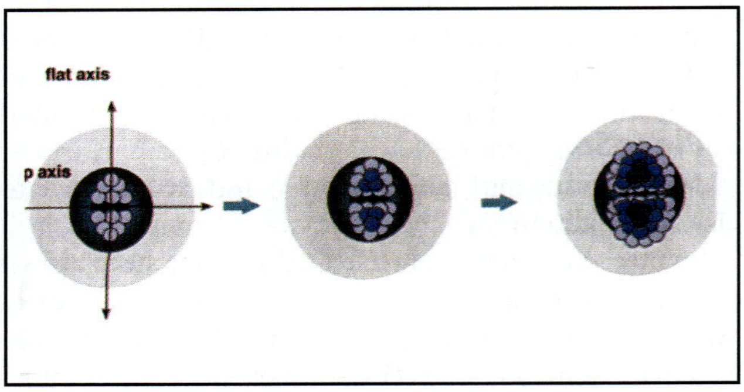

Figure 11-3. Scarring system of Bausch & Lomb. Excimer laser correction for hyperopic astigmatism. The laser beam moves over the cornea and steepens the flat axis. (Reprinted with permission from Slade SG, Doane JF. Treatment of astigmatism. In: Buratto L, Brint SF, eds. *LASIK Principles and Techniques*. Thorofare, NJ: SLACK Incorporated; 1998:251.)

is made of a material with a known ablation rate, and shaped to deliver a graded ablation of the cornea, with the flatter area of the corneal surface receiving more treatment to increase its curvature (Figure 11-2).

The mask systems have been virtually replaced by scanning laser systems. Scanning lasers rapidly pattern the cornea and use a high rate of ablation pulses. A main advantage of scanning lasers with regard to hyperopic astigmatism is that these lasers are capable of steepening as well as flattening the desired corneal meridians.

The Bausch & Lomb (Rochester, NY) Technolas Planoscan excimer laser delivers laser pulses (2 mm) at a relatively high frequency (25 Hz) in a circular pattern over the cornea and an optical zone of 6 to 9 mm (Figure 11-3).[13]

The VISX Star (Santa Clara, Calif) S2-S4 laser utilizes 7 scanning beams over the cornea to treat hyperopia and astigmatism. These beams are offset to effect an ablation out to 9.0 mm. Doane et al[14] presented data on 100 eyes with hyperopia from 0.5 to 6.00 D (mean, +2.08) and a cylinder from 0.50 to 4.00 D (mean, 0.74 D) treated with the VISX S2 laser. They utilized the Hansatome and microkeratome and an external fixation device to reduce decentration. The results were satisfactory with an effective reduction of the hyperopic sphere and cylinder. The vast majority of eyes maintained, or gained one line of best-corrected visual acuity (BCVA). In another study by Manche[15] using the same laser, good results were obtained with a mean pre- and post-cycloplegic spherical equivalent of +3.23 and -0.21, respectively. There was a 70% reduction in mean astigmatism as measured by vector analysis and no loss of BCVA. Newer versions of the VISX laser (S3 and S4) utilize similar systems, with the added advantage of a tracking system.

The LADARVision (Alcon, Fort Worth, Tex) is a scanning laser with a smaller spot laser beam of 0.8 mm. This small beam allows for a more precise and gradual reshaping of the cornea. In addition, a tracking system is incorporated in the laser. The Nidek, Meditec, and MEL lasers have also incorporated a scanning approach. Most of these lasers incorporate the hyperopic astigmatic correction with spherical hyperopic correction, but the option of combining myopic astigmatism with hyperopic spherical correction remains available.

Azar and Primack[9] reported comparisons of the theoretical ablation profiles and depth of tissue removal. They showed that treatment strategies that combine myopic cylindrical and hyperopic spherical corrections for hyperopic astigmatism or mixed astigmatism incur the greatest amount of corneal tissue ablation.

Until recently the treatment compound hyperopic astigmatism consisted of the combined use of hyperopic spherical and myopic cylindrical corrections. In contrast to the principle of equivalency, when combining cylindrical and spherical spectacle corrections, the amount of tissue removed during LASIK for hyperopic astigmatism may vary according to the treatment approach.

Four approaches can be used (either sequentially or concomitantly) for the treatment of compound hyperopic astigmatism:

1. Combined hyperopic spherical and myopic cylindrical treatments.
2. Combined spherical (plus or minus) and hyperopic cylindrical treatment.
3. Combined cylindrical treatments.
4. Combined cross cylinder and spherical equivalent (SE) treatment.

These 4 strategies may result in different depths of corneal tissue ablation for the same diameters of the optical zones. Deeper ablations may increase the risk of ectasia after LASIK; therefore, strategies that remove less corneal tissue are preferable in the treatment of hyperopic astigmatism. To understand why this is so, a basic understanding of the depth and the profiles of ablated lenticules for myopic cylinder and hyperopic cylinder must be gained.[8-10]

Myopic Cylinder Ablation

Figure 11-4 shows the ablation lenticules of myopic cylinder is of convex shape, along the initial steeper meridian and the tissue ablation deepest in the center. However, the flattening of this initial "steeper" meridian cannot be performed selectively. (It implies that there must be also a plano ablation of the "flat" principal meridian.) For example, a cylindrical treatment of plano -1.00 x 180 is equivalent in terms of optical results and the amount of ablated tissue to the sequential of plano +1.00 x 90 and -1.00 sphere.

Thus the lenticules ablated for the cylindrical myopic treatment can be considered as two successive treatments—first, a positive cylindrical treatment on the initial "flatter" meridian (to steepen its curvature until it equals that of the opposite principal meridian). Then myopic spherical treatment of similar magnitude aims to flatten both meridians to the desired radius of curvature.

This approach with two successive ablations preserves the curvature of the cornea. Thus a myopic cylindrical treatment removes more corneal tissue than a myopic spherical correction with the greatest amount of ablation in the flatter meridian.

Hyperopic Cylinder Ablation

Figure 11-5 shows the shape of the ablated lenticule for pure cylindrical hyperopia. This involves the ablation of a lenticule of concave shape along the initial "flatter" meridian and of null thickness along the orthogonal steeper meridian. The maximal thickness of the hyperopic cylindrical lenticule occurs at the outer edge of the optical zone. Argento et al reported a series in which steepening the flattest meridian was attempted by utilizing a variety of techniques using the keracor 116/117 laser.[16] This technique produced steepening in the flattest meridian with almost no effect on the opposite meridian.

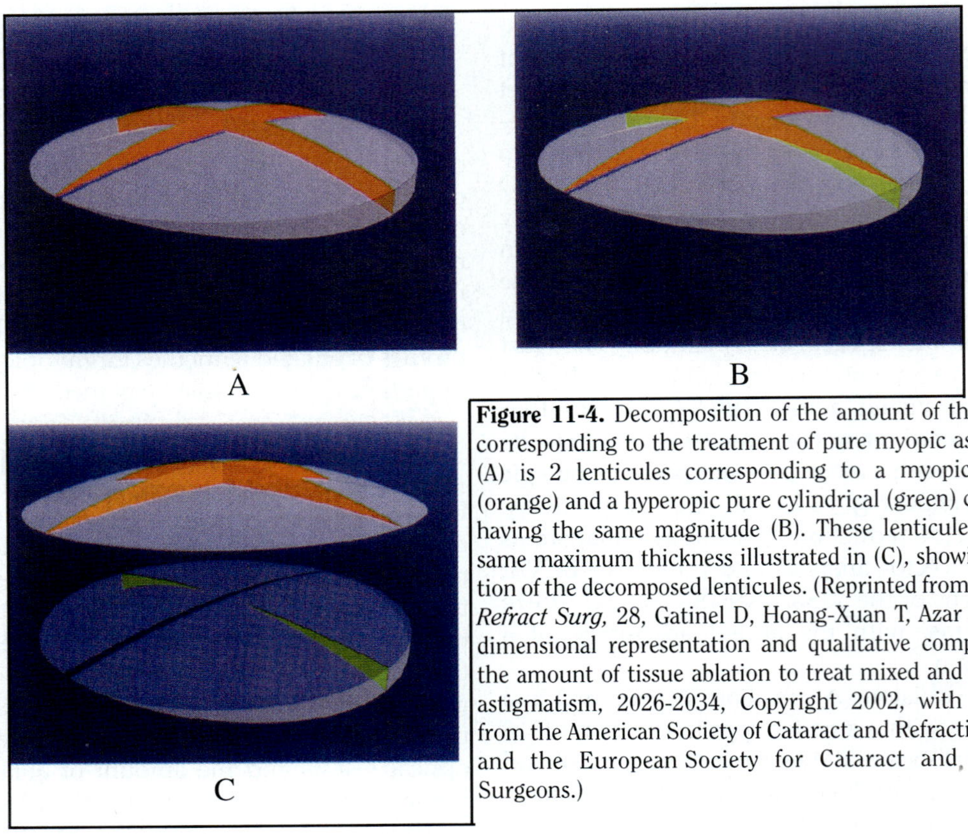

Figure 11-4. Decomposition of the amount of the lenticule corresponding to the treatment of pure myopic astigmatism (A) is 2 lenticules corresponding to a myopic spherical (orange) and a hyperopic pure cylindrical (green) component having the same magnitude (B). These lenticules have the same maximum thickness illustrated in (C), showing separation of the decomposed lenticules. (Reprinted from *J Cataract Refract Surg,* 28, Gatinel D, Hoang-Xuan T, Azar DT, Three-dimensional representation and qualitative comparisons of the amount of tissue ablation to treat mixed and compound astigmatism, 2026-2034, Copyright 2002, with permision from the American Society of Cataract and Refractive Surgery and the European Society for Cataract and Refractive Surgeons.)

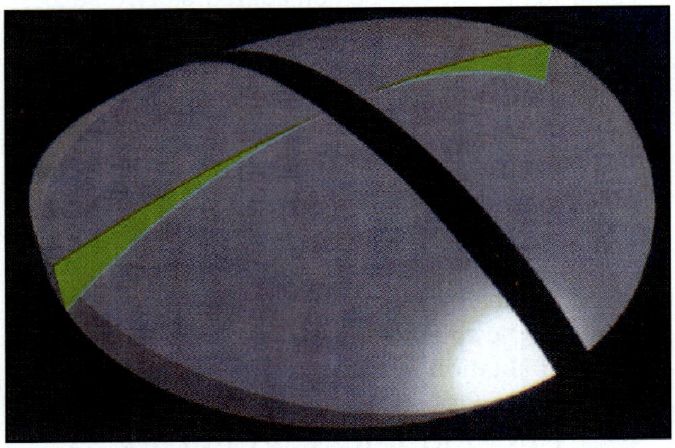

Figure 11-5. Schematic representation of the lenticule ablated for correction of pure cylindrical hyperopia. The cross-section corresponding to the direction of the principal meridians is outlined in green. The lenticule thickness is zero along the direction of the initial steeper meridian. (Reprinted from *J Cataract Refract Surg,* 28, Gatinel D, Hoang-Xuan T, Azar DT, Three-dimensional representation and qualitative comparisons of the amount of tissue ablation to treat mixed and compound astigmatism, 2026-2034, Copyright 2002, with permision from the American Society of Cataract and Refractive Surgery and the European Society for Cataract and Refractive Surgeons.)

The hyperopic cylindrical treatment removes less tissue than the hyperopic spherical correction. Neither hyperopic ablation pattern affects the central cornea.

The deductions that can be derived from the two diagrams are:

1. Hyperopic cylindrical correction ablates less tissue than a myopic cylindrical treatment.
2. The hyperopic cylindrical correction preserves central corneal thickness.

The four different approaches of the ablation depths and profiles in compound hyperopic astigmatism can be best explained by an example.

A hypothetical situation of with-the-rule (WTR) astigmatism is cited in which the combined cylindrical notation was +5.00 x 90 and +2.00 x 180 (equivalent to +2.00 + 3.00 x 90 or +5.00 – 3.00 x 180). In this example the depth of ablation per diopter, h, is approximated by Munnerlyn's equation: S2/3, where S=diameter of optical zone.

Combination of hyperopic spherical and myopic cylindrical excimer laser ablation.

As shown in Figure 11-6, the hyperopic sphere of +5.00 and a myopic cylinder of -3.00 X 180 have been done. The hyperopic spherical correction has steepened all meridians (green profile in diagram). The myopic cylindrical correction then creates a new horizontal meridian (blue ablation profile). To preserve corneal curvature, for myopic cylindrical treatment a lenticule of constant thickness along the

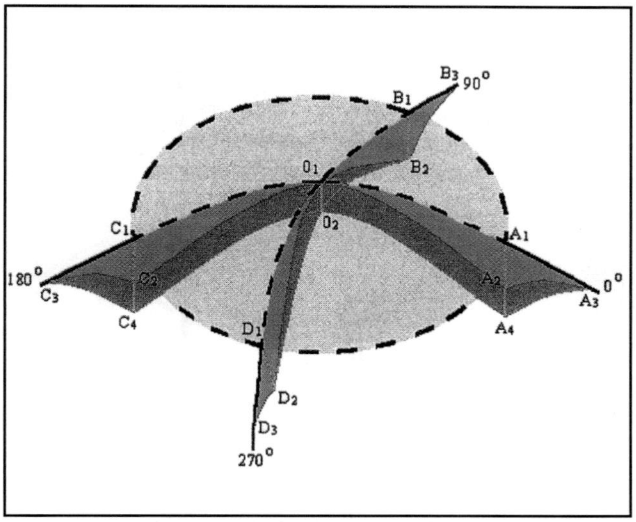

Figure 11-6. Hyperopic WTR astigmatism corrected with a +5.00 D hyperopic spherical (green) and a -3.00 D myopic cylindrical (blue) laser ablation pattern applied to the LASIK bed (resulting in greatest central ablation and volume of tissue removed). (Reprinted from *J Cataract Refract Surg,* 26, Azar DT, Primack JD, Theoretical analysis of ablation depths and profiles in laser in situ keratomileusis for compound hyperopic and mixed astigmatism, 1123-1136, Copyright 2000, with permision from the American Society of Cataract and Refractive Surgery and the European Society for Cataract and Refractive Surgeons.)

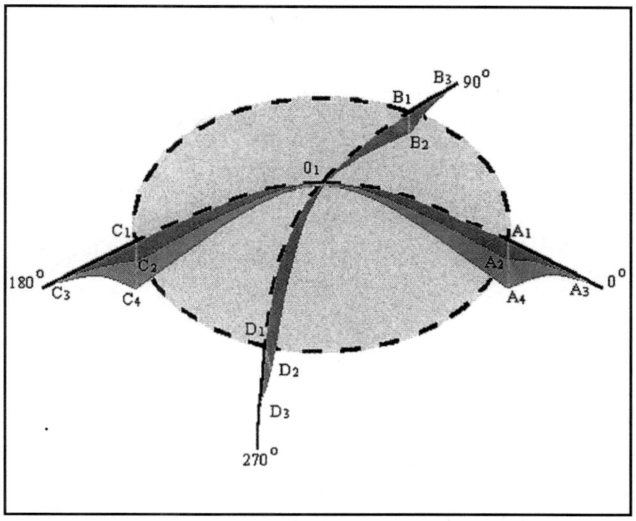

Figure 11-7. Hyperopic WTR astigmatism corrected with a +2.00 D hyperopic spherical (dark green) and +3.00 D hyperopic cylindrical (green) laser ablation pattern applied to the LASIK bed). Note absent ablation in central cornea. (Reprinted from *J Cataract Refract Surg,* 26, Azar DT, Primack JD, Theoretical analysis of ablation depths and profiles in laser in situ keratomileusis for compound hyperopic and mixed astigmatism, 1123-1136, Copyright 2000, with permision from the American Society of Cataract and Refractive Surgery and the European Society for Cataract and Refractive Surgeons.)

initial "flatter" meridian is created (blue profile in vertical meridian, Figure 11-6).

The hyperopic spherical correction resulted in an ablation depth of 5 h. As mentioned above h is approximately S2/3. The myopic cylindrical correction resulted in a tissue ablation of 3 h. The extent of central corneal ablation was proportional to the degree of myopic cylinder being treated. Thus the ablation depth was 3 h centrally, 5 h at each vertical meridian, and 8h at the horizontal meridian.

Combination of Hyperopic Spherical and Hyperopic Cylindrical Excimer Laser Ablation

Figure 11-7 shows the ablation profiles and depths of the hyperopic sphere of +2.00 D and a hyperopic cylinder of +3.00 x 90 applied to the LASIK bed. This has the same optical outcome as Figure 11-6. The hyperopic spherical correction steepens both meridians (green ablated area in vertical and horizontal meridians).

The hyperopic cylindrical correction creates a new ablation lenticule (dark green area Figure 11-7). This meridian is now steeper than the post-hyperopic spherical ablation meridian. The vertical meridian remains untouched by the hyperopic cylindrical ablation and maintains its post-hyperopic spherical ablation profile (light green ablation profile Figure 11-7).

Thus more tissue ablation has occurred peripherally, tapering toward the center of the optical zone, which maintains its preoperative central corneal thickness. In comparison to Figure 11-6, the approach of hyperopic spherical and cylindrical correction results in no ablation of the central cornea and less ablation of the peripheral cornea.

An ablation depth of 2 h at the vertical meridian, 5 h at the horizontal meridian, and no ablation in the center of the cornea occurs in Figure 11-7.

Combination of Two Hyperopic Cylindrical Excimer Laser Ablations.

Figure 11-8 shows 2 hyperopic cylindrical corrections of +5.00 x 90 and +2.00 x 180 (the equivalent of 2 spherocylindrical equations mentioned previously). The formula +2.00 x 1810 creates a new horizontal meridian (green area on Figure 11-8). This area is steeper than the preoperative horizontal meridian.

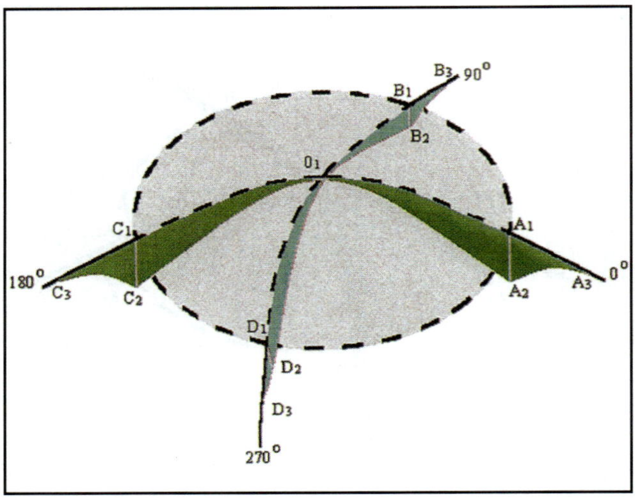

Figure 11-8. Hyperopic WTR astigmatism corrected with a +2.00 x 180 (green) and +5.00 x 90 (dark green) combined hyperopic cylindrical laser ablation pattern applied to the LASIK bed). Note absent ablation in central cornea. (Reprinted from *J Cataract Refract Surg,* 26, Azar DT, Primack JD, Theoretical analysis of ablation depths and profiles in laser in situ keratomileusis for compound hyperopic and mixed astigmatism, 1123-1136, Copyright 2000, with permision from the American Society of Cataract and Refractive Surgery and the European Society for Cataract and Refractive Surgeons.)

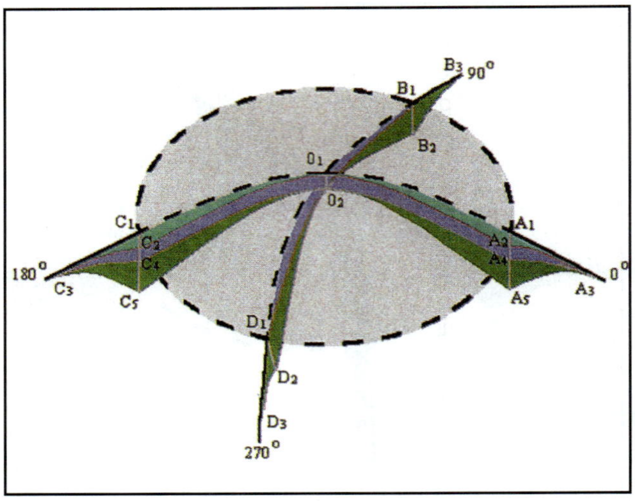

Figure 11-9. Hyperopic WTR astigmatism corrected with a combined cross-cylinder (+1.50 x 90 [green] and -1.50 x 180 [blue]) and +3.50 D SE (dark green) laser ablation pattern applied to the LASIK bed). Note absent ablation in central cornea. (Reprinted from *J Cataract Refract Surg,* 26, Azar DT, Primack JD, Theoretical analysis of ablation depths and profiles in laser in situ keratomileusis for compound hyperopic and mixed astigmatism, 1123-1136, Copyright 2000, with permision from the American Society of Cataract and Refractive Surgery and the European Society for Cataract and Refractive Surgeons.)

The vertical meridian is untouched by the first hyperopic cylindrical ablation and maintains its preoperative curvature. The second hyperopic cylindrical correction of +5.00 x 90 creates a new vertical meridian (dark green area on Figure 11-8). This new vertical meridian is steeper than the preoperative horizontal meridian but less deep than the postoperative horizontal meridian. The horizontal axis is untouched by the second hyperopic cylindrical ablation.

There is preservation of the central corneal tissue, and the maximal amount of ablation occurs in the periphery. The final corneal contour results in an ablation depth of 2 h vertically and 5 h at the horizontal meridian. Thus there is a similar amount of theoretical tissue ablation, as in Figure 11-7.

Combination of Cross Cylinder and SE Excimer Laser Ablation

Figure 11-9 shows the ablation profiles and depths of a cross-cylinder correction of +1.50 x 90 and –1.50 x 180 followed by a SE ablation of +3.50 D.

The hyperopic cylindrical correction of +1.50X90 removes a lenticule and creates a new horizontal meridian (dark green area on Figure 11-9). This meridian is steeper than the preoperative horizontal meridian.

The myopic cylindrical correction of –1.50 x 180 removes lenticules in both the horizontal and vertical meridians (blue area on Figure 11-9). This vertical meridian is flatter than the preoperative meridian.

The cross-cylinder ablation has flattened the steep meridian and steepened the flat meridian. This is followed by a hyperopic spherical ablation of +3.50 D which steepens both meridians (light green area Figure 11-9).

Thus the final corneal contour results when there is an ablation depth of 1.5 h centrally, 3.5 h at each vertical meridian, and 6.5 h at each horizontal meridian.

It can be seen from the preceding discussion and Figure 11-3 that the maximal amount of tissue ablation occurs in Figure 11-6, followed by Figure 11-9, and the minimal in Figures 11-7 and 11-8.

Thus the combined use of hyperopic spherical and myopic cylindrical correction for the treatment of hyperopic astigmatism incurs the greatest amount of central and peripheral corneal tissue ablation and therefore may be the sub-optimal treatment alternative.

Using this approach Ibrahim[17] had to increase the degree of spherical ablation by 50 percent of the cylindrical correction, because of the hyperopic shift that occurs with myopic cylindrical correction. (This varies with different laser software.) Thus the previous estimate of excessive tissue ablation is actually an underestimation of the real in-vivo tissue loss.

In contrast to the hyperopic spherical and myopic cylindrical approach, reports of studies in which hyperopic cylindrical ablation was done to correct hyperopic compound astigmatism, no shift in the spherical component of the correction was observed. However, regression has been shown to increase with the magnitude of the positive cylinder error. The mechanism of regression may be epithelial thickening. This was demonstrated by Reinstein et al, using high-frequency ultrasound.[18] This thickening begins at a point precisely coincident with the beginning of the doughnut-shaped zone of stromal tissue removal. It reverses the contouring effect of the laser ablation. This might be triggered by the abrupt transition along the initial flatter meridian created by the pure hyperopic correction.

An additional advantage of the above approach is that the myopic component of the refractive error is expressed as a sphere, which in these ametropes will be of a lower value than the amount of myopic error expressed as a cylinder in an equivalent spherocylindrical equation. This is important because it results in less myopic laser correction, which is what determines the amount of central corneal ablation.

As noted above, the use of cross cylinder (Figure 11-9) does not warrant the minimal amount of tissue removal but might increase the refractive outcome by reducing the overcorrection on non-principal meridians and favors the induction of prolate asphericity.[19]

Encouraging results have been reported by Vinciguerra et al,[20] who treated compound astigmatism in LASIK procedures using cross-cylindrical ablation.

Molina and coauthors[21] performed LASIK in 123 eyes using a Nidek (Japan) EC-5000 laser, treating 52 eyes with a myopic cylindrical and hyperopic spherical ablation and 71 eyes with combined cylinder ablation. The tissue study concluded that a marked reduction of stromal tissue ablation occurred with the combined cylinder program.

Although the final optical result may be the same, different strategies vary in depth, profile, and amount of tissue ablation. Thus it is important to avoid the negative cylinder treatment for the sequential correction of compound hyperopic astigmatism. It minimizes the amount of corneal tissue ablation for hyperopic astigmatism, subsequently prevents complications like ectasia, and preserves the corneal biochemical stability and the possibility of retreatment, and results in optimization of the corneal shape.

Reports by Ditzen et al,[22] Göker et al,[23] and Argento et al[24] showed encouraging results with various excimer lasers. Predictability after hyperopic LASIK was only moderate; it lagged behind myopic LASIK in predictability. One problem in assessing results in hyperopic surgery is the measurement of uncorrected visual acuity. Unlike myopia, this parameter is very age dependent.

Complications

With the earlier studies the complication rates were relatively high, indicating a learning curve for the new LASIK procedure and keratomes that were not as reliable as the ones now available. Some complications seemed higher in hyperopic LASIK. This included higher rates of decentration than in myopia and resulted in loss of BCVA. However, with the introduction of laser tracking of ocular movements, decentration may be avoidable.

Probst et al[25] and Özdamar et al[26] reported an epithelial pigmentation ring pattern, that they called a pseudo-Fleischer ring, after hyperopic LASIK. A case of acute angle-closure glaucoma after H-LASIK has been reported.[27] Otherwise the complications in H-LASIK were similar to those in myopia.

Future of Hyperopic Astigmatism Treatment With Topography-Assisted Laser

The future of laser hyperopic astigmatism correction is almost completely dependent on the increased sophistication of the laser design and ways to measure the cornea. These two components must be coordinated so that the laser is directed in its ablation to whatever is presented to it by the topographer. A combination of real-time feedback loop between the laser and the measuring device, so that the progress of ablation is measured and the laser is directed accordingly, would be the most desirable combination.

References

1. Hoffmann F, Schüler A. Indications, results, and complications of refractive corneal surgery with mechanical methods. *Curr Opin Ophthalmol.* 1995;6(IV):67-72.
2. Bores LD. Refractive surgery. *J Fla Med Assoc.* 1994;81(4):272-277.

3. Sher NA. Hyperopic refractive surgery. *Curr Opin Ophthalmol*. 2001;12(4):304-308.
4. Lyle WA, Jin GJC. Hyperopic automated lamellar keratoplasty: complications and visual results. *Arch Ophthalmol*. 1998;116:425-428.
5. Friedlander MH, Rich LF, Werblin TP, Kaufman HE, Granet N. Keratophakia using preserved lenticules. *Ophthalmology*. 1980;87:687-692.
6. Troutman RC, Swinger C. Refractive keratoplasty: keratophakia and keratomileusis. *Trans Am Ophthalmol Soc*. 1978;76:329-339.
7. Sher NA, ed. *Surgery of Hyperopia and Presbyopia*. Baltimore, MD: Williams & Wilkins; 1997.
8. Munnerlyn CR, Koons SJ, Marshall J. Photorefractive keratectomy: a technique for laser refractive surgery. *J Cataract Refract Surg*. 1988;14:46-52.
9. Azar DT, Primack JD. Theoretical analysis of ablation depths and profiles in laser in situ keratomileusis for compound hyperopic and mixed astigmatism. *J Cataract Refract Surg*. 2000;26:1123-1136.
10. Gatinel D, Hoang-Xuan T, Azar DT. Three-dimensional representation and qualitative comparisons of the amount of tissue ablation to treat mixed and compound astigmatism. *J Cataract Refract Surg*. 2002;28:2026-2034.
11. Gimbel H, Basti S, Kaye GB, Ferensowicz M. Experience during the learning curve of laser in situ keratomileusis. *J Cataract Refract Surg*. 1996;22:542-550.
12. Gulani A. *Hyperopic LASIK*. Emedicine.com. Jan 2003. Available at http://www.emedicine.com. Accessed January 27, 2003.
13. Arbelaez MC. Hyperopic LASIK with the Chiron Technolas excimer laser. In: Machat JJ, Slade SG, Probst LE, eds. *The Art of LASIK*. 2nd ed. Thorofare, NJ: SLACK Incorporated; 1999:311-315.
14. Doane JF, Morris SB, Border AD, Denning J. Presented at American Society of Cataract and Refractive Surgery, April 1999.
15. Manche EE. *Hyperopic LASIK for simple hyperopia and compound hyperopic using the VISX Star S2 Smoothscan*. Presented at American Society of Cataract and Refractive Surgery, April 1999.
16. Argento CJ, Cosentino MJ, Biondini A. Treatment of hyperopic astigmatism. *J Cataract Refract Surg*. 1997;23:1480-1490.
17. Ibrahim O. Laser in situ keratomileusis for hyperopia and hyperopic astigmatism. *J Cataract Refract Surg*. 1998;14(suppl):S179-S182.
18. Reinstein DZ, Silverman RH, Sutton HFS, Coleman DJ. Very high frequency ultrasound corneal analysis identifies anatomic correlates of optical complications of lamellar refractive surgery: anatomic diagnosis in lamellar surgery. *Ophthalmology*. 1999;106:474-482.
19. Vinciguerra P, Camesasca FI. Cross cylinder ablation. In: MacRae SM, Krueger RR, Applegate RA, eds. *Customized Corneal Ablation: The Quest for Super Vision*. Thorofare, NJ: SLACK Incorporated; 2001:319-327.
20. Vinciguerra P, Epstein D, Azzolini M, Radice P, Sborgia M. Algorithm to correct hyperopic astigmatism with the Nidek EC-5000 excimer laser. *J Refract Surg*. 1999;15(suppl):S186-S187.
21. Molina R, Monasterio R, Soliz E, Foianini J. Correction of astigmatism using positive and negative cylinder programs with the Nidek EC-5000 excimer laser. *J Refract Surg*. 1999;15(suppl):S159-S196.
22. Ditzen K, Nadimi H. *Mid-Summer Symposium and Scientific Exhibition. International Society of Refractive Surgery*. Minneapolis, Minn: July 1996.
23. Göker S, Er H, Kahvecioglu C. Laser in situ keratomileusis to correct hyperopia from +4.25 to +8.00 diopters. *J Refract Surg*. 1998;14:26-30.
24. Argento CJ, Cosentino MJ. Laser in situ keratomileusis for hyperopia. *J Cataract Refract Surg*. 1998;24:1050-1058.
25. Probst LE, Almasswary MA, Bell J. Pseudo-Fleischer ring after hyperopic laser in situ keratomileusis. *J Cataract Refract Surg*. 1999;25:868-870.
26. Özdamar A, Aras C, Sener B, Karaçorlu M. Corneal iron ring after hyperopic laser-assisted in situ keratomileusis. *Cornea*. 1999;18:243-245.
27. Paciuc M, Velasco CF, Naranjo R. Acute angle-closure glaucoma after hyperopic laser in situ keratomileusis. *J Cataract Refract Surg*. 2000;26:620-623.

Chapter Twelve

Optimizing the Hyperopic Ablation Profile

Paolo Vinciguerra, MD and Fabrizio I. Camesasca, MD

Why Treating Hyperopia Can Be So Frustrating

More or less consciously, the novice refractive surgeon may consider the treatment of hyperopia as a situation opposite to but similar, almost specular, to myopia. Disappointingly, laser refractive surgery for hyperopia has often led to more unsatisfactory results and complications than for myopia.[1-4]

Apparently, hyperopia treatment just increases the physiological characteristics of the cornea, with a center more curved than the periphery. Moreover, ablation is applied peripherally, where the cornea is thicker. However, if we carefully examine a corneal surface after hyperopic ablation, we may notice some important peculiarities. An important one concerns the transition zones: Treating myopia we create just one transition zone, while in the treatment of hyperopia, the central corneal curvature is increased and two transition zones are needed, featuring a double change in curvature and a median flexus point (Figure 12-1). This double transition zone is the most critical point of hyperopia treatment.[5] The most central of these two transition zones cannot be considered as part of the optical zone (Figure 12-2). This portion of the induced curvature is used to generate a refractive effect, but it features a flexus with a variation in curvature, and is connected to the peripheral corneal curvature through the second curvature zone. Therefore, when comparing myopic and hyperopic treatments with the same ablation diameter, the hyperopic optical zone will be smaller than the myopic one. This makes a hyperopic treatment more sensitive to decentration, with decreasing quality of vision if the treatment is not perfectly centered.

The ablation diameter must be planned to fit the zone of curvature inversion right where the normal peripheral corneal flattens. Using the elevation map, the surgeon must calculate the maximal corneal diameter, and place the flexus on the flat peripheral cornea, thus preserving the normal corneal physiology (Figure 12-3). If the flexus area is positioned centrally, far from this peripheral area of physiological corneal flattening, multifocality and high order optical aberrations will be induced. Also, hyperopic ablation generates a negative longitudinal spherical aberration with a degraded vision quality due to the fact that para-axial light rays will pass through the first curvature flexus that imparts a hyperopic shift (Figure 12-4).

However, it is important to remember that these problems are sometimes reduced by the anatomical characteristics of hyperopic eyes. Generally speaking, the size of the optical zone is less important for a hyperopic patient than for a myopic one. The hyperopic eye features smaller axial length, anterior

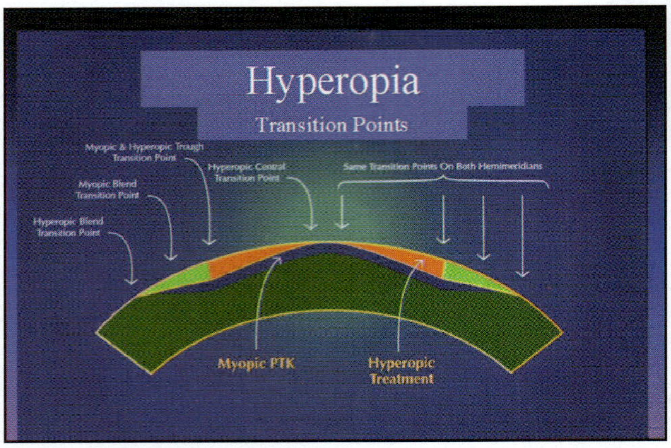

Figure 12-1. Hyperopic ablation. Central corneal curvature is increased and two transition zones are induced, leading to a double change in curvature.

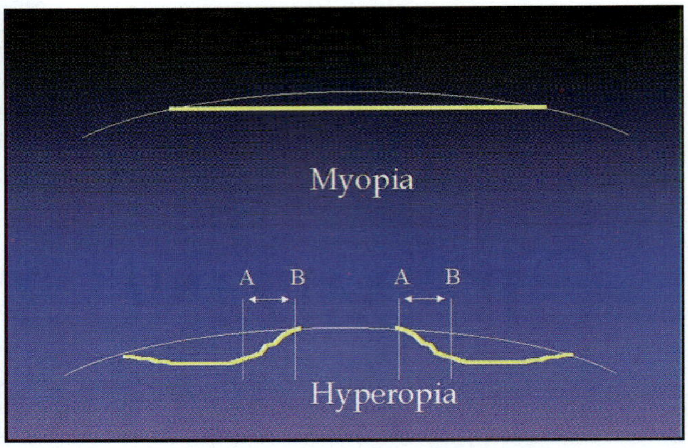

Figure 12-2. Hyperopic ablation. Central part of transition zone (A-B) cannot be considered part of the optical zone.

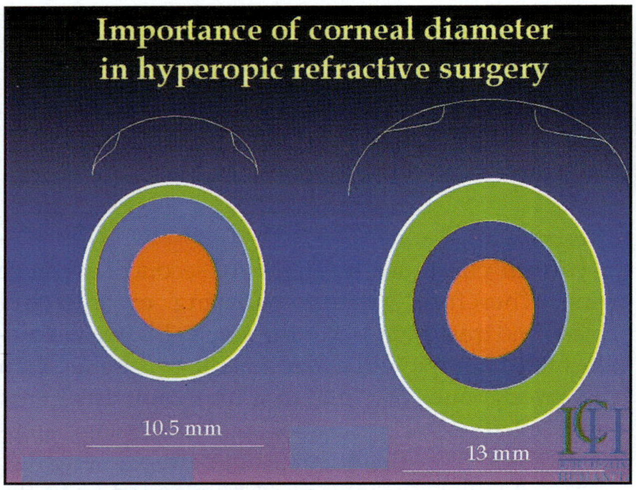

Figure 12-3. Importance of corneal diameter in hyperopic refractive surgery.

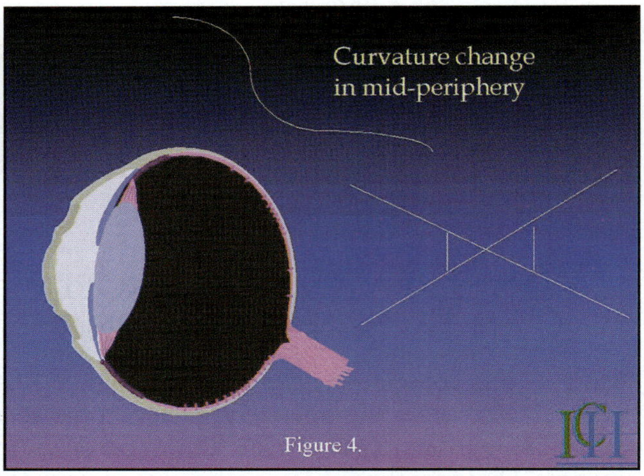

Figure 12-4. Hyperopic ablation. When the optical zone is small, para-axial light rays will pass through the first curvature flexus with consequent hyperopic shift, negative longitudinal spherical aberration, and worse vision quality.

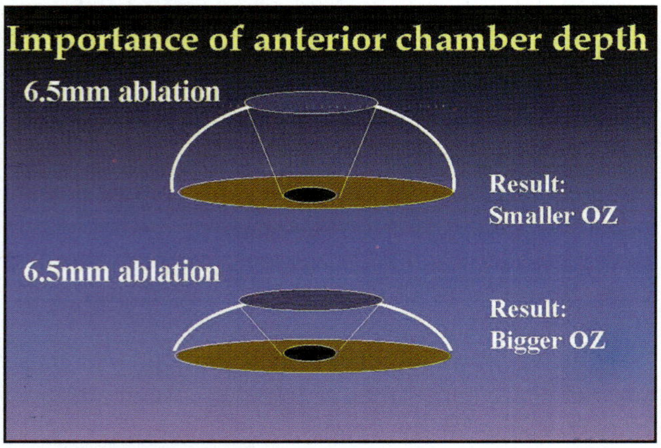

Figure 12-5. Given a 6.5-mm optical zone ablation, an eye with a shallow chamber will enjoy a larger optical zone than one with a deep chamber, and even a small size optical zone may sufficiently cover the pupillary area.

chamber, and corneal diameter. Given the same ablation diameter, an eye with a shallow chamber will enjoy a larger optical zone than one with a deep chamber (Figure 12-5), and will have a larger portion of corneal surface involved by the treatment. Moreover, the two above-mentioned transition zones will lay peripherally, positioned in a corneal area with lesser curvature and lesser influence on refraction. In a hyperopic eye with a shallow anterior chamber the treatment results will be less influenced by pupil diameter. A smaller optical zone may sufficiently cover the pupillary area, because the treated corneal arc will be closer to the pupillary area, and thus able to cover the pupil halos during mydriasis (see Figure 12-5).

These and the following observations can be assumed to be valid for photoreactive keratotomy (PRK), laser-assisted epithelial keratomileusis (LASEK), and laser-assisted in-situ keratomileusis (LASIK) treatments. Therefore, hereafter we will refer to refractive treatment as including PRK, LASEK and LASIK, with some important exceptions that will be detailed.

Analyzing Hyperopia Treatment: Optical Zone, Corneal Eccentricity, Spherical Aberration

Optical Zone and Ablation Zone

In refractive surgery, it is mandatory to understand the difference between ablation zone and optical zone, as two are often mistakenly attributed the same meaning. The ablation zone is the diameter of the area where the tissue has been removed, but the obtained refractive effect is expressed by the diameter of the optical zone. The peripheral limit of the ablation zone is often marked by the presence of a "red ring" that indicates a sharp variation in corneal curvature. Topographically, the instantaneous algorithm highlights the ablation zone, while the axial algorithm the useful optical zone, although the latter is represented more accurately by a wavefront map.

Corneal Eccentricity

Corneal eccentricity is the measure of corneal asphericity; it expresses the degree of change in corneal curvature (corneal curvature gradient), from a flatter periphery to a more curved central portion. Eccentricity values are positive when the cornea is prolate (ie, flatter around the periphery and more curved centrally), and negative when it is oblate (more curved around the periphery and flatter centrally). Normal eccentricity values (e values) range between +0.4 and +0.6 (normally prolate cornea: curved in the center, flat in the periphery).[6] A hyperopic treatment increases the e value, thus approaching a keratoconus-like situation. Central keratoconus, featuring a high eccentricity, with e values of +1.5 or more, amplifies the physiological situation of transition from a curved central cornea to a flat periphery. On the contrary, a myopic treatment induces negative eccentricity, inverting the normal morphology.

Spherical Aberration

Spherical aberration is the property of a spherical optic medium, which causes peripheral rays to be focused before axial rays (rays are only focused in the same point in aplanatic surfaces, where the dioptric power is identical in every point). From the point of view of subjective perception, the effect is a point-like image surrounded by a halo of variable width depending on the magnitude of the spherical aberration. The difference in diopters between the central and the marginal power of the pupil is called longitudinal spherical aberration (LSA). The spherical aberration of a normal eye is approximately 0.50 D. LSA expresses the aberration induced by corneal multifocality. It is a measure of spherical aberration; its increase indicates a decrease in contrast sensitivity.

Spherical Aberration After Refractive Surgery

Spherical aberration is commonly observed after refractive surgery, and is due to a marked change in the corneal profile, in the portion which demarcates the transition area between the ablated area and the untreated area. The red ring in the topographic map of myopic treatment, as well as the blue ring in the hyperopic treatment, both highlighted by the instantaneous algorithm. Like other eye aberrations, spherical aberrations are influenced by many variables—eg, they increase as the pupil diameter expands, and also vary according to age, accommodation, vitreous body properties, retina morphology, and probably other factors unknown so far.[7,8] The aberrometer is presently the ideal tool for the study of eye errors and aberrations through the analysis of the emerging wavefront. However, a spherical aberration can be suspected through other investigation methods—for example, corneal topography: In the instantaneous map, when the red ring is visible, in the elevation map, and if corneal eccentricity values are negative.

Spherical aberrations impair vision to variable extents, depending on their degree of severity. Minor spherical aberrations scarcely reduce vision quality, as they cause a slight loss of sensitivity to contrast, and contribute to give greater depth of field and focus. Conversely, more substantial spherical aberrations interfere with the optical quality of the retinal image, and manifest themselves with an excessive reduction of perceived contrast and with night halos. Spherical aberrations have an influence on the size of the optical zone and the quality of vision, and this influence can be clearly observed by subtracting only spherical aberrations from wavefront maps. The greatest weight is attributable to spherical aberrations (Figures 12-6A and B).

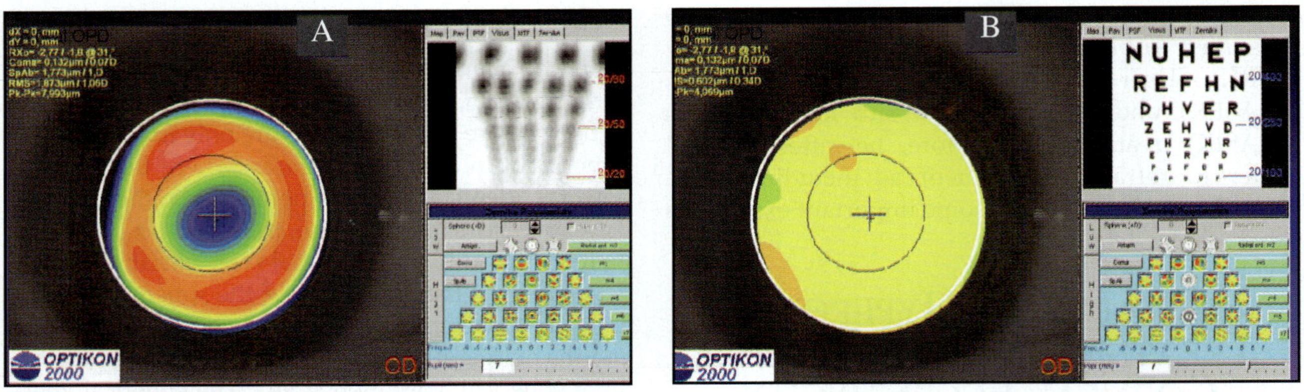

Figures 12-6A and B. Corneal wavefront map before (A) and after (B) subtracting spherical aberrations only. It can be noted how the optical zone becomes suddenly larger, resulting in better visual quality.

Several methods have been suggested to widen optical zones and essentially reduce spherical aberrations. Among them, selective ablations in some corneal areas performed with masks, and compound ablations (ablations that combine myopia and hyperopia, though maintaining the same spherical equivalent [SE]).

For example, if we wanted to widen an optical zone of 5 mm after a correction for -5.00 D maintaining the central power unaltered, the selective ablation system performed with masks proposes to place a contact lens cut to 5 mm, so as to mask the original ablation area, perform an ablation of 7 mm for -5.00 D (removing approximately 80 µm) followed by a PTK neutral ablation, to keep the 2 areas connected. The residual corneal tissue is often too thin; it is difficult to place the contact lens over the main optical zone and obtain perfect overlapping between these areas with the diameter of the PTK ablation. It is often difficult to seamlessly join the 2 ablation areas.

Indeed, several authors have proposed composed ablation as an alternative technique to reduce the spherical aberrations of myopia: myopic ablation with a 25% increase of the pre-surgery sphere, followed by a hyperopic ablation (25% of the pre-surgery sphere). The assumption underlying this technique is that the optical zone increases beyond the technical limits of the laser; theoretically, peripheral ablation would eliminate the large red ring, which causes spherical aberrations. In a study we conducted, 8 eyes of 4 patients with moderate bilateral myopia underwent LASEK with a NIDEK EC-5000 excimer laser (Japan). In each patient, 1 eye was treated with composed ablation (group 1), while the other was treated with standard ablation (group 2) with the cross cylinder technique.[9]

In the relative and elevation topographic maps of eyes, which received composed ablation, we found a large red ring with a high dioptric gradient and a central island, which caused significant optical aberrations. This was because the hyperopic ablation removed tissue not only in the area marked by the red ring, where the spherical aberration is located, but also in the center, thus obtaining a change of the central cornea curvature. Moreover, we had to remove tissue also in the centre in order to overcorrect the myopic component. In all cases (group 1) we had a worse wavefront, and all the patients were satisfied with the eye subjected to standard ablation (group 2).

Optical Zone and Spherical Aberration in Hyperopic Ablation

If the optical zone is planned merely as a function of the diameter of the ablation zone, without taking into account spherical aberration, the results may be frustrating. Actually, if spherical aberration has a high value, even a treatment with a very wide ablation zone may actually feature a small optical zone on the axial map. High spherical aberration in myopic treatment is indicated by red ring that is intense (high gradient), wide (larger cornea involved), and closer to the corneal apex (small transition zone). The same red ring pattern will show both on the topographic (instantaneous algorithm) and aberrometric map. Hyperopic ablation may induce more spherical aberration than myopic, because spherical aberration will be induced by two rings (blue in hyperopic) indicating the two abovementioned corneal curvature gradients. The external ring is harder to highlight on maps because it is positioned on the flatter, more peripheral cornea.

A high corneal curvature gradient, with blue ring closer to the corneal apex, and thus high spherical aberration, will induce a small optical zone, with the optical situation of a central keratoconus, which is notoriously poor. This may easily explain the scarce popularity of this treatment among hyperopic patients. A correction of 3.00 D on a hyperopic patient often will be qualitatively poor, with reduced night vision and significant halo perception. Furthermore, a corrected myopic patient will experience an enlargement of the retinal image, while a hyperopic patient will see it reduced.

In the past, it was generally thought that excessively high corneal curvature values would lead to a keratoconus-like situation. From our studies, it appears that an important factor for this complication is the eccentricity. Interestingly, we may meet patients with corneal curvature values of 46.00 D that show good visual acuity, while others with, for example, 45.00 D do not enjoy such good vision. In a patient with 46.00 D and normal eccentricity, there is no marked peripheral flattening and visual acuity will be good. Another patient, with a keratoconus and a corneal curvature within normal values, such as 45.00 D, will inevitably show a high eccentricity, therefore marked spherical aberrations, and a very small homogeneous optical zone and reduced vision quality.

High eccentricity after a wrongly performed hyperopic treatment might lead to an optical situation resembling a central keratoconus: It sports a central dioptrically homogeneous area, but featuring a small diameter, so the patient enjoys bearable optical quality situation only in miosis, while when the pupil dilates multifocality becomes unbearable (see Figure 12-4). The corneal periphery features high dioptrical gradient form center to periphery (high eccentricity). This situation is typical of old-style treatments for hyperopia.

Correction of Hyperopia With LASIK, LASEK, and PRK

Correction of hyperopia with LASIK is more successful, even in the presence of high eccentricity values. As a matter of fact, the flap does not follow perfectly the new shape of the stromal bed, thus reducing the eccentricity created by the ablation. In LASEK and PRK, corneal epithelium follows faithfully the new imparted morphology. However, above certain values of eccentricity, even LASIK fails.

Retreatment with PTK of these fibrotic areas in hyperopia leads to limited or no result at all, if corneal eccentricity remains positive (e = 1.0 – 1.5), with recurrence of the scar on the point of greatest corneal curvature. On the opposite, when eccentricity is decreased—ie, with corneal excimer laser smoothing, recurrence is prevented. A key point of hyperopic ablation is thus to maintain a corneal eccentricity as much as possible close to physiological values.

Corneal topography offers the advantage of an accurate evaluation of the quality of hyperopic ablation. A wide, homogeneous central area is necessary for a better vision quality and surgeon must strive to achieve it, as well as topographically monitor the result. The aberrometric map allows evaluation of central corneal dioptrical homogeneity, as well as detection of irregularities that may generate aberrations. The more peripheral is treatment, the less important is the second, peripheral part of the transition zone (see Figures 12-1 and 12-2). Our experience with the optical path difference (OPD) aberrometer shows that with good topographical indexes we have a satisfactory aberrometric map: more than 80% of optical aberrations are caused by the first corneal surface.

The future is represented by a wider optical zone (in relation to corneal diameter), of 6.5 mm or greater, with a first, more smooth and homogeneous transition zone up to 9 mm, and a second, limbal transition zone, of more than 9 mm. Let us remember that the corneal periphery offers also the advantage of a greater thickness (Figure 12-7).

Complications of Hyperopia Treatment

Several possible causes may be considered responsible for complications in the treatment of hyperopia:

Decentration

The hyperopic patient usually has more problems in fixating the target light, due to the accommodative effort for focusing on this near target, with possible loss of fixation. Because the real optical zone is smaller in the hyperopic treatment than in the myopic treatment, decentration leads to more severe consequences. The effect of the same amount of decentration in mm from the visual axis is quite different according to corneal curvature: Steeper corneas are more affected. The greater the corneal curvature, the more the decentration is increased due to a prismatic effect (Figure 12-8). Correction of decentration is possible, but difficult, and nevertheless induces relevant optical aberrations (ie, coma).

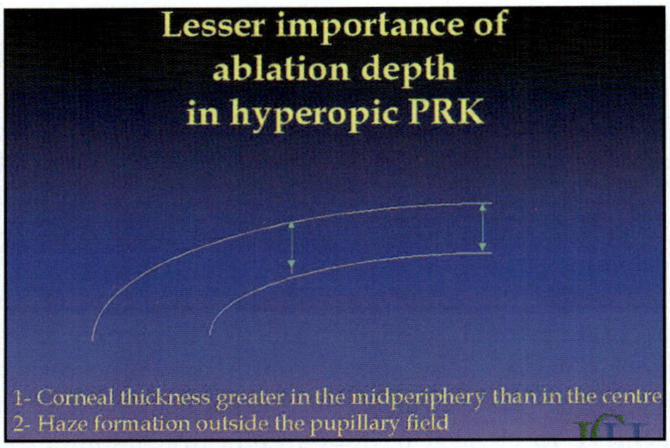

Figure 12-7. Hyperopic ablation. The corneal periphery offers the advantage of a greater thickness allowing deeper ablations. Haze in the periphery will not hamper visual acuity.

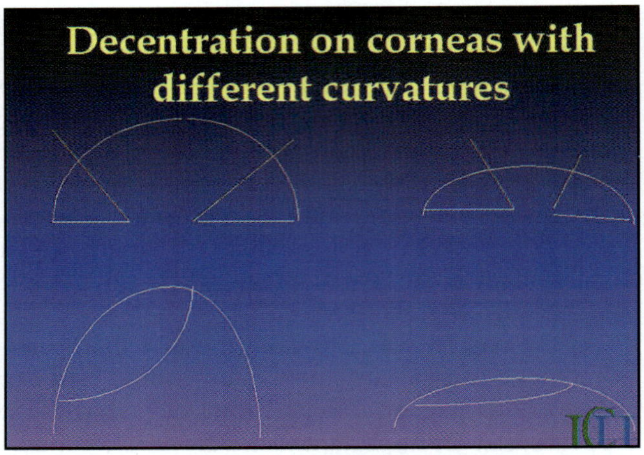

Figure 12-8. Influence of corneal curvature on decentration. The greater the corneal curvature, the more decentration is increased due to prismatic effect.

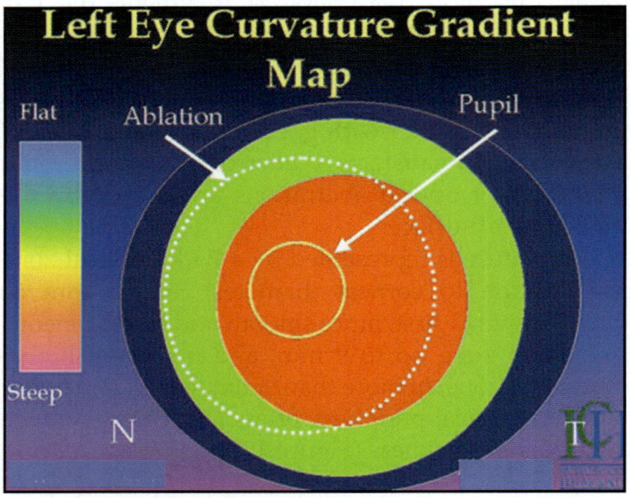

Figure 12-9. Influence of the transition zone in the temporal corneal region. In an eye with nasal pupil, the transition zone will involve temporally a paracentral, steeper corneal portion with consequent postoperative high dioptrical gradient. Nasally, the transition zone will involve a flatter peripheral cornea.

Let us examine the keratoscopic appearance of an improperly administered treatment for hyperopia. The rings will show extremely inhomogeneous intermediate spaces; some rings will show sudden, intermediate space increase, expression of a sudden change in the ray of curvature. These curvature changes, especially if asymmetrical, induce aberrations of 1st, 2nd, 3rd, and 4th order. Maintaining a constant ray of curvature is mandatory to achieve good visual quality. Conversely, an elevated spherical aberration reduces the contrast perceived by the patient. Furthermore, if this condition is asymmetrically distributed on the cornea, coma and other aberrations will be present, reducing the quality of vision and causing monocular ghosting and double vision.

Lack of Adequate Transition Zone

This may be caused by inadequate analysis of the preoperative corneal topography, error in surgical strategy and limits of possible transition zone size with a particular type of laser. The resulting complications include dimensionally insufficient optical zone, with fluctuations in visual acuity, as well as rapid postoperative dioptrical variations induced by focal 4th order optical aberrations, and regression. The width of the transition zone must be defined considering the amount of correction to impart and the topographical features of the eye. The transition zone has more influence in high corrections and in more "spherical" corneas, as well as in the temporal corneal region (Figure 12-9). In LASIK patients, an inadequate transition zone causes loss of vision quality, with occurrence of halos and glare, more regression, and loss of vision.

Hyperopic White Scar

Highly positive eccentricity values (above 1.0 – 1.2) are typical of keratoconus cases and of some cases of hyperopic ablations that share the presence of a subepithelial (PRK) or sub-flap (LASIK) whitish scar.[10,11] This scar corresponds topographically to the point of maximal corneal curvature (Figures 12-10 and 12-11). In these cases there is always a high eccentricity value, and thus high spherical aberration. Presently, the etiology of this scar remains uncertain, and includes an inhomogeneous lachrymal film, as well as lid trauma on the affected cornea. In the past, the scar has been considered the consequence of the selective denervation of the central corneal area due to the depth of the peripheral ablation. Nowadays, this hypothesis is no longer

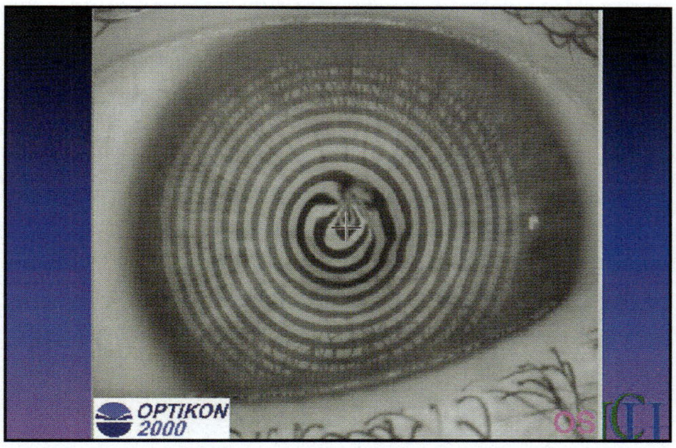

Figure 12-10. Keratoscopy of an eye with a subepithelial (PRK) whitish scar, corresponding topographically to the point of maximal corneal curvature.

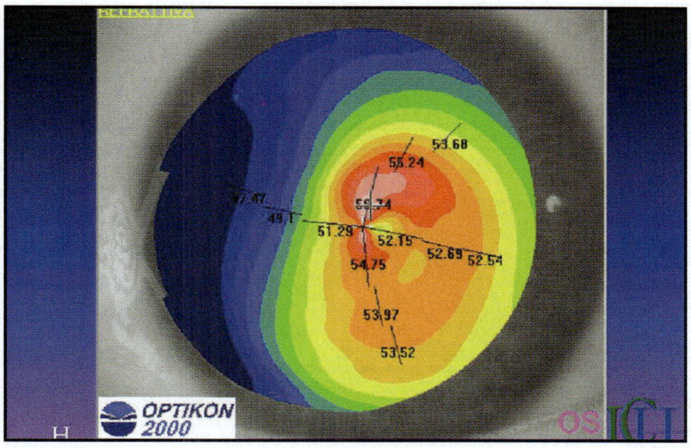

Figure 12-11. Topography of same eye seen in Figure 12-10.

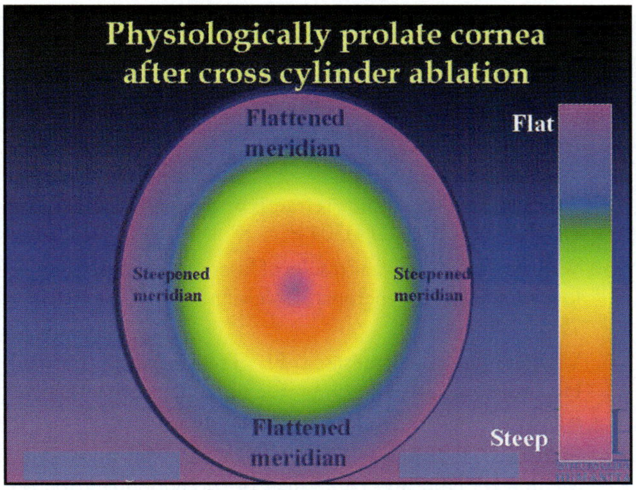

Figure 12-12. Scheme of physiologically prolate cornea after cross cylinder ablation for hyperopic astigmatism.

sustainable, because the scar is observed in the point of greatest corneal curvature and not in that of maximal corneal ablation. Furthermore, the scar is not observed with a greater frequency in LASIK eyes, where central corneal denervation is more complete. However, a similar scar is present in post-traumatic corneal leukomas, always in the point of greatest corneal curvature. Very often, in these cases of corneal leukoma, topographic analysis may be misleading, due to problems with the elaboration of the map. Keratoscopy must always be obtained and examined.

Retreatments

It is necessary to ablate selectively the corneal apex, after precise identification with the pachymetric map. The diameter must be carefully measured, and then the ablation performed. Then, it is important to reduce the eccentricity. The ablation must be myopic, in order to substantially widen the optical and transition zones. The use of a masking fluid (usually a viscoelastic solution) is frequently helpful. Successful treatment of white scars features reduction of corneal eccentricity.

Hyperopic Astigmatism

The goal of custom ablation is to achieve a corneal surface that is as much as possible symmetrical and similar to a physiological corneal surface. Symmetry is an essential factor in order to prevent high-order optical aberrations (ie, coma, a 3rd-order aberration). Correction of hyperopic astigmatism with traditional techniques may lead to the onset of a central keratoconus with leukoma, especially if the spherical equivalent is positive.

Cross-Cylinder Technique

A valid alternative is represented by the cross-cylinder technique.[12-17] If the spherical equivalent is negative, eccentricity does not increase but decreases, becoming negative and no leukoma will appear. If the mean ray of curvature is preserved, mean eccentricity remains constant. Therefore, cross-cylinder techniques do not increase eccentricity, and a corneal situation closer to normal physiology can be obtained (Figures 12-12 and 12-13).

If the spherical equivalent is positive and the postoperative increase in curvature is sudden, we will have a corneal area featuring an extreme curvature, just like a keratoconus. This area is more easily exposed to lid trauma, as well as to an inhomoge-

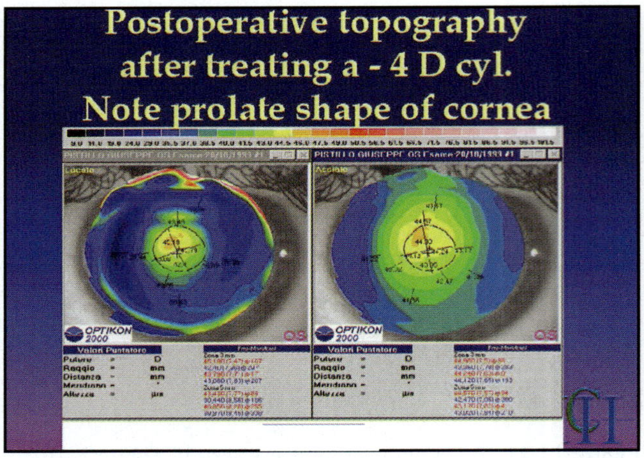

Figure 12-13. Postoperative topography after treatment for hyperopic astigmatism of -4.00 D. Cornea shows a prolate shape.

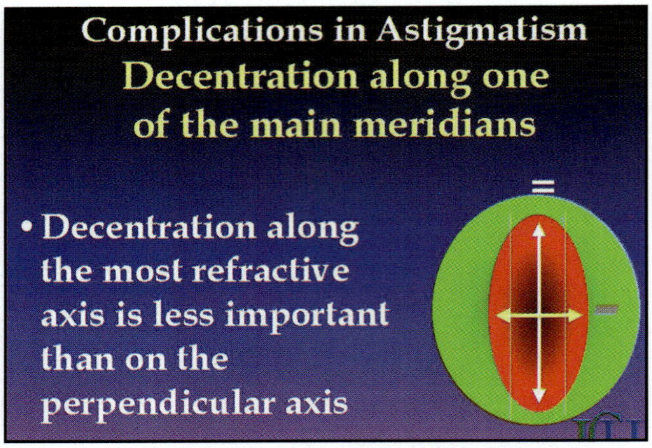

Figure 12-14. Decentration along the most steep axis is less troublesome than decentration along the less refractive axis. This last case may lead to hypocorrection, induction of 4th order optical aberrations with loss in visual acuity, monocular diplopia, and halos.

neous distribution of the tear film, with risk of leukoma occurrence.

Complications of Hyperopic Astigmatism Treatment

Decentration Along One of the Two Main Meridians

This situation differs depending on the axis of decentration: Decentration along the most steep axis is less troublesome than decentration along the less refractive axis. This last may lead to hypercorrection, and induction of 4th-order optical aberrations, leading to loss in visual acuity, monocular diplopia, and halos (Figure 12-14).

Axis variation

This can be induced by incorrect patient positioning, errors in the laser setting of the astigmatism axis (TABO versus international), differences in objective versus subjective axis, or a tracking problem. Axis variation may result in postoperative hyper-hypocorrection of sphere, hypocorrection of astigmatism, mixed astigmatism, irregular astigmatism, and pseudo-decentration.

References

1. Tabbara KF, El-Sheik HF, Monowarul-Islam SM. Laser in situ keratomileusis for the correction of hyperopia from +0.50 to +11.50 diopters with the keracor 117C laser. *J Refractive Surg.* 2001; 17:123-128.
2. Ditzen K, Huschka H, Pieger S. Laser in situ keratomileusis for hyperopia. *J Cataract Refract Surg.* 1998;24:42-47.
3. Zadok D, Maskaleris G, Montes M, Shah S, Garcia V, Chayet A. Hyperopic laser in situ keratomileusis with the Nidek EC-5000 excimer laser. *Ophthalmology.* 2000;107:1132-1137.
4. Sher NA. Hyperopic refractive surgery. *Curr Opin Ophthalmol.* 2001; 12(4)304-8
5. Williams DK. One-year results of laser vision correction for low to moderate hyperopia. *Ophthalmology.* 2000; 107:72-75.
6. Vinciguerra P, Camesasca FI. Treatment of corneal Hyperopia: a new ablation profile to reduce corneal eccentricity. *J Refractive Surgery.* 2002 May-Jun (suppl).
7. Martinez CE, Applegate RA, Klyce SD, McDonald MB, Medina JP, Howland HC. Effect of papillary dilatation on optical aberration after keratectomy. *Arch Ophthalmol.* 1998 Aug;116(8):1053-62.
8. McLellan JS, Marcos S, Burns SA. Age related changes in monochromatic wave aberration of human eye. *Invest Ophthalmol Vis Sci.* 2001 May;42(6):1390.
9. Vinciguerra P, Torres Munoz MI, Camesasca FI. Reduction of spherical aberration: experimental model of photoablation. *J Refractive Surg.* 2002 May-Jun; 18(3 suppl):S366.
10. Nagy Z, Krueger RR, Suveges I. Central bump-like opacity as a complication of high hyperopic photorefractive keratectomy. *Am J Ophthalmol.* 1999;128:636-638.
11. Sener B, Özdamar A, Aras C. Apical nodular subepithelial corneal scar after retreatment in hyperopic photorefractive keratectomy. *J Cataract Refract Surg.* 2000;26:352-357.
12. Vinciguerra P, Epstein D, Radice P, Azzolini M. Long-term results of photorefractive keratectomy for hyperopia and hyperopic astigmatism. *J Refract Surg.* 1998;14:2 Suppl, S183-S185.
13. Vinciguerra P, Sborgia M, Epstein D, Azzolini M, MacRae S. Photorefractive keratectomy to correct myopic or hyperopic astigmatism with a cross-cylinder ablation. *J Refract Surg.* 1999;15:2 Suppl,S183-S185.

14. Azar DT, Primack JD. Theoretical analysis of ablation depths and profiles in laser in situ keratomileusis for compound hyperopic and mixed astigmatism. *J Cataract Refract Surg*. 2000;26:1123-1136.
15. Vinciguerra P. Cross-cylinder ablation for the correction of myopic or hyperopic astigmatism. In: Gimbel HV, Anderson Penno EE, eds. *Refractive Surgery. A Manual of Principles and Practice*. Thorofare, NJ: SLACK Incorporated; 2000;105-113.
16. Epstein D, Vinciguerra P, Camesasca FI, et al. Cross Cylinder ablation in LASIK and PRK—a new tissue-sparing, accuracy-enhancing strategy for correcting astigmatism. *Invest Ophthalmol Vis Sci*. 2000;41:S690.
17. Vinciguerra P, Camesasca FI. Cross cylinder ablation. In: MacRae SM, Krueger RR, Applegate RA, eds. *Custom Corneal Ablation: The Quest for Super Vision*. Thorofare, NJ: SLACK Incorporated; 2001.

Section Three

Enhancement After Overcorrected Myopic Refractive Surgery

Chapter Thirteen

Management of Hyperopia After Radial Keratotomy

Laura T. Muller, MD and Parag A. Majmudar, MD

Introduction

History of RK

Since the late 19th century, ophthalmic surgeons have attempted to treat refractive errors by making incisions into the cornea.[1] Originally performed to correct astigmatism and keratoconus, radial keratotomy was popularized for the treatment of myopia in the 1970's by Russian ophthalmologists Durnev and Fyodorov and American ophthalmologist Bores.[2,3] The safety, efficacy, and predictability of radial keratotomy (RK) were evaluated in the Prospective Evaluation of Radial Keratotomy (PERK) Study.[4] The PERK study demonstrated a 100% decrease in the level of myopia with 88% of all subjects achieving an uncorrected acuity of 20/40 or better. In the group that had fewer than or equal to 6.33 D of myopia, 90% of the subjects achieved uncorrected acuity of 20/40 or better.[5] However, only 58% of patients maintained a stable refraction between 6 months and 4 years after RK. Many patients drifted back toward myopia, while others became increasingly hyperopic.

Manifestation of Consecutive Hyperopia After RK

The conversion of a myopic to a hyperopic refractive error is one of the most frequent and significant complications of RK.[6] The clinical manifestations of hyperopia after RK can be seen in the immediate postoperative setting, or years after the initial surgery. Hyperopia in the immediate post-RK period can be due to corneal edema and wound gape leading to greater flattening of the cornea. In addition, there are several other stresses on the functioning of the visual system in the early postoperative period. In general, myopes tend to have less accommodative demand than emmetropes. When converted abruptly to hyperopia, there is an increased accommodative demand. Moreover, there is also an effect on the vergence of the eyes. Myopes usually exert fusional convergence in order to maintain binocular vision, but if converted to a hyperope, functional *divergence* is now required to maintain fusion. This sudden stress on vergence is probably more significant in producing symptoms than is the sudden stress on accommodation.[7]

The more common manifestation of hyperopia after RK is a gradual onset in the late postoperative period. The ongoing effect of the procedure over time results in progressive hyperopia referred to as the "hyperopic shift." In the PERK study, 43% of patients had a hyperopic shift of +1.00 D or more over a 10-year follow-up period. The greatest rate of change occurred between 6 months and 2 years postoperatively at a rate of +0.21 D per year, with a smaller rate of change of 0.06 D per year between years 2 and 10.[8] The degree of hyperopic shift is closely correlated to higher degrees of preoperative myopia rather than the number, depth, and length of incisions. Other factors contributing to progressive hyperopia after RK include radial incisions that extend to the limbus, multiple enhancement procedures, peripheral redeepening procedures, use of a metal rather than diamond blade,[9] lack of preoperative cycloplegia with undiscovered latent hyperopia, postoperative contact wear and postoperative ocular massage.[8] In addition, it has been found that travel to a high altitude can cause a hyperopic shift.[10] Since the 1970s over 1.2 million RK procedures have been performed and it is estimated that 20% to 30% of these patients may now be hyperopic.[11]

Evaluation of the Hyperopic Post-RK Patient

Clinical History

An accurate clinical evaluation of the hyperopic post-RK patient is essential in order to plan the best potential surgical or non-surgical intervention. Previous records including preoperative findings and the original operative plan are extremely helpful in order to evaluate refractive stability and help to differentiate between individuals with progressive hyperopia and those who were initially overcorrected and lost the ability to accommodate. When young patients undergo RK, they may be very happy with an initial outcome of +0.75 but as the years pass and accommodative amplitudes decrease, they may have increasing visual complaints. Patients with progressive hyperopia due to wound gape often have associated symptoms of ghosting and decreased contrast sensitivity.[12] A medical history is important in discerning the presence of systemic disease or medications that may influence corneal wound healing and help guide in management decisions. History of contact lens usage should be elicited. RK patients are exquisitely sensitive to contact lens warpage. It is generally recommended that patients remain out of soft contact lenses for at least 2 weeks and hard contact lenses for at least 1 month prior to evaluation and treatment.[13]

Refraction

Diurnal fluctuation in visual acuity after RK is well documented and may occur in up to 60% of patients.[3,14] The fluctuation is likely multifactorial involving corneal hydration and intraocular pressure. Therefore, intraocular pressure (IOP), topography and refraction must be obtained at different times of the day, with documentation of the time of the evaluation.[15,16] Some clinicians have noted as much as a 2-D change between morning and evening cycloplegic refractions.[16] It is not uncommon for a patient to be more hyperopic early in the day. In addition, it is important to "push plus" during the refraction as younger hyperopes have a strong tendency to accommodate. It is interesting to note that during refraction one may note a lower level of add than expected for patients after RK due to the multifocality of a cornea after RK.

Irregular Astigmatism

The presence of irregular astigmatism can lead to a decrease in best-corrected visual acuity (BCVA). Observation of the mires during manual keratometry can uncover microscopic irregularity of the anterior refractive surface of the cornea. This micro-irregularity may not be revealed on topography.[12] Laranjera et al describes that a "breaking of the mires" on keratometry can be a sign of poor wound healing of the RK incisions.[17]

Rigid gas permeable (RGP) contact lens (CTL) over refraction can help to neutralize irregular astigmatism and aid in attaining the BCVA.

Other Testing

In patients who have undergone recent RK, a hyperopic shift can occur simply due to corneal edema. With as little as 7 to 10 µm of epithelial thickening, a diopter of hyperopia may be induced. Pachymetry of greater than 520 µm is essential in considering additional corneal surgery. Corneal sensation should be tested to evaluate for possible hypesthesia, particularly if transverse incisions have been used in conjunction with the initial RK procedure.[18] During slit lamp biomicroscopy, special attention should be made in evaluating the epithelium for map dot fingerprint changes,[19] for the presence of epithelial cysts in the incisions, observation of micro dehiscence or wound gape (Figure 13-1), evaluating for the presence and degree of ectasia of the RK incisions, noting the presence of sub epithelial fibrosis or iron deposition, and the presence of neovascularization in the RK incisions. Evaluating the number of RK incisions as well as the presence or absence of astigmatic keratotomy (AK) incisions is important when considering LASIK as the "pie pieces" may separate after the microkeratomes pass. The presence and location of epithelial cysts should be noted as they may be a sign of incomplete healing of RK incisions. Some authors suggest removing epithelial cysts and allowing the cornea to heal prior to performing the microkeratomes pass of the LASIK procedure.[20]

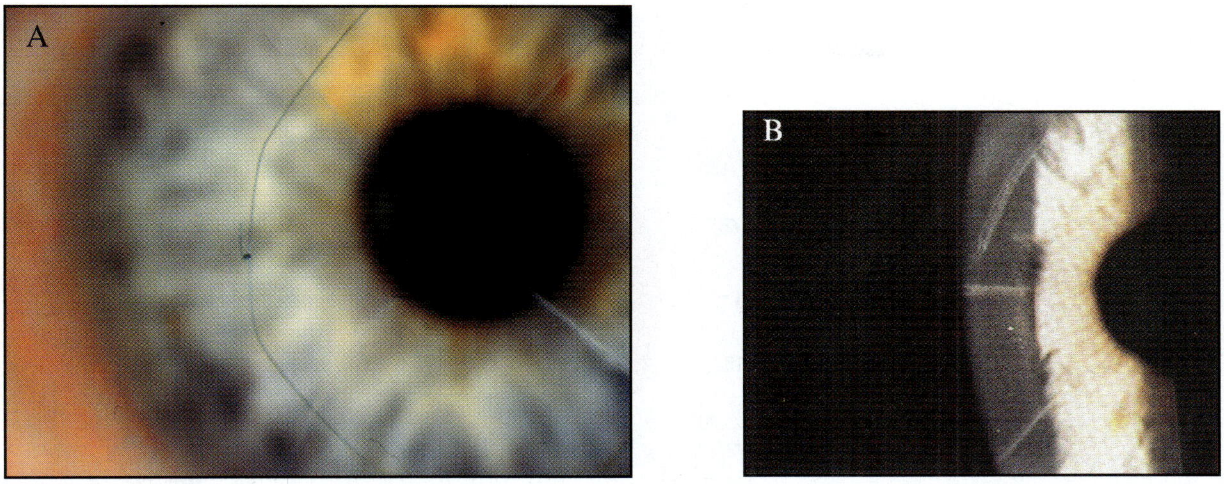

Figure 13-1A and B. Comparing RK wound gape. A) Shows RK with wound gape and Grene Lasso suture in place. B) shows RK with no wound gape. (Courtesy of Ethicon Brochure for the Grene Lasso Procedure and Bruce Grene, MD.)

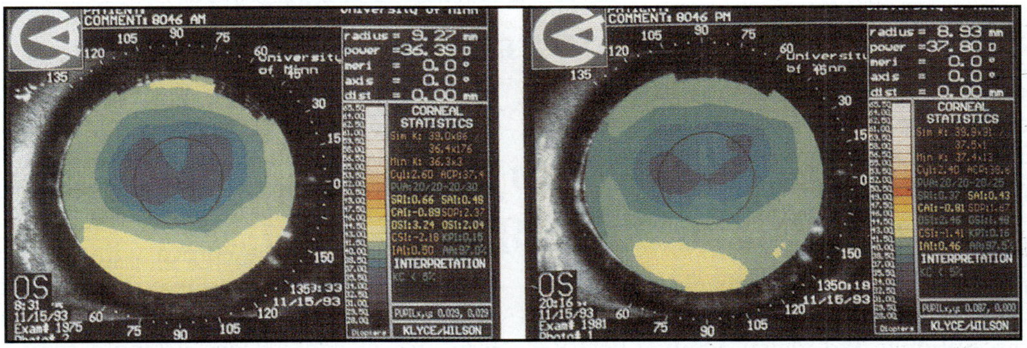

Figure13-2. Diurnal fluctuation of topography in patients after RK . (Reprinted with permission from Kemp JR, Martinez CE, Klyce SD, et al. Diurnal fluctuations in corneal topography 10 years after radial keratotomy in the prospective evaluation of radial keratotomy study. *J Cataract Refract Surg.* 1999;25:904-910.)

Topography

Serial topography can be helpful in determining the fluctuations that occur with diurnal variation.[15,21] The cornea is often flatter in the morning and steepens throughout the day. One theory for this change is the pressure exerted by the eyelids while the eyes are closed at night (Figure 13-2). It is also important to make note of the central and peripheral keratometry readings as many post-RK patients are quite flat centrally, yet have a normal peripheral keratometry reading. Orbscan (Bausch & Lomb, Rochester, NY) topographic evaluation can be helpful in determining posterior elevation, anterior elevation, and pachymetry. It can also help to assess the presence and degree of ectasia.

Wavefront

Wavefront analysis may be useful in determining higher order aberrations induced by the initial RK procedure. Evaluation of a wavefront error can help to quantify the quality of the optical image. With a larger pupil, if the RK incisions are within the clear zone, the dissatisfaction of a hyperopic patient can be increased by aberrations.[22] The potential future integration of wavefront evaluation with a refractive plan may be useful in post-RK patients, but it has the potential to be inaccurate in patients with diurnal variation. The diurnal evaluation of wavefront aberrations would add to the body of clinical knowledge in understanding the optics of the post-RK eye.[23]

Non-Surgical Management

There are a variety of non-surgical options for patients with hyperopia following RK with the use of spectacles being the most obvious choice. This is a viable option with low levels of hyperopia in the absence of irregular astigmatism. In presbyopia,

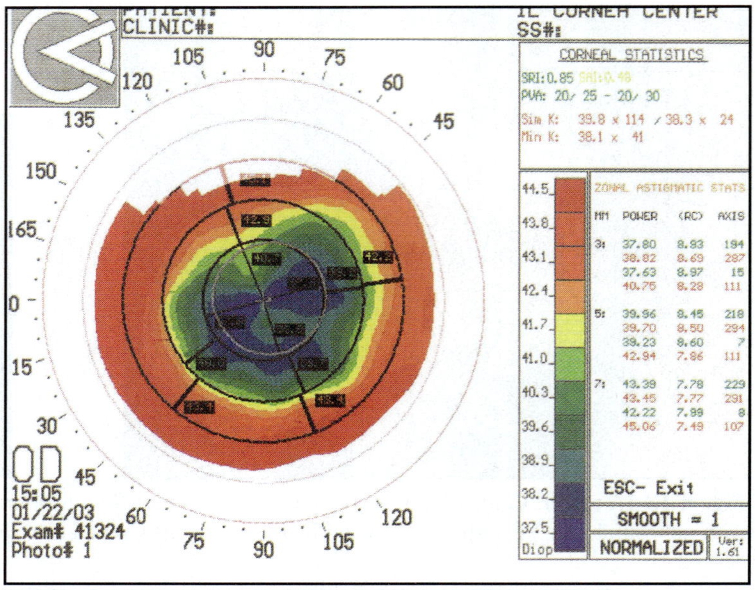

Figure 13-3. Typical appearance of topography after RK. Note alternating steep and flat areas.

spectacles may be required despite surgical intervention. In addition, spectacles may be required for refractive instability, and the patient may need to use multiple spectacles to optimize the vision.[24-26]

Contact Lens Fitting

RGP CTLs are very helpful in managing refractive error; they are a good solution for irregular astigmatism and can optimize the visual acuity.[27] Post-RK corneas are flat in the center and steep in the mid periphery, leading to the potential need for specialized lenses including aspheric lenses or scleral lenses. Soft CTLs do not generally play a role in managing hyperopia after RK due to the risk for corneal neovascularization and vascularization of the incisions. They may also carry an increased risk of microbial keratitis, because patients often have abnormal epithelium overlying the keratotomy incisions.[28] However, soft CTLs may be used in special circumstances. Damiano and Forstot advocated the use of soft CTLs for 6 months to induce "molding" of the cornea.[29]

Corneal topography may be a valuable tool in RGP CTL fitting. Corneal topographic changes after RK are typified by central flattening and paracentral steepening (Figure 13-3). A CTL fit requires a paracentral bearing and peripheral edge lift. The lens must pivot over the paracentral break points, sometimes referred to as "knees," often decentering superonasally or inferotemporally (over the steepest portion of the cornea). Difficulty in centration is increased when transverse incisions are present. The tear lens in this situation is thicker, creating more plus power that must be offset by adding correction nearly equal to the original myopia.[30] In addition, the large tear pool can be stagnant leading to hypoxia and consequent stromal and epithelial edema.

Orthokeratology or corneal refractive therapy (CRT) to steepen the cornea with a gas permeable hard contact lens is endorsed by some optometric practices. The effect is temporary and requires long-term use of contact lens. Using a semi-scleral lens such as the Macrolens (C & H, Dallas, Tex) is helpful in vaulting the entire cornea to provide a generous tear meniscus to neutralize the astigmatism.[31]

Pharmacologic Treatment

Pharmacologic manipulation of accommodation with low-dose pilocarpine has been used to treat mild cases of hyperopia, taking advantage of the myopic shift associated with pilocarpine. Pilocarpine also induces miosis, which creates a larger depth of field. One study demonstrated a mean myopic shift of -0.71 D with doses titrated between 1% and 4%.[17] Interestingly, patients demonstrated an average keratometric steepening of 2.18 D. The authors hypothesize that pilocarpine stimulated corneal wound healing with the added short-term benefit of inducing accommodation to reduce the hyperopia. Although the mechanism is unclear, the effect of pilocarpine seems to have more effects on the corneal wound in the initial phase after surgery, and it is probably not an appropriate treatment modality for most hyperopic post-RK patients seen in clinic several years postoperatively. In addition, the effect of pilocarpine is often unpredictable and can be short

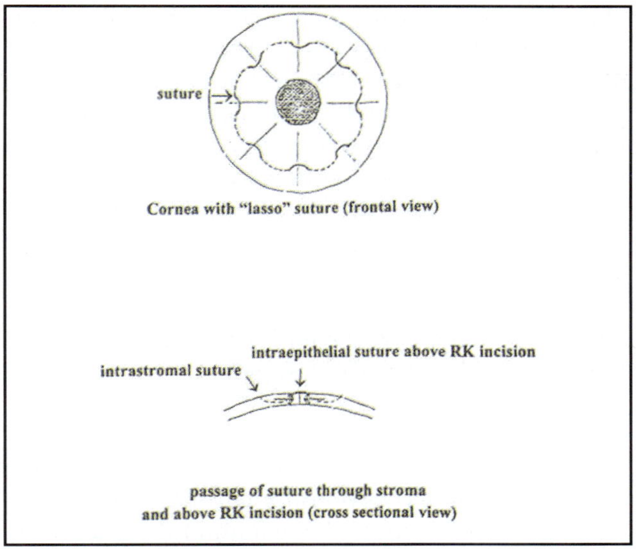

Figure 13-4A. Technique of Grene lasso placement (courtesy of AJO 1998:126:825-827).

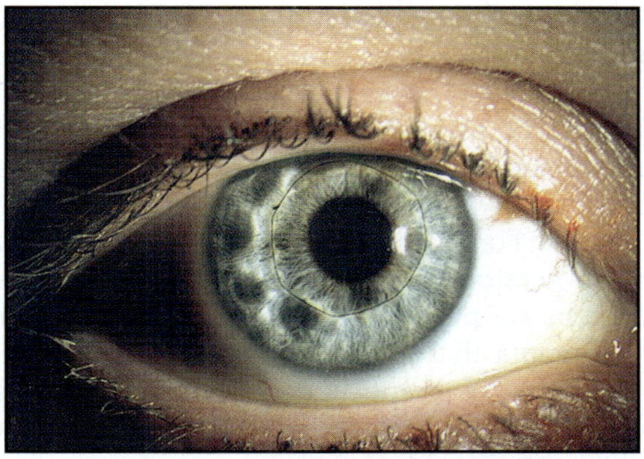

Figure 13-4B. Appearance of Grene lasso upon completion.

lived and there is the risk of brow ache, increased rate of cataract progression, and the risk of a retinal tear.[31]

Surgical Options

The goal of many patients initially undergoing RK is to be free of glasses or CTLs; therefore, many post-RK consecutive hyperopes desire a more permanent or surgical solution. In general, corneal surgery for hyperopia is more complicated than in myopia. The ophthalmologist must create complex compound curves with a steeper central area and a flatter paracentral area. With corneal surgery for hyperopia, there is an increased chance of decentration and unwanted optical aberrations.

A variety of techniques can be used to manage the hyperopic post-RK patient. Included in these options are compression sutures (interrupted or lasso), excimer laser refractive surgery (including LASIK, PRK, or LASEK), Holmium-YAG laser thermokeratoplasty (LTK), conductive keratoplasty (CK), intraocular lenses (IOLs), or corneal transplantation.

Compression Sutures

Compression sutures are particularly useful in patients with diurnal fluctuation in vision. The surgeon may opt for single interrupted sutures, especially in the setting of a patient with asymmetrical incisions. When placing single interrupted sutures, one must choose an optical zone for suture placement. A 7-mm optical zone appears to be optimal, as sutures placed in smaller optical zones can induce higher amounts of astigmatism. A disadvantage to the interrupted suture technique is the loss of effect (by up to 70%) over time.[32]

Lasso sutures are best for symmetrical incisions. Hofman reported the use of a single continuous purse-string suture of merseline as a management for overcorrection in 1987.[33] The Grene lasso was developed to better address wound gape by forcing the corneal "knee" posteriorly.[34] It was first described in 1994 and refined in subsequent years for management of post-RK hyperopia. The technique of the Grene lasso utilizes 10-0 nylon on a compound J-curve needle (Ethicon CS-B-6, Johnson and Johnson, Sommerville, NJ) needle with a "steep and deep" suture path. Each suture bite enters and exits adjacent to a radial incision to a depth of 70% to 80% (Figures 13-4A and B). The suture is superficial over the RK incisions and deep within the stroma between the RK incisions. This is in contrast to traditional continuous suturing where the superficial portion of the suture is over the intervening stroma and the suture is passed through the cornea adjacent and beneath the RK incision. When the lasso is completed, the knot is triple-tied and buried as deeply as possible. Nylon is the preferred suture material over merseline or prolene. Approximately half of patients receiving the merseline sutures developed inflammatory keratitis and prolene tended to stretch, resulting in less effective compression. Dr. Grene considers the Grene lasso technique to affect three factors that contribute to hyperopia: wound gape, microirregular astigmatism, and overcorrection.[34] Lindstrom modified the Grene Lasso into the "over and under" technique instead of the "steep and deep" as described by Grene.[32] In an 8-

cut RK, the first bite goes under or through an incision and the next goes over an incision, alternating under and over 4 times.[12,34] With either technique, the effect can be titrated quantitatively with a surgical keratometer. Lindstrom recommends steepening the cornea by twice the amount of the consecutive hyperopia. For example, if the patient is +2.00 D with a mean keratometry reading of 40.00 D, the cornea should be steepened 4.00 D to 44.00 D. This induces mild myopia that slowly drifts toward plano over time. In the "over and under" technique, there is a possibility of loosening of the sutures, which can lead to irritation. Multiple lasso sutures may also be placed at various optical zones to titrate the effect.[35] In general, intrastromal circular sutures (lasso sutures) are not highly predictable. Risks with this procedure are decreased predictability and difficulty in titrating refractive error correction. Over time, the steepening effect may be lost; and there is also the potential for suture erosion.

Automated Lamellar Keratoplasty

Several studies in the late 1980's and early 1990's evaluated hyperopic automated lamellar keratoplasty (ALK) in post-RK eyes. Induction of irregular astigmatism with concomitant loss of best spectacle-corrected visual acuity (BSCVA) and glare was found to be among the complications in undergoing these procedures.[36]

Photorefractive Keratectomy

The excimer laser has been used after RK for nearly a decade.[37,38] In the early 1990's the Summit therapeutic refractive trial proved excimer photorefractive keratectomy (PRK) was safe and effective in treating residual myopia after RK. However, it had a tendency to be imprecise and risked loss of BCVA due to irregular astigmatism and haze.[37,39] In a virgin cornea, PRK has also been proven to be safe, effective, and predictable in correcting hyperopia with a larger optical zone (5.0 mm) and ablation zone (9.0 mm).[40] These results have been extrapolated to the use of PRK after RK to treat hyperopia. Several studies have found that PRK can be successfully used to treat hyperopia after RK.[41] The use of PRK after RK can be a challenge and certain nuances should be noted during the procedure. When debriding the epithelium, consideration must be given to removal of epithelial cysts within the wound. One may also consider the use of a masking agent such as celluvisc if irregular astigmatism is present. LASEK, a modification of PRK, may also be an option for treating hyperopia after RK. Some studies have found that although PRK can be useful after RK, there is an increased risk of subepithelial fibrosis.[37] The use of adjunctive mitomycin-C should be considered when performing PRK over RK as it has been shown to be beneficial in preventing haze in a variety of clinical settings. MMC has been shown to be a useful adjunct in preventing post-PRK haze,[42] primary prevention of haze in high-risk surface ablation,[43] and following surface ablation over buttonholed LASIK flaps.[44] Although experience with MMC in the specific circumstance of hyperopia after RK is limited, this technique warrants further investigation.

LASIK

Laser-assisted in-situ keratomileusis (LASIK) is one of the most popular options for correcting hyperopia after RK. Several studies have found LASIK after RK to be safe and effective.[20,45] Francesconi et al, in a study of 69 eyes, found 65% to achieve an UCVA of 20/40 or better. This and other studies noted that the reduction of refractive cylinder was poor in H-LASIK after RK.[20,46]

There are risks associated with the creation of a LASIK flap in a cornea with previous RK incisions. Special notation should be made of the K readings as especially flat Ks (39.00 D to 41.00 D) increase the chance of a smaller or "free cap" microkeratome flap which leads to a smaller ablation zone and increases the risk of regression. However, it should be kept in mind that although the central curvature is flatter post-RK, the peripheral curvature is often normal. There is also the possibility for the RK incisions to rupture when building to high IOP during the suction phase.[47] Using a thicker plate on the microkeratome and use of generous lubrication when passing the microkeratome can help prevent dehiscence of the RK incisions within the LASIK flap. Careful preoperative assessment of the RK incision is important in preventing wound dehiscence. Epithelial cysts within the incisions may indicate less than adequate tensile strength and may result in splaying of the incisions during the creation of the LASIK flap. When lifting the flap, a wide spatula should be used and one should avoid grabbing the flap edge with forceps to prevent the RK incisions from opening in a pizza pie fashion. Chung et al describe a technique using a Sinskey hook to roll the flap to prevent dehiscence of the RK incisional scars (Figure 13-5).[48] Additionally efforts should be directed toward protecting the epithelium and avoiding epithelial scraping. This decreases the risk of keratocyte activation and helps to lower the incidence of corneal haze and epithelial ingrowth. This is illustrated in Figure 13-6,

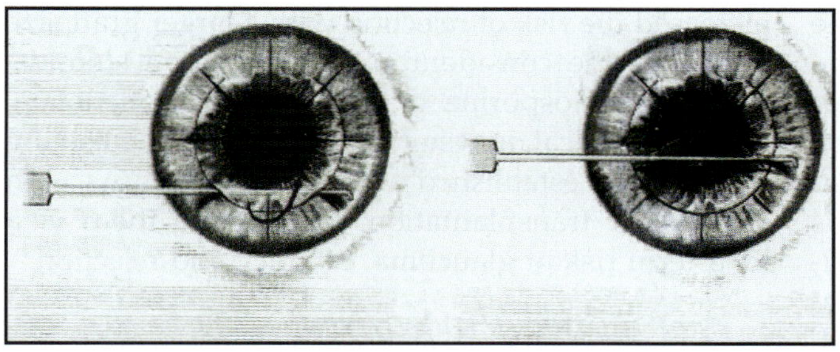

Figure 13-5. Technique to decrease risk of splaying RK incision. (Reprinted with permission from Chung MS, Pepose JS, Manche EE. Management of the corneal flap in laser in situ keratomileusis after previous radial keratotomy. *Am J Ophthalmol.* 2001;132:252-253.)

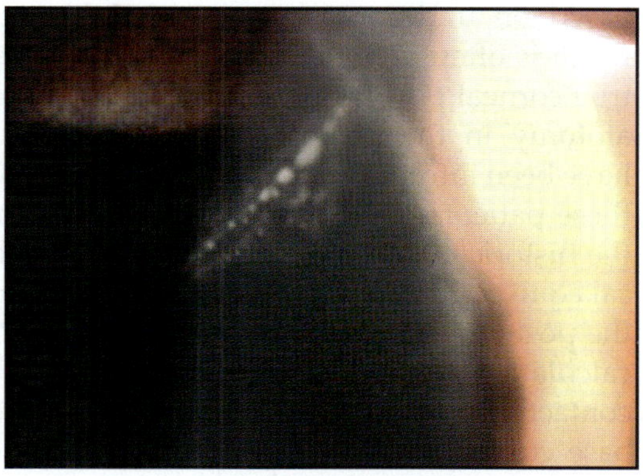

Figure 13-6. Epithelial ingrowth in the interface after LASIK for overcorrected RK (photo courtesy of Neal A. Sher, MD).

which shows epithelial ingrowth after LASIK on an eye with prior RK. At the end of the procedure when the flap is replaced, care should be taken to reconstruct the proper anatomical position of the flap so that all segments are properly aligned.[40] Postoperatively, there is a risk of epithelial ingrowth beneath the LASIK flap or through the RK incisions, risk of irregular astigmatism, and risk of further destabilization of the cornea.

Despite these increased risks, LASIK does have the advantage over PRK of faster visual recovery and less haze following the procedure. LASIK has been proven to be safe and effective for moderate hyperopia ranging from +1.00 D to +4.00 D, whereas in greater levels of hyperopia, loss of BCVA may be more likely. As with other hyperopic LASIK procedures, an initial overcorrection is preferred as the treatment will inevitably regress. Due to the added problems of lifting a post-RK LASIK flap, there is the strong possibility that the patient must be counseled "this is the last refractive procedure that they can have on their cornea."

Laser Thermal Keratoplasty and Conductive Keratoplasty

In the last several years, minimally invasive collagen shrinking procedures such as laser thermokeratoplasty (LTK) and RK have received FDA approval for the treatment of low hyperopia. LTK (Sunrise Technologies International, Fremont, Calif) uses a Holmium-YAG laser via a patented process for shrinking collagen. Two concentric rings of 8 simultaneous spots of laser energy are applied to the periphery of the cornea, resulting in increased central curvature and a myopic shift. After RK, this procedure has some degree of efficacy, but as in most uses of LTK, it has been found to have significant regression.[49] This is especially true in eyes that are more than +3.00 D hyperopic and in patients younger than 40 years old.[50] Early studies with Summit Technology's Holmium laser and the diode laser as well as Sunrise Technologies' LTK procedure all showed that due to collagen shrinkage there was a tendency for the RK incisions to become splayed apart, worsening the hyperopia.[51]

Conductive keratoplasty (CK) (Refractec, Inc., Irvine, Calif) is a collagen-shrinking procedure that uses radiofrequency energy to reshape the cornea and adjust its refractive characteristics. The probe tip serves as an RF antenna while the speculum holding the eye open serves as the return path. CK may be a viable option for some post-RK patients.[52] CK may be a better choice than LTK due to the cylindrical footprint of CK providing energy more consistently to the deep corneal stroma than the conical profile that results from LTK. This may result in less regression of effect. On a virgin cornea, the technique for CK is with a 450-µm radio frequency probe placed to 80 percent depth of the cornea. There are options to place the probe within the RK incision or adjacent to the RK incision.[53] CK has been shown to be useful in sealing gaping AK incisions, which may reduce the fluctuation in vision by decreasing the ectasia. With CK, however, there is the same potential for induced astigmatism as seen with LTK.

Refractive Lensectomy and Phakic Intraocular Lenses

Refractive lensectomy is a surgical alternative that has been shown to be successful in correcting hyperopia after RK.[50] Depending on the degree of hyperopia, it may require 1 or 2 IOLs in the capsular bag or ciliary sulcus.[49] Special care must be taken when performing IOL calculations as corneal refractive surgery of any kind, including RK and LASIK, changes the effective power of the cornea. If a lens is selected based on traditional lens calculation methods the result is often more hyperopic than expected, as the true corneal power is overestimated by manual keratotomy in the post-RK patient. Several methods have been introduced to perform IOL calculations on these patients. The most commonly used method is the historical method in which the change in spherical equivalent before and after RK is subtracted from the postoperative manual keratometry. Another IOL calculation method involves performing a RGP lens contact over-refraction. Using a RGP of a known base curve, the patient is refracted and the corneal power is estimated. Whichever method is used, selecting the highest power lens of any of the estimations often yields an accurate result.[55] Once an appropriate lens has been selected and the operation is performed, during the procedure the surgeon must pay special attention to the incision as there have been reported cases of splaying of RK incisions with cataract surgery.[56]

Phakic IOLs for hyperopia are already in use in many parts of the world and are currently being studied in FDA clinical trials in the United States. Models under current investigation include the STAAR implantable contact lens, the Ophthec (Netherlands) Artisan lens, and the CIBA Vision (Duluth, Ga) PRL. For hyperopia, the implantable lens has a relatively high vault, preventing contact with the crystalline lens to decrease the chance of secondary cataract formation. The Ophthec PMMA Artisan lens,[57] which is fixated to the anterior surface of the iris by a clip (iris-claw). It has been used in hyperopic patients and has the benefit over clear lens extraction (CLE) in preserving accommodation.[58] There is a risk of corneal edema due to endothelial damage, which may require a penetrating keratoplasty.[59]

Penetrating Keratoplasty

Penetrating keratoplasty is not a widely used technique for hyperopia following RK and is considered a last resort. Indications for hyperopic post-RK patients requiring penetrating keratoplasty include uncorrectable irregular astigmatism, ectasia, and multifocal scarring. These complications are more common with small optical zones (less than 2.75 mm) or incisions numbering greater than 16. During penetrating keratoplasty, a purse-string suture may help to stabilize the cornea prior to trephination.[59] Corneal transplantation may be necessary in cases of scarring or irregular astigmatism with small optical zones or deep and multiple incisions, all of which are risk factors for progressive hyperopia as well. Post-RK patients often require a larger graft. The increased the risk of rejection with a larger graft size mandates the consideration of long term steroids, systemic cyclosporine or systemic mycophenolate, although topical or systemic medications are usually reserved for established allograft rejection. As with all corneal transplantation procedures, there is a long-term risk of glaucoma, cataract, and rejection.

Abandoned Procedures

Other procedures that have been unsuccessful, and ultimately abandoned in the past to cure hyperopic shift following RK include hexagonal keratotomy (HK) which has unpredictable results and may lead to irregular astigmatism, hyperopic automated lamellar keratoplasty (ALK), which led to progressive corneal ectasia in 26% of eyes, and hot-needle TK, which produced focal corneal necrosis and an unstable refraction.[60] Intracorneal lenses, which often had a high index of refraction and small diameter, have not been successful in correcting hyperopia and aphakia.[61,62] Their use led to decreased quality of vision, interface scarring, and to termination of the research.

Summary

The management of hyperopia in general can be very challenging. This is especially true in the subset of patients with consecutive or progressive hyperopia following RK. As technology progresses we will have the potential to refine our current techniques, and potentially integrate wavefront analysis. As phakic IOLs are approved, they may also be an increasingly utilized option in managing hyperopia after RK. Ophthalmologists and researchers will continue to improve diagnostic and management techniques, which might enable these patients to improve their quality of life.

References

1. Bates WH. A suggestion of an operation to correct astigmatism. *Arch Ophthalmol.* 1894;23:9-13.
2. Fyodorov SN, Durnev VV. Anterior keratotomy method application with the purpose of surgical correction of myopia. In: *Pressing Problems of Ophthalmosurgery*. Moscow 1977:47-48.
3. Bores LD, Myers W, Cowden J. Radial keratotomy: An analysis of the American experience. *Ann Ophthalmol.* 1981;12:941-8.
4. Waring GO III, Lynn MJ, Nizam A et al. Results of the prospective evaluation of radial keratotomy (PERK) study five years after surgery. *Ophthalmology*. 1991:98:1164-1176.
5. Rowsey JJ, Balyeat HD, Rabinovitch B, et al. Predicting the results of radial keratotomy. *Ophthalmology*. 1983; 90:642-54.

6. Arrowsmith PN, Marks RG. Visual, refractive and keratometric results of radial keratotomy: a two-year follow up. *Arch Ophthalmol.* 1987;105:76-80.
7. Rashid ER, Waring GO. Complications of Radial and Transverse Keratotomy. *Survey of Ophthalmology.* 1989: 34(2):73-106.
8. Waring GO III, Lynn MJ, McDonnell PJ. Results of the prospective evaluation of radial keratotomy (PERK) study 10 years after surgery. *Arch Ophthalmol.* 1994;112:1298-1308.
9. Deitz MR, Sanders DR, Raanan MG. Progressive hyperopia in radial keratotomy. Long-term follow-up of the diamond-knife and metal-blade series. *Ophthalmology.* 1986; 93(10):1284-1289.
10. Mader TH, Blanton CL, Gilbert BN, et al. Refractive changes during 72-hour exposure to high altitude after refractive surgery. *Ophthalmology.* 1996;104:1188-1195.
11. Hardten DR. *Correction of progressive hyperopia after radial keratotomy.* Refractive Surgery Subspecialty Day. American Academy of Ophthalmology;2002.
12. Miyashiro MJ, Yee RW, Patel G, et al. Lasso procedure to revise overcorrection with radial keratotomy. *Am J Ophthalmology.* 1998;126:825-827.
13. Wilson SE, Klyce SD. Screening for corneal topographic abnormalities before refractive surgery. *Ophthalmology.* 1994;101:147-152.
14. Hoffer KJ, Darrin JJ, Pettit TH, et al. UCLA clinical trial of radial keratotomy; preliminary report. *Ophthalmology.* 1981;88:729-736.
15. Kemp JR, Martinez CE, Klyce SD, et al. Diurnal fluctuations in corneal topography 10 years after radial keratotomy in the prospective evaluation of radial keratotomy study. *J Cataract Refract Surg.* 1999;25:904-910.
16. Schanzlin DJ, Santos VR, WaringGO III, et al. Diurnal change in refraction, corneal curvature, visual acuity and intraocular pressure after radial keratotomy in the PERK study. *Ophthalmology.* 1986;93:167-175.
17. Laranjera E, Buzard KA. Pilocarpine in the management of overcorrection after radial keratotomy. *J Refract Surg.* 1996;12:382-390.
18. Shivitz IA. Arrowsmith PN. Corneal sensitivity after radial keratotomy. *Ophthalmology.* 1988;95(6):827-32.
19. Nelson JD, Williams P, Lindstrom RL, et al. Map-finger-dot changes in the corneal epithelium basement membrane following radial keratotomy. *Ophthalmology.* 1985;92:199-205.
20. Francesconi CM, Nose RAM, Nose W. Hyperopic Laser-assisted in situ keratomileusis for radial keratotomy-induced hyperopia. *Ophthalmology.* 2002;109:602-605.
21. Kwitko S, Gritz DC, Garbus JJ, et al. Diurnal variation of corneal topography after radial keratotomy. *Arch Ophthalmol.* 1992;110:351-356.
22. Alpins NA. Wavefront technology: a new advance that fails to answer old questions on corneal vs. refractive astigmatism correction. *J Refract Surg.* 2002;18(6):737-9.
23. Nagy ZZ, Palagyi-Deak I, Kovacs A, Kelemen E, Forster W. First results with wavefront-guided photorefractive keratectomy for hyperopia. *J Refract Surg.* 2002;18(5):S620-3.
24. Wyzinski P, O'Dell LW. Diurnal cycle of refraction after radial keratotomy. *Ophthalmol.* 1987;94:120-124.
25. Santos VR, Waring GO III, Lynn MJ, et al. Morning to evening change in refraction, corneal curvature and visual acuity 2 to 4 years after radial keratotomy in the PERK study. *Ophthalmol.* 1988;95:1487-1493.
26. MacRae S, Rich L, Phillips D, Bedrossian R. Diurnal variation in vision after radial keratotomy. *Am J Ophthalmol.* 1989; 107:262-267.
27. Zadnik K. Contact lens management of patients who have had unsuccessful refractive surgery. *Curr Opin Ophthalmol.* 1999;10(4):260-3.
28. Wilhelmus KR, Hamburg S. Bacterial keratitis following radial keratotomy. *Cornea.* 1983;2:143-146.
29. Damiano RE, Forstot SL. Extreme corneal flattening after radial keratotomy. [Letter]. *Am J Ophthalmol.* 1991;112(6):738.
30. Hofmann RF, Starling JC, Masler W. Contact fitting after radial keratotomy: one year results. *J Refract Surg.* 1986;2:155-162.
31. Lim L, Siow KL, Sakamoto R, Chong JS, Tan DT. Reverse geometry contact lens wear after photorefractive keratectomy, radial keratotomy, or penetrating keratoplasty. *Cornea.* 2000;19(3):320-4.
32. Lindquist TD, Williams PA, Lindstrom RL. Surgical treatment of overcorrection following radial keratotomy: evaluation of clinical effectiveness. *Ophthalmic Surg.* 1991;22:12-15.
33. Hoffman RF. Reoperations after radial keratotomy and astigmatic keratotomy. *J Refract Surg.* 1987;3:119-128.
34. Grene RB. Use of the Grene lasso following radial keratotomy. *Rev Ophthalmol.* 1996;11:31-42.
35. Miyashiro MJ, Yee RW, Patel G, Karas Y, Grene RB. Lasso procedure to revise overcorrection with radial keratotomy *Am J Ophthalmol.* 1998;126(6):825-7.
36. Manche EE, Judge A, Maloney RK. Lamellar keratoplasty for hyperopia. *J Refract Surg.* 1996;12: 42-9.
37. Burnstein Y, Hersh PS. Photorefractive keratectomy following radial keratotomy. *J Refract Surg.*1996;12(1):163-70.
38. Probst LE, Machat JJ. Conservative photorefractive keratectomy for residual myopia following radial keratotomy. *Can J Ophthalmol.* 1988;33(1):20-7.
39. Maloney RK, Chan WK, Steinert R, et al. A multicenter trial of photorefractive keratectomy for residual myopia after previous ocular surgery. *Ophthalmology.* 1995;102: 1042-1052.
40. Jackson WB, Casson E, Hodge WG, et al. Laser vision correction for low hyperopia; an 18 month assessment of safety and efficacy. *Ophthalmology.* 1998; 105:1727-1737.
41. Venter JA. Photorefractive keratectomy for hyperopia after radial keratotomy. *J Refract Surg.* 1997;13(5 Suppl):S456.

42. Majmudar PA, Forstot SL, Dennis RF, et al. Topical Mintomycin-C for sub epithelial fibrosis after refractive corneal surgery. *Ophthalmology*. 2000;107:89-94.

43. Carones F, Vigo L, Scandola E, Vacchini L. Evaluation of the prophylactic use of Mitomycin-C to inhibit haze formation after photorefractive keratectomy. *J Cataract Refract Surg*. 2002;28:2088-2095.

44. Lane HA, Swale JA, Majmudar PA. Prophylactic use of Mitomycin-C in the management of a buttonholed LASIK flap. *J Cataract Refract Surg*. 2003; 29:000.

45. Clausse MA, Boutros G, Khanjian G, Wagner C, Garabet AL. A retrospective study of laser in situ keratomileusis after radial keratotomy. *J Refract Surg*. 2001;17(2 Suppl):S200-1.

46. Buzard KA, Fundingsland BR. Excimer laser assisted in situ keratomileusis of hyperopia. *J Cataract Refract Surg*. 1999;25:197-204.

47. Lipshitz I, Man O, Shemesh G, Lazar M, Loewenstein A. Laser in situ keratomileusis to correct hyperopic shift after radial keratotomy. *J Cataract Refract Surg*. 2001;27:273-276.

48. Chung MS, Pepose JS, Manche EE. Management of the corneal flap in laser in situ keratomileusis after previous radial keratotomy. *Am J Ophthalmol*. 2001;132:252-253.

49. Eggink CA, Meurs P, Bardak Y, Deutman AF. Holmium laser thermal keratoplasty for hyperopia and astigmatism after photorefractive keratectomy. *J Refract Surg*. 2000;16(3):317-22.

50. Nano HD, Muzzin S. Noncontact Holmium-YAG laser thermal keratoplasty for hyperopia. *J Cataract Refract Surg*. 1998;24:751-757.

51. Gore C, Rosen ES. Overcorrected radial keratotomy treated with posterior chamber phakic intraocular lens and laser thermal keratoplasty. *J Refract Surg*. 1999;15(6):683-6.

52. Haw WW, Manche EE. Conductive keratoplasty and laser thermal keratoplasty. *Int Ophthalmol Clin*. 2002 Fall;42(4):99-106.

53. McDonald M. CK after RK. AAO *Refractive Surgery Discussion Group*. 2002.

54. Siganos DS, Pallikaris IG. Clear lensectomy and intraocular lens implantation for hyperopia from +7 to +14 diopters. *J Refract Surg*. 1998;14:105-113.

55. Speicher L. Intraocular lens calculation status after corneal refractive surgery. *Curr Opin Ophthalmol*. 2001;12(1):17-29.

56. Chen L, Mannis MJ, Salz JJ, et al. Analysis of intraocular lens power calculation in post-RK eyes. *J Cataract Refract Surg*. 2003;29:65-70.

57. Pesado PM, Ghiringhello MP, Tagliavacche P. Posterior chamber collamer phakic intraocular lens for myopia and hyperopia. *J Refract Surg*. 1999;15:415-423.

58. Fechner PU, Singh D, Wulff K. Iris-claw in phakic eyes to correct hyperopia. Preliminary study. *J Cataract Refract Surg*. 1998;24:48-56.

59. Sanders DR, Martin RG, Brown DC, Shepherd J, Deitz MR, DeLuca M. Posterior chamber phakic intraocular lens for hyperopia. *J Refract Surg*. 1999;15:309-315.

60. McNeill JI, Wilkins DL. A purse-string suture for penetrating keratoplasty following radial keratotomy. *Refractive & Corneal Surgery*. 1991;7(5):392-4.

61. Steinert RF, Storie B, Smith P, et al. Hydrogen intracorneal lenses in aphakic eyes. *Arch Ophthalmol*. 1996;114:135-141.

62. Waring GO. A cautionary tale of innovation in refractive surgery. *Arch Ophthalmol*. 1999;117:1069-1073.

Chapter Fourteen

Management of Residual Hyperopia After Myopic LASIK and PRK

Neal A. Sher, MD, FACS

Introduction

Residual or consecutive hyperopia after attempted myopic correction can be a difficult clinical problem leading to patient dissatisfaction. The management of this overcorrection can be more problematic than the treatment of residual myopia.

Etiology of Overcorrection

Because there are multiple causes, determining the precise factors that lead to overcorrection is important in preventing it. It is especially critical for the surgeon to rule out laser calibration errors as well as environmental factors such as humidity. These may lead to multiple cases of overcorrection operated on the same day or within a short period of time.

Laser Calibration

Calibration issues are critical to the outcome of a laser ablation procedure. There has been a marked improvement in the reliability and accuracy of excimer lasers in the last decade. Despite that, it is important to check the laser ablation rate prior to surgery.

Torres, Ang, and Azar recently reviewed the issue of excimer laser calibration.[1] Calibration methods are based on measurement of energy (energy models) or measurement of ablation (ablation models). Energy models use direct measurement of the energy output of the laser with meters, which is accurate only with ±25% due to the extraordinarily high output of lasers.

Furthermore, meter calibration requires sophisticated equipment. For these reasons, the ablation models, which include the ablation of Wratten (Kodak, Rochester, NY) filters, PMMA blanks, and scanning profilometry are used most frequently.

The VISX (Santa Clara, Calif) laser is calibrated by the preoperative ablation of a standardized PMMA sheet of plastic. The laser is programmed to ablate a myopic lens, which is then read in a lensometer. The readouts are then fed back into the calibration program and the fluence is adjusted accordingly.

The Chiron-Technolas (Bausch & Lomb, Rochester, NY) laser is reprogrammed after ablating a special foil and determining how may pulses are needed to perforate one layer. The Coherent-Schwind laser uses a gelatin film for calibration.[1]

The surgeon should be especially careful after any change of optics or other mechanical overhauls of the laser. Increased throughput of laser energy has been known to cause overcorrections. This is made particularly distressing with the common use of bilateral simultaneous surgery.

Ablation algorithms in broad beam lasers depend upon the even distribution of laser energy across the beam diameter. The presence of hot or cold spots within this distribution can lead to uneven ablation patterns and the inducement of irregular astigmatism, central islands, under- and overcorrections, and other unpredictable findings. The causes of this include degradation of laser optics as well as interference with the beam itself. The latter can be caused by blockage from the laser plume of subsequent pulses of laser energy.

The shift to scanning lasers or rasterization of a smaller beam laser has made a significant improvement in preventing the sequelae from a lack of homogeneous energy distribution.

Environmental Issues

The normal thickness and transparency of the cornea depends on its relative hydration. In a recent study,[2] patients who had LASIK with temperature levels between 25.1 ± 1.4°C and humidity levels between 45.1 ± 4.2% had better refractive results on the 15th day after surgery. It is extremely important to control humidity and temperature in the laser suite. Each manufacturer has humidity and temperature recommendations. In general, humidity from 30% to 40% and temperatures of 65 to 72°F are ideal. At the Phillips Eye Institute, the facility in which I do my procedures, the following type of system was created to modulate the humidity and temperature extremes seen in our geographic region.

The air handling unit is a constant volume system that re-circulates air within the room and brings in a minimum amount of outside air. The unit has a 30% pre-filter and a 95% final filter to eliminate dust and dirt particles. It is also equipped with a humidifier and a dehumidification cycle. There is a thermostat and a humidistat in the space to control the temperature and humidity levels. The following describes the sequence on a call for humidification or dehumidification.

Humidification

When the humidistat calls for humidification, a control valve opens and allows low pressure steam to flow to a steam wand located in the ductwork. As the humidity level in the space rises, the control valve modulates until the humidistat closes the valve.

Dehumidification

When the humidistat calls for dehumidification, the cooling comes on and removes moisture as the air passes over the cooling coil. An electric reheat coil that is installed in the ductwork heats the air back up as required to maintain the space temperature. After the humidity level drops to the humidity set point, the cooling shuts off. The electric duct coil will continue to operate as needed to maintain the space temperature.

Nomograms

It is important for each surgeon to develop a nomogram to improve the accuracy and quality of surgical outcomes and prevent overcorrections.

There are several commercially available database programs, which will develop a nomogram for the surgeon. These include products by Jack Holladay, MD, and Guy Kezarian, MD, (www.refractiveconsultants.com), and by Perry Binder, MD (Outcome Analysis Software, LASIKsupport@aol.com).

Despite large advances in manufacturing, each excimer laser—even the same model by the same manufacturer—should be considered unique and efforts made to determine refractive outcomes on a small number of eyes before using the laser on a wider group of patients.

When to Consider Retreatment

Retreatment can be considered when the patient is dissatisfied due to the presence of residual refractive error or induced refractive error. The necessity for treatment depends on a number of factors and is influenced by subjective factors such as patient expectations and demands. The patient's age and residual accommodative capacity are significant factors in determining which patients to retreat.

Retreatment using medical modalities can be done very early in the postoperative course, usually within the first month. Surgical modalities need to wait until refractive stability is obtained. One rule of thumb suggests waiting 1 month per diopter of attempted correction with a minimum of 4 to 6 months for any surgical retreatment. This guideline should be tempered by the clinical situation. In general, retreatments for under correction and residual myopia can be done earlier than for induced hyperopia.

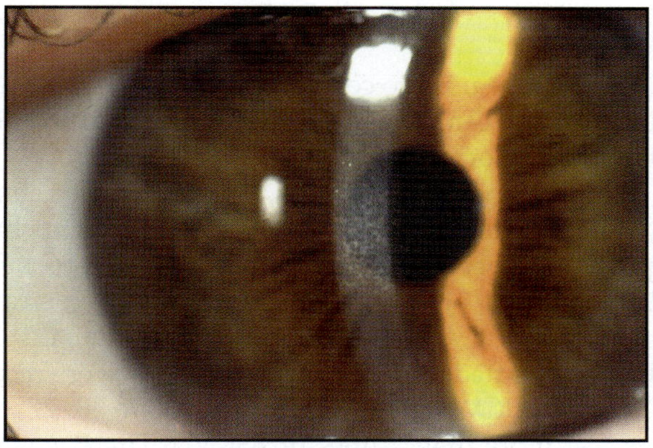

Figure 14-1. Corneal haze 8 weeks post-PRK Grade 2 to 3.

Treatment of Overcorections After PRK and LASEK

Healing Patterns

To better understand the healing process after PRK and possibly LASEK, a simple classification of healing patterns has been described. Durrie describes 3 basic healing patterns after excimer PRK for myopia differentiated by the amount of subepithelial haze.[3] This classification, although overly simplified, is useful in understanding the healing process.[4] It represented the healing patterns of the earlier generation of excimer lasers that did not have scanning technology. These lasers produced more overcorrection. Despite this, the classification still has some value.

Type I healing is observed in over 90% of eyes. These eyes have an initial hyperopic overcorrection and then a gradual regression toward emmetropia. The hyperopic overshoot is dependent on a number of factors including laser type, patient age, attempted correction, beam diameter, corneal hydration and a number of other variables. There is a minimal haze, which peaks at 3 months after surgery.

For the overwhelming majority of patients who have Type I healing patterns, a tapering regimen of 0.1% fluorometholone, beginning at QID and dropping down each 3 or 4 weeks until discontinued in the third or fourth month. The IOP should be monitored. As discussed above, topical corticosteroids after the first week may not be needed at all after epithelial healing in the lower myopic corrections.

Type II healing is associated with a minimal healing response. The usual hyperopic overshoot does not regress. Patients typically have manifest refraction +1.00 D to +2.00 D at one month. This may be even higher in larger attempted corrections. There is an absence of corneal haze. If the refractive error is 1.00 D more hyperopic than predicted outcome at the one month visit, and there is minimal or no corneal haze, steroids should be quickly tapered and discontinued over the next 2 to 4 weeks.

Type III healers have an over aggressive healing response with significant corneal haze at 1 to 3 months and regression of the refractive correction (Figure 14-1). These patients typically end up undercorrected and with corneal haze or scarring.

Early Treatment of Overcorrections After PRK and LASEK

The easiest way to adjust PRK or LASEK outcomes is to alter the corticosteroid taper. The healing pattern should be determined as described above. Corticosteroids can be tapered quickly for an over correction. I personally prefer the contact lens-assisted pharmacologically induced kerato steepening (CLAPIKs) technique described by Dr. Jay MacDonald in detail in Chapter 15. This requires the use of a tight-fitting soft contact lens worn continuously with the use of topical ketorolac. Any of these techniques require close follow-up of the patient.

Late Treatment of Overcorrections After PRK and LASEK

Surface Ablation

Retreatment using surface ablation for overcorrection after prior PRK is possible but presents the surgeon with significant challenges. Early indications show that LASEK can be repeated in a similar manner but raising an epithelial flap after prior LASEK would be challenging. PRK can be repeated. However, hyperopic photoreactive keratotomy (H-PRK), requires a large optical zone, up to 9 mm, and a large epithelial defect with a prolonged healing time. There is a significant risk of inducing corneal haze as the keratocytes in the ablated cornea remain activated for many months after prior PRK. One should consider the use of 0.02% mitomycin C, as proposed by Majmudar et al, to reduce the risks of corneal haze and irregular astigmatism.[5]

The use of LASIK after prior PRK does not present the haze risk of PRK after prior LASIK. The standard prerequisites for LASIK still exist, with special care regarding residual bed thickness. In a series of 36 eyes treated with LASIK that had undergone prior PRK, only two developed any significant haze.[6]

Conductive Keratoplasty

Conductive keratoplasty (CK) is a radiofrequency-based technique for steepening the central cornea to reduce low to moderate hyperopia. Comaish and Lawless[7] followed 4 patients for at least 6 months after they had CK to correct hyperopia after LASIK. There was an overcorrection noted after the CK procedure in all patients, but no sight-threatening complications. They concluded that the CK algorithm needed to be refined. In another small series,[8] Gomez presented a series of patients who underwent CK to correct residual hyperopia after prior LASIK, PRK, or laser thermokeratoplasty (LTK). The results were mixed. More recently, surgeons have been having better success with CK after LASIK for consecutive hyperopia. Dr. Jonathan Davidorf and Dr. Forrest P. Murphy have demonstrated that CK can safely reduce hyperopia in these eyes. There was a consensus that the amount of energy applied should be cut back by approximately one-third. For example, if two rings of 8 mm are indicated in the nomogram, one ring should be applied. Theoretically uneven shrinkage of the LASIK flap—near the edge—may result in irregular astigmatism or even ingrowth. Flap problems such as edge lift or ingrowth have not been described in the limited number of cases performed to date (personal communication, Dr. J. Davidorf and Dr. F. Murphy, March 2003). It is not known what the minimum interval of time after the primary LASIK procedure is before the CK procedure.

Holmium LTK, using a contact method and the Technomed Holmium-YAG laser (Holmium 25, Technomed, Baeswller, Germany) has been evaluated. The laser uses a probe with an optic fiber (diameter 55 μm) to make contact with the cornea to produce a thermal effect. Eggink et al[9] used this device to treat 16 eyes for hyperopia or astigmatism after prior PRK. The procedure did not produce much effect at 9-mm diameter treatment zone and mild to moderate effect at an 8-mm zone. The follow up was 11 months.

LTK (formerly Sunrise Technologies, Fremont, Calif) has been advocated for the treatment of hyperopia after myopic surgery or as a primary technique.[10] Anecdotal reports have shown unpredictability and overcorrection. This technique has been largely abandoned.

LASIK

LASIK can be used to correct consecutive hyperopia. Retreatment can sometimes be done by lifting the flap and performing a hyperopic ablation.

This may not be possible in the presence of a small LASIK flap. In one study,[11] 54 eyes of 47 patients had spherical hyperopic LASIK by multiple surgeons for the treatment of significant consecutive hyperopia after myopic LASIK. In 42 eyes, the initial LASIK flaps were lifted and in 12 eyes, the flaps were recut. The mean UCVA improved from 20/38 to 20/27. No eye lost more than 2 lines of BSCVA. There was no difference in patients who had lifts versus recuts. There was a tendency toward overcorrection.

Mulhern, Condon, and O'Keefe reported on 17 eyes undergoing LASIK for consecutive hyperopia.[12] The results were also satisfactory and stable. Interface haze was minimal. Occasional epithelial cells nests were noted. A peripheral scar was noticed at the margins of the flap in some eyes. Progressive ectasia was noted in one patient. In another study, Rojas, Haw, and Manche[13] reported on 36 eyes of 30 patients with consecutive hyperopia after myopic LASIK that underwent retreatment. No eye lost 2 or more lines of BSCVA. One eye developed DLK, which resolved without serious sequelae. Two eyes developed epithelial ingrowth that did not require intervention. The location of the hinge and axis is important in planning the retreatment. If a treatment is performed with inadequate bed size, astigmatism can be induced.

There are significant risks in recutting a flap, even after 12 months. The biggest problem with recutting a flap (either for myopic or hyperopic correction) is the dislodgement of a sliver of corneal tissue. This small piece of tissue may be displaced during the keratome pass. It represents tissue between the "healed" original cut and the new cut. It may be impossible to replace and cause irregular astigmatism. Figure 14-2 shows a "sliver" of tissue after a recut enhancement seven months after the original surgery. This required a flap lift in an effort to smooth the dislodged tissue.

Summary

Consecutive hyperopia after attempted myopic correction is a difficult clinical problem leading to patient dissatisfaction. Fortunately, a number of modalities including pharmacologic modification, hyperopic LASIK, PRK, and conductive keratoplasty offer relief for these distressed patients.

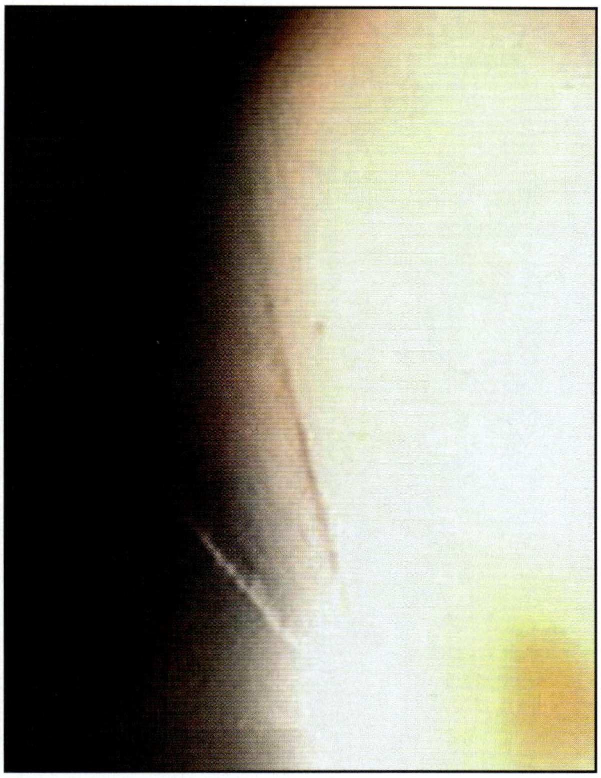

Figure 14-2. LASIK recut enhancement with lamellar "sliver" dislodged after keratome passed. When present in visual axis, these slivers can cause irregular astigmatism (photo courtesy of Neal A. Sher, MD).

References

1. Torres R, Ang RT, Azar DT. Lasers in LASIK: basic aspects. In: Azar DT and Koch DD, eds. *LASIK Fundamentals, Surgical Techniques, and Complications*. New York: Marcel Dekker, Inc; 2002:52.
2. de Souza IR, de Souza AP. Influence of temperature and humidity on laser in situ keratomileusis outcomes. *J Refractive Surgery*. 2001;17(supplement): S202-S204.
3. Durrie DS, Lesher MP, Cavanaugh TB. Classification of variable clinical response after photorefractive keratectomy for myopia. *J Refract Surg*. 1995;11(5),341-7.
4. Sher NA. Postoperative care of the PRK patient: Focal point module. *American Academy of Ophthalmology*. December 1998.
5. Majmudar PA, Forstot SL, Nirankari VS, et al. Topical mitomycin-C for subepithelial fibrosis after refractive corneal surgery. *Ophthalmology*. 107:89-94,2000.
6. Lazaro C, Castillo A, Hernandez-Matamoros JL, et al. Laser in situ keratomileusis enhancement after photorefractive keratectomy. *Ophthalmology*. 2001 Aug;108(8):1423-9.
7. Comaish IF, Lawless MA. Conductive keratoplasty to correct residual hyperopia after corneal surgery. *J Cataract Refract Surg*. 2003;29(1):202-6.
8. Gomez, J. *Eurotimes*. Originally presented at Sixth Winter Refractive Surgery Meeting of the ESCRS, Barcelona Spain, 2002.
9. Eggink CA, Meurs P, Bardak Y, Deutman AF. Holmium laser thermal keratoplasty for hyperopia and astigmatism after photorefractive keratectomy. *J Refract Surg*. 2000;16:317-322.
10. Koch DD, Kohnen T, McDonnell PJ, Menefee R, Berry M. Hyperopia correction by noncontact Holmium-YAG laser thermal keratoplasty: US phase IIA clinical study with 2-year follow-up. *Ophthalmology*. 1997 Nov;104(11):1938-47.
11. Jacobs JM, Sanderson MC, Spivack LD, et al. Hyperopic laser in-situ keratomileusis to treat overcorrected myopic LASIK. *J Cataract Refract Surg*. 2001;27:389-395.
12. Mulhern MG, Condon PI, O'Keefe M. Myopic and hyperopic laser in-situ keratomileusis retreatments. Indications, techniques, limitations, and results. *J Cataract Refract Surg*. 2001;27:1278-1287.
13. Rojas MC, Haw WW, Manche EE. Laser in-situ keratomileusis enhancement for consecutive hyperopia after myopic Overcorrection. *J Cataract Refract Surg*. 2002;28: 37-43.

Chapter Fifteen

Contact Lens-Assisted Pharmacologically Induced Keratoshaping

J.E. "Jay" McDonald II, MD; Allyson Mertins, OD; and David Deitz, Research Assistant

Introduction

Even the most successful refractive surgeons have patients who experience hyperopia following excimer laser procedures. Until recently, a hyperopic enhancement was the only option to restore emmetropia. Surgical outcomes with hyperopic enhancements for undercorrected hyperopia or consecutive myopia are not as predictable as surgical outcomes with primary hyperopic excimer laser surgery.[1,2] The previous chapter by Dr. Sher points out some of the modalities used to treat hyperopia following excimer laser procedures and some of the pitfalls. Thus, there has not existed a consistent mode of treatment for consecutive hyperopia.

Contact lens-assisted pharmacologically induced keratoshaping (CLAPIKS) is rapidly becoming a very effective tool in the management of consecutive hyperopia. This non-surgical approach involves changing the corneal contour with a steep contact lens worn on an extended wear schedule used in conjunction with a nonsteroidal anti-inflammatory drug (NSAID). Although not 100% effective, CLAPIKS provides the refractive surgeon with a tool other than excimer laser enhancement to permanently titrate the refractive status to the desired level. In the authors' experience, patients are generally more receptive to this non-surgical approach than to additional surgical intervention.

CLAPIKS has many applications. In addition to helping overcorrected myopes and undercorrected hyperopes, it can be used to fine tune monovision, and "reverse CLAPIKS" can be used in the overcorrected hyperope or undercorrected myope.

Historical Review

In the earliest days of PRK, increasing or decreasing steroid drops in the early postoperative period was utilized to titrate over or undercorrection. The ability to induce changes in overcorrected LASIK patients without the use of contact lenses was first brought to attention by Dr. Tal Raviv. Raviv used an NSAID in postoperative excimer laser patients to induce a myopic refractive shift and experienced very good results (American Society of Cataract and Refractive Surgery, 1999).

Cognizant of the success Raviv experienced with his patients, and in order to satisfy our patients' desire for instant relief, we began to combine the use of the NSAID with a soft disposable contact lens (CTL). Our success in early reversal was consistent with Tal Raviv's results.

The author attended the International Society of Refractive Surgery in 1999 and heard a talk by Henry Edelhauser, PhD, on the ability of NSAIDS to cause morphologic changes in the cornea stroma. Edelhauser showed that an NSAID (he used diclofenac sodium 0.1% (Voltaren, CibaVision, Duluth, Ga) was able to induce not only pleomorphic changes in the basal epithelial cells but a thickening of the anterior stroma of over 50 μm. However, these changes only occurred when the superficial epithelium was removed. When the NSAID was applied to an intact corneal epithelium, it did not penetrate to induce any remarkable anatomical changes in either the epithelium or the anterior stroma. The author then realized that the contact lens could serve a dual purpose: molding the cornea (his original intent for adding the CTL to the regimen) and possibly altering the epithelial barrier. Obviously, removing the epithelium to increase penetration was not an option, but using a tight-fitting, continuous wear CTL might work. This compromise of the epithelial barrier allows the NSAID to reach its target tissue.

Impairment of The Epithelial Barrier

There are several factors associated with the CTL fit that would assist in breaking down the tight junctional complexes that form the epithelial barrier. For this technique to work, the CTL must possess three essential properties: tight-fitting (steep), low dk/L value, and overnight, uninterrupted wear. Minimal lens movement achieved with a tight-fitting lens, the low dk/L value of the CTL, and the use of an extended wear regimen all induce prolonged hypoxia.[3-5] This hypoxia leads to a chronic inhibition of epithelial metabolism, which in turn increases the penetration of the epithelial barrier. Extended wear use has been associated with a decreased rate of mitosis and a decrease in desmosomal connections between epithelial cells. This has been shown to also increase drug penetration.[6]

Alternative Explanations for Refractive Shifts

It can be argued that emmetropization would have taken place naturally without intervention, particularly in the undercorrected hyperope. This argument is particularly strong for patients that are treated at 1 to 2 weeks postoperatively. The authors do not have any controls, as most cases were unilateral, and all patients with a significant refractive error desired treatment. We found it difficult to convince a patient to sit idly when vision was compromised. Several patients were treated outside of the 3-month time frame when "normal" postoperative refractive transitions typically occur, refuting the argument for natural progression.[7,8]

It can also be argued that the CTL itself induced the refractive shift. This has been described as "myopic creep" associated with low dk/L CTL worn on an extended wear basis. The refractive change is secondary to corneal hypoxia that causes a change in the posterior corneal curvature. It is typically seen in extended wear, low dk/L lenses, but does not appear in the new high dk/L silicone hydrogels.[9] However, this phenomenon is typically associated with patients who use CTLs on an extended wear basis for many years; most CLAPIKS patients show a refractive effect within a few weeks of initiating treatment. Also, this myopic progression seen with extended wear contact lenses appears to be reversible with removal of the contact lens; almost all CLAPIKS patients retain the refractive effect upon cessation of lens wear.[10]

Morphologic changes in CLAPIKS may take place at the stromal level, as suggested by the work of Edelhauser. However, there is also the possibility that changes take place at the epithelial level. It is well known that compensatory hyperplasia of the corneal epithelium is a contributory factor in refractive regression after excimer laser photoablation.[11] Studies were initially done on photorefractive keratectomy (PRK) eyes, and there are additional studies that demonstrate the same hyperplasia in laser-assisted in-situ keratomileusis (LASIK) eyes.[12] It has been suggested that after lamellar refractive surgery the epithelium appears to possess the ability to remodel itself to compensate for stromal surface abnormalities caused by either flap irregularity or irregular stromal resection.[13] Small ablation zones, greater attempted corrections, and deeper ablations are all factors associated with an increase in epithelial thickness and corresponding increase in myopic refractive error.[14] Hyperplasia has been successfully modulated postoperatively with the use of steroids. It could also be that epithelial hyperplasia is the etiology of the morphological changes seen in CLAPIKS. Perhaps the NSAID somehow enhances this hyperplasia at the epithelial level. However, the course of hyperplasia over time refutes, for some cases, this theory. In cases of hyperplasia, the epithelium shows a tendency toward hyperplasia starting from the first day, increasing up to the third month postoperatively and subsequently stable.[15] The authors have achieved statistically significant refractive shifts well after 3 months postoperatively. Also, patients who experience epithelial hyperplasia after PRK or LASIK demonstrate a significant increase of myopia within weeks of surgery that progressively increases; our patients demonstrate a hyperopic refractive error that shifts toward emmetropia. Perhaps the process is the same; further studies need to be done to delineate the level of change.

Table 15-1

Contact Lens Options for CLAPIKS

Low dk/L Contact Lenses	*Manufacturer*	*Base Curve for CLAPIKS (Reverse CLAPIKS)*
Acuvue	Johnson and Johnson, New Brunswick, NJ	8.4 (8.8)
Acuvue 2	Johnson and Johnson	8.3 (8.7)
Optima FW	Bausch & Lomb	8.4 (9.0)
Focus 1-2 week	Ciba Vision	8.4 (8.8)

Additional Applications

The fact that the process is almost as successful in post-LASIK patients where the epithelium is not exposed to "raw stroma" suggests that the process may take place entirely in the stroma. We started CLAPIKS on postoperative excimer laser patients, and the results were statistically significant. We then tried CLAPIKS on postoperative radial keratotomy and astigmatic keratotomy patients, but were not nearly as successful and the results were not statistically significant. We also tried CLAPIKS on low hyperopes with no prior history of refractive surgery, and again, there was little success. Most likely, the cornea must require some type of prior insult to the stromal tissue before CLAPIKS can result in any shift in refractive error.

Current Technique

CLAPIKS can be initiated at any time after the 1-week postoperative visit. It is usually initiated when there is a significant difference in the postoperative refraction and the intended refraction, and/or when the patient is unhappy with the visual outcome. For example, a postoperative myopic LASIK patient with a goal of plano that refracts +2.00 with an uncorrected visual acuity of 20/70, or a postoperative myopic LASIK patient with a goal of -1.50 that refracts plano with an uncorrected near visual acuity of J10 would warrant treatment. However, a postoperative myopic LASIK patient with a goal of plano that refracts +0.50 with an uncorrected visual acuity of 20/25 would not necessarily be started on CLAPIKS if early in the postoperative period. The clinician should use his or her judgment as to when treatment should be initiated. The authors have initiated treatment as far as 18 months postoperative with statistically significant results.

A soft disposable CTL with a steep base curve (8.4 or steeper) is fit on an extended wear schedule. A relatively low dk/L value is preferred, as oxygen deprivation is desirable to compromise the epithelial barrier (Table 15-1). Lenses such as Ciba Vision (Duluth, Ga) Focus Night and Day that provide a high dk/L should be avoided. Most soft disposable CTLs only offer a few base curves, the steepest possible should be chosen. A slight amount of movement is desirable. If the lens appears to have no movement whatsoever, the patient should be monitored very closely for the first few days. The lens should cover the limbus 360 degrees.

Baseline pre-treatment measurements should include uncorrected visual acuity at distance and near, manifest refraction, corneal topography, and slit lamp examination. A contact lens with the desired prescription is inserted and inspected for adequate movement. The patient is instructed to use Keratolac tromethamine 0.50% (Acular, Allergan, Irvine, Calif) QID. Preservative-free artificial tears may be used as needed for dryness.

Follow-up visits should be at 7- to 10-day intervals. The CTL is removed and discarded. Uncorrected visual acuities at distance and near are measured, and manifest refraction and slit lamp examination is performed. Corneal topography may be obtained, as the surgeon deems necessary. A new CTL in the desired prescription is inserted, and Acular may be continued four times daily. If there has not been any change in the uncorrected visual acuity (UCVA) or manifest refraction, Acular may be increased to 6 times daily.

The patient is seen at 1-week intervals until the desired refractive error is obtained. At this point, the CTLs and Acular are continued for 10 days to 2 weeks to prevent regression. The patient may return to the office to have the CTL removed, or may remove the lens themselves if comfortable doing so. Acular is stopped when the CTL is discontinued (Figure 15-1).

The patient is reassessed 2 weeks after treatment has stopped to ascertain stability. Post-treatment measurements should include uncorrected visual acuity at distance and near, manifest refraction, corneal topography, and slit lamp examination. If the patient is stable, the surgeon can consider CLAPIKS to have been successful and see the patient for annual examination.

Autorefraction may be used in addition to manifest refraction to assess stability and ensure reliability. This is particularly useful when the ophthalmologist will not be doing the refraction, as there can be variation between technicians.

The Astigmatic Patient

When a patient refracts greater than 1.00 D of cylinder, CLAPIKS should not be attempted. The risk of inducing irregular astigmatism or higher order aberrations is considered to be too great at this time. Patients that exhibit less than 1.00 D of cylinder may be treated with a spherical equivalent lens. Toric lenses are not recommended. Toric lenses have been shown to change the shape of the cornea and reversibly alter refractive error, which would affect measurements. Also, if a toric lens rotates off axis, the reshaping of the cornea could result in inducement of higher order aberrations.

The Typical Patient

Most patients will take an average of 2 weeks to show any effect, either in UCVA or manifest refraction. Do not give up if there is not any change for the first few visits.

Due to the NSAID, most patients are able to tolerate CLAPIKS with no discomfort. Even patients that could never wear CTLs due to dry eye irritation are able to do CLAPIKS comfortably. It is important to counsel these patients as they may be reluctant to try CLAPIKS due to past history with CTLs, particularly extended wear.

The Atypical Patient

When there is no change in manifest refraction or uncorrected visual acuity after a few weeks of treatment, Acular can be increased to 6 times per day. If there is no effect after a few weeks of using Acular 6 times per day, the treatment should be considered unsuccessful and stopped.

Occasionally, a patient will experience dry eye symptoms, most often noted in the morning upon awakening. This can be solved by increasing the use of preservative-free artificial tears, preservative-free gels at bedtime, and/or punctal occlusion. The authors have only had one patient discontinue CLAPIKS due to ocular discomfort.

Improvement in Acuity Without Corresponding Improvement in Refraction

It is not uncommon to achieve an increase in visual acuity without the expected change in manifest refraction. For example, a patient may start with manifest refraction of +1.25 D, UCVA of 20/50. The follow-up visit may yield UCVA of 20/30 with no change in manifest refraction. When this occurs, treatment should be continued with no change in contact lens power. The authors propose the treatment procedure itself could aid in the cornea surface "smoothing" with elimination of higher order optical aberrations.

Reverse CLAPIKS

"Reverse CLAPIKS" can be used to flatten the cornea and induce a hyperopic shift. This can be useful in fine tuning the overcorrected hyperope or the undercorrected myope. The process is identical as that used for CLAPIKS with 1 exception: a CTL with a flat base curve (8.7 or flatter) is used; of course, the appropriate myopic refraction is used.

Criteria for Patient Selection

CLAPIKS can be initiated at any time after the first week after surgery. Patients should have complaints of decreased vision, and there should be a significant difference between the current and target refraction.

Patients need to be willing to return to the office on a weekly basis for follow-up examination. This may be extended to an every other week visit once the surgeon feels comfortable that the patient is tolerating the treatment. However, it is not recommended to let the patient go for more than 2 weeks unchecked. Most disposable lenses are only approved for 2 weeks maximum wear; thus the lens needs to be replaced at least every 2 weeks. Some patients will have a shift of 1.00 D or more from week to week, therefore requiring this close monitoring to avoid overcorrection.

Patients need to be informed that CLAPIKS is not 100% effective. Some patients do not respond at all, while other patients respond but not enough to reach the target refractive error.

Patients who have not tolerated CTLs in the past are not necessarily poor candidates for CLAPIKS. Because of the anti-inflammatory properties of Acular, patients are usually able to comfortably wear the lens. It is thought that the effect of the NSAID is similar to the effect of topical anesthetics used in initial diagnostic and dispensing of rigid gas permeable

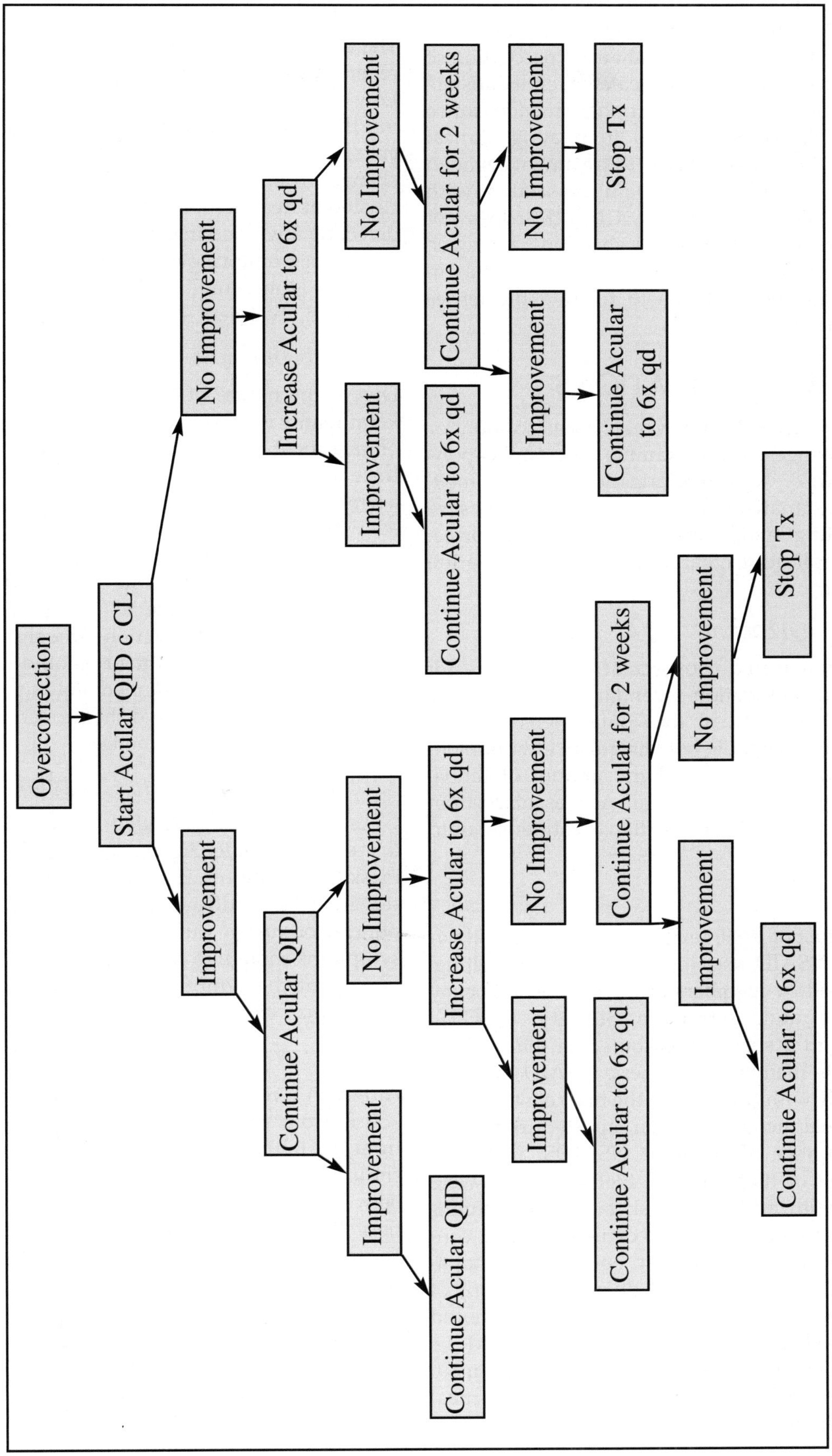

Figure 15-1. CLAPIKS treatment flow chart.

(RGP) lenses. Topical anesthetics used during initial fitting visits result in significantly fewer dropouts, improved initial comfort, an enhanced perception of the adaptation process and greater overall satisfaction with RGP lenses.[16] A similar phenomenon can be seen when NSAIDS are used in treating corneal defects; addition of an NSAID to treatment regimen significantly decreases the pain associated with corneal abrasions.[17] Obviously, CLAPIKS does not involve RGP lenses or corneal abrasions; however, inferences can be made to the effect Acular has in allowing CLAPIKS patients to tolerate the lenses very comfortably.

Complications

Patients are checked on a weekly basis to monitor refractive changes and to examine for complications that may arise. Neovascularization, corneal melt, induced astigmatism, keratopathy, dry eye syndrome creating intolerance to wear, and overcorrection are complications that may necessitate cessation of treatment.

Neovascularization

It is well known that neovascularization can result from oxygen deprivation secondary to contact lens wear. The low dk/L of the contact lens and the extended wear schedule both create an environment of oxygen deprivation. A slight amount of limbal injection is normal, however if neovascularization encroaches on the edge of the flap, treatment should be stopped.

Corneal Melt

During August of 1999, severe complications following topical NSAID use, including corneal melting, were reported by members of the American Society of Cataract and Refractive Surgery (ASCRS) responding to a survey distributed in letters from ASCRS to its members. A generic NSAID that was subsequently withdrawn from the market was implicated. Corneal melts have been reported in patients using a number of different NSAIDS, including Acular. Most of these corneal melts reported were associated with additional risk factors: conditions that predisposed the patient to corneal melting, concurrent topical steroid use, and epithelial keratopathy.[18-20] Most CLAPIKS patients do not possess any of these risk factors; however, corneal integrity should be monitored closely, and treatment should be stopped immediately at the first sign of corneal melt. The authors have never encountered any corneal melt issues in any of their patients.

Induced Astigmatism

The cornea may not steepen (or flatten in the case of reverse CLAPIKS) at the same rate in each meridian. Low (<1.00 D) amounts of cylinder may refract during the course of treatment. In the authors' experience, this astigmatism is fleeting and usually changes from visit to visit with resolution by the conclusion of treatment. Corneal topography is useful in detecting any trend in progression of astigmatism, as well as in monitoring irregular astigmatism. If a progression is measured and/or visual acuity is compromised, treatment should be stopped.

Keratopathy

Due to the nature of the CTL wear schedule, mild keratopathy is most likely to occur during the course of treatment. Slit lamp examination may reveal a trace to 1+ amount of keratitis. Patients may be asymptomatic, or they may have symptoms associated with dry eye syndrome. Symptomatic patients can be managed quite effectively with preservative-free artificial tears, flax seed oil, and/or punctal occlusion. If a moderate to severe keratopathy is observed, the risk of infection outweighs the benefit of treatment and treatment should be stopped. Treatment should stop immediately upon the observance of any infiltrate, and the proper treatment for the infiltrate should commence.

Dry Eye Syndrome—Intolerance

CTLs, particularly extended wear, can exacerbate dry eye syndrome. Again, the NSAID will help to mask the symptoms. If a patient is symptomatic, preservative-free artificial tears, flax seed oil, and/or punctal occlusion can, in most cases, alleviate the symptoms enough to continue with treatment. In the rare event the symptoms cannot be alleviated, the patient may elect to stop treatment.

Overcorrection

Although rare, it is possible to get changes of over -.50 D from week to week. Patients are instructed from the initiation of treatment to call immediately should vision become significantly blurred in between visits, indicating a rapid change in refraction. This is particularly important as the changes approach the target refraction. If the change in refraction does exceed the target, treatment is stopped immediately and the patient is monitored. The authors have never experienced an overcorrection. This is most likely due to the close monitoring and generally slow refractive shift (Table 15-2).

Table 15-2

Contraindications for Continuing Treatment

Absolute Contraindications	Relative Contraindications
Corneal melt	Neovascularization
Infiltrates	Patient discomfort
Overcorrection	Induced astigmatism
Grade 3 or above corneal staining	Trace to Grade 2 corneal staining

Future Plans and Developments

There are many questions that remain unanswered as to the actual mechanism of the refractive shift. Very high frequency (VHF) ultrasound scanning would help elucidate the corneal level of anatomical change. Orbscan (Bausch & Lomb, Rochester, NY) measurements and wavefront technology would also be of great benefit in understanding the mechanism of corneal change. More studies incorporating these measurements need to be undertaken.

The authors have proposed that the cornea needs to have had some prior stromal insult for CLAPIKS to be effective. CLAPIKS has not produced statistically significant results in the radial keratotomy/astigmatic keratotomy patient, nor has it been effective in the surgically untreated eye. If we can understand why excimer laser patients respond in particular, this may shed some light on the mechanism of action.

As mentioned previously, the authors have patients that have experienced an increase in visual acuity without a corresponding change in manifest refraction. Wavefront analysis would certainly help to explain the underlying process seen in these patients.

CLAPIKS is a time-intensive process for both patient and practitioner. The visits are relatively short and straightforward; however, the frequency of the visits adds up to a good deal of chair time. Methods to streamline the process of each visit would assist in decreasing chair time for the ophthalmologist. This may be achieved from large scale data pooling across the country. As we learn more about the frequency of side effects of CLAPIKS, we may be more comfortable letting the patient go for a longer period of time in between visits.

Summary

We have used CLAPIKS to successfully treat just shy of 100 patients to date, and surgeons across the country are adding CLAPIKS to their menu of refractive options as the word spreads about its efficacy. We have found it to be a safe, non-invasive technique that can be presented to the patient as an alternative to hyperopic LASIK.

It can be particularly useful in the early postoperative period when the patient may be concerned about the uncorrected vision. By actively treating the patient's immediate complaints, both the patient and doctor feel in control of the refractive outcome. In the clinical setting, this has the effect of alleviating the tension of a perceived mediocre outcome by directly addressing the refractive outcome shortfall. Because the residual refractive error can be incorporated into the CTL, the patient will see better as soon as treatment is started.

Although it does require more time of both the doctor and patient, the authors have found most patients to be very receptive to this nonsurgical approach.

References

1. Mulhern MG, Condon PI, O'Keefe M. Myopic and hyperopic laser in situ keratomileusis retreatments: indications, techniques, limitations, and results. *J Cataract Refract Surg.* 2001;27(8):1278-87.
2. Choi RY, Wilson SE. Hyperopic laser in situ keratomileusis: primary and secondary treatments are safe and effective. *Cornea.* 2001;20(4):388-93.
3. Jalbert I, Stapleton F. Effect of lens wear on corneal stroma: preliminary findings. *Aust N Z J Ophthalmol.* 1999;27(3-4):211-3.
4. Efron N, Mutalib HA, Perez-Gomez I, Koh HH. Confocal microscopic observations of the human cornea following overnight contact lens wear. *Clin Exp Optom.* 2002;85(3):149-55.
5. Efron N, Perez-Gomex I, Morgan PB. Confocal microscopic observations of stromal keratocytes during extended contact lens wear. *Clin Exp Optom.* 2002;85(3):156-60.
6. Adler. The cornea. In: Hart W, ed. *Adler's Physiology of the Eye.* 9th ed. St. Louis, MO: Mosby; 1992:62-63.
7. Lyle WA, Jin GJ. Retreatment after initial laser in situ keratomileusis. *J Cataract Refract Surg.* 2000;26(5):625-6.

8. Han HS, Song JS, Kim HM. Long-term results of laser in situ keratomileusis for high myopia. *Korean J Ophthalmol.* 2000;14(1):1-6.
9. Nichols J. Extended wear update. *CL Spectrum.* 2001;16(7):33-37.
10. Dumbleton KA, Chalmers RL, Richter DB, Fonn D. Changes in myopic refractive error with nine months' extended wear of hydrogel lenses with high and low oxygen permeability. *Optom Vis Sci.* 2000;77(6):285.
11. Dillon EC, Eagle RC Jr, Laibson PR. Compensatory epithelial hyperplasia in human corneal disease. *Ophthalmic Surg.* 1992;23(11):729-32.
12. Lohmann CP, Guell JL. Regression after LASIK for the treatment of myopia: the role of the corneal epithelium. *Semin Ophthalmol.* 1998;13(2):79-82.
13. Reinstein DZ, Silverman RH, Sutton HFS, Coleman DJ. Very high-frequency ultrasound corneal analysis identifies anatomic correlates of optical complication of lamellar refractive surgery. *Ophthalmology.* 1999;106:474-482.
14. Gauthier CA, Holden BA, Epstein D, Tengroth B, Fagerholm P, Hamberg-Nystrom H. Factors affecting epithelial hyperplasia after photorefractive keratectomy. *J Cataract Refract Surg.* 1997;23(7):1042-50.
15. Spadea L, Fasciani R, Necozione S, Balestrazzi E. Role of the corneal epithelium in refractive changes following laser in situ keratomileusis for high myopia. *J Cataract Refract Surg.* 2000;16(2):133-9.
16. Bennett ES, Smyth J, Henry VA, Bassi CJ, Morgan BW. Effect of topical anesthetic use on initial patient satisfaction and overall success with rigid gas permeable contact lenses. *Optom Vis Sci.* 1998;75(11):800-5.
17. Donnenfeld ED, Selking BA, Perry HD, et al. Controlled evaluation of a bandage contact lens and a topical nonsteroidal anti-inflammatory drug in treating traumatic corneal abrasions. *Ophthalmology.* 1995;102(6):979-84.
18. Flach AJ. Corneal melts associated with topically applied nonsteroidal anti-inflammatory drugs. *Trans Am Ophthalmol Soc.* 2001;99:205-12.
19. Hargrave SL, Jung JC, Fini ME, Gelender H. Possible role of the vitamin E solubilizer in topical diclofenac on matrix metalloproteinase expression in corneal melting: an analysis of postoperative keratolysis. *Ophthalmology.* 2002; 109(2):343-50.
20. Guidera AC, Luchs JI, Udell IJ. Keratitis, ulceration, and perforation associated with topical nonsteroidal anti-inflammatory drugs. *Ophthalmology.* 2001;108(5):936-44.

Section Four

Intrastromal Techniques

Chapter Sixteen

Non-Contact Laser Thermal Keratoplasty

Peter G. Kansas, MD; Shula Luck, BA; and Neal A. Sher, MD, FACS

Introduction

Thermal keratoplasty (TK) is a surgical technique of heating corneal collagen and shrinking it, thus producing corneal steepening to reduce hyperopia. The concept of changing the shape of the cornea is one of the oldest in refractive and corneal surgery, originating from the work of Lans in 1898.[1] It evolved from heating with metal probes[2] to heating with a laser.[3] The latter procedure was called laser thermokeratoplasty or LTK.

The technique has presented surgeons with a technical challenge. Over time, heated collagen reverts to its original shape, thus regressing the correction. LTK, developed over a decade ago by Sunrise Technologies (Fremont, Calif), has proved disappointing to many surgeons and the company ceased operations. We feel it is valuable to recount LTK's history, technique, and complications for the purpose of exploring its future, including new methods and technologies, which anticipate the advancement of variations on LTK.

Historical Overview

TK, a system of heat-generated corneal shaping, is not a modern concept. In the 1980's, well after the importation of radial keratotomy (RK) to the United States from the former Soviet Union, Fyodorov described and produced an instrument and technique to heat, shrink, and steepen the cornea.[4] Fyodorov's instrument was a hand-held cylindrical device with large footplates similar to an RK hand piece. It had a hot tip that would plunge between the footplates into the cornea to a preset depth. The pattern was one of 2 or 3 rows orientated along 8 radially placed lines [similar to RK] placed in the mid periphery. This technique did in fact steepen the cornea but it caused stromal necrosis and irregular healing, so it never was accepted outside the Soviet Union. Rowsey et al worked on this in the late 1970s and early 1980 using an instrument developed with the Los Alamos labs.[2] Lasers were suggested as a means of performing TK.[5,6] After a hiatus of some years, TK resurfaced with the advent of holmium lasers, both contact and non-contact devices.[7-10]

Relevant Anatomy and Physiology

LTK was recently reviewed by Parag Majmudar, MD, in a Web-based publication.[11] All forms of TK hinge on the reaction of corneal collagen fibers to the effects of heat. The heat energy must only be directed at the stromal collagen fibers without effecting the epithelium or endothelium.

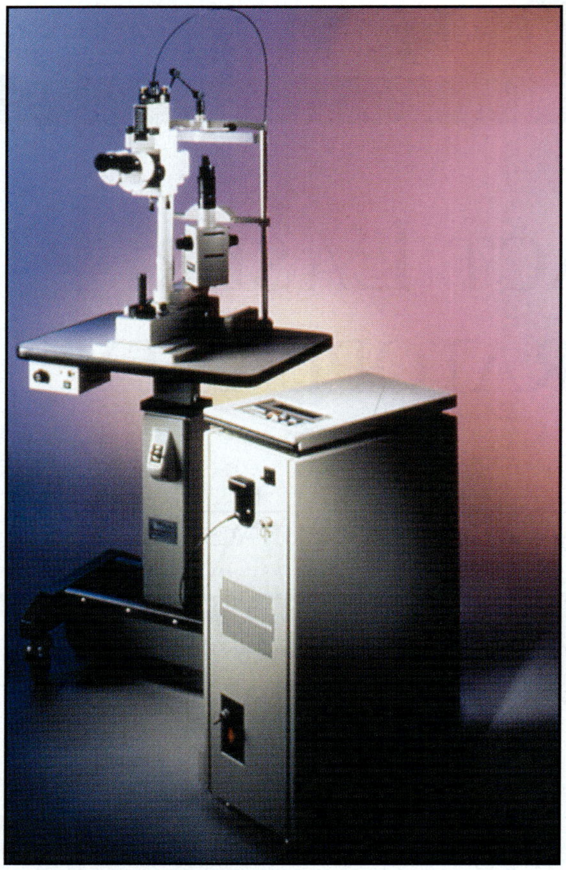

Figure 16-1. The Holmium-YAG Laser Corneal Shaping system (courtesy of Sunrise Technologies, Fremont, Calif).

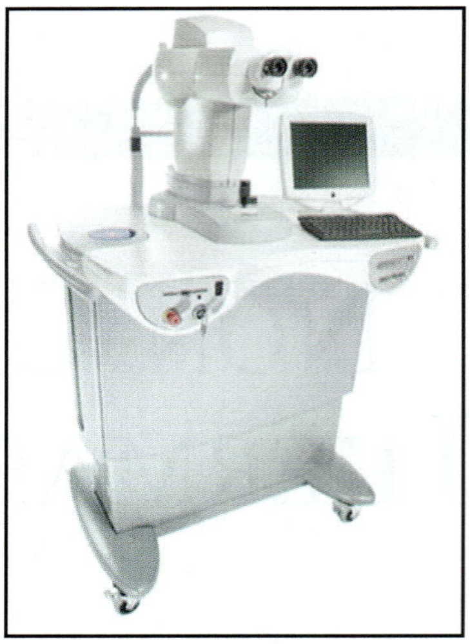

Figure 16-2. Hyperion Holmium-YAG laser system (courtesy of Sunrise Technologies, Fremont, Calif). This laser emits an invisible infrared beam with a 2120 nm wavelength. It delivers its energy in a series of focused beamlets to the mid periphery of the cornea where the thickness is in the 600 μm range.

Human collagen can shrink by 66% when exposed to temperatures of 55 to 85°C. On a biochemical level, the heat induces disruption of hydrogen bonds in the super coiled tertiary structure of collagen, allowing it to partially unwind and develop new bonds. At higher temperatures (65 to 78°C), hydrolysis of the heat-labile cross-links occurs and the collagen will relax. Further heating above 78°C induces necrosis.

Koch et al[12] conducted LTK using 10 pulses and a range of radiant energies on 3 human corneas 1 day prior to their removal at penetrating keratoplasty. Koch treated rabbit corneas with 10 and 5-pulse LTK with a 3-month follow-up. He found that the more pulse radiant energy, the greater acute tissue injury. Three weeks after LTK, epithelial hyperplasia and stromal contraction were present. At follow-up, the epithelial attachment complex in the rabbit corneas was repaired. Also keratocyte activation, synthesis of type I collagen, partial restoration of stromal keratin sulfate and type VI collagen, and retro-corneal membrane formation all occurred. The 5-pulse treatments produced less acute tissue injury than 10-pulse and normal stromal architecture restored itself more quickly. Koch concluded that the corneal tissue changes produced by non-contact LTK prompt rabbit corneas to respond with rapid wound healing. This could contribute to postoperative regression observed in human eyes treated with LTK.

Surgical Technique

From the surgeon's point of view, LTK requires learning no new surgical skills. Aligning the patient correctly is the most crucial technical point and is not much different than aligning a patient for fundus photography. The learning curve is shallow and short.

After a series of earlier prototypes (Figure 16-1), Sunrise Technology introduced the Hyperion LTK system (Figure 16-2). The Hyperion LTK system is a Holmium-YAG laser emitting an invisible infrared beam with a 2120 nm wavelength. It delivers its energy in a series of focused beamlets to the mid periphery of the cornea where the thickness is in the 600-μm range. The Hyperion is an optical delivery system that splits the emitted beam into eight equal beams. A red aiming beam of 635 nm projects 8 spots corresponding to the 8 holmium spots to be delivered. Another laser source provides two converging green focusing beams (532 nm) that, when exactly superimposed on the epithelium at the pupil center,

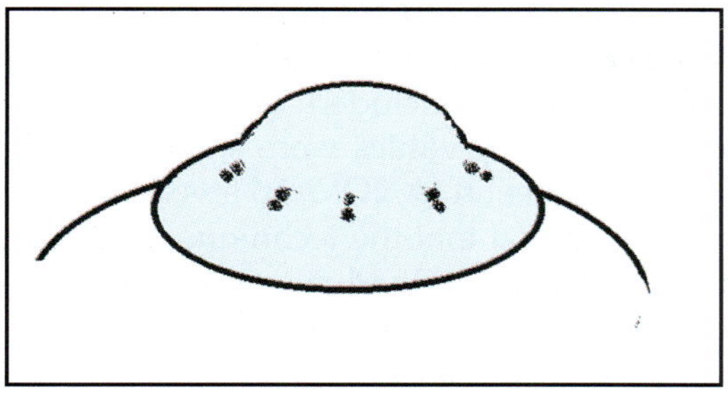

Figure 16-3. Schematic of the cornea after LTK. The stroma is heated to 60°C causing shrinking of the cornea collagen in a circular manner thus steepening the central cornea (courtesy of Peter Kansas, MD).

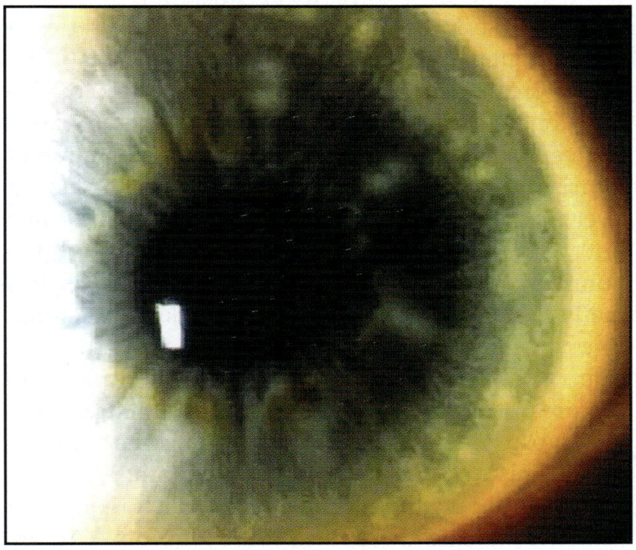

Figure 16-5. The appearance of LTK lesions at approximately one month after treatment, which have faded but are still visible.

provides final focus. It lays down 2 rings of 8 spots each ring with 6- and 7-mm diameters respectively. Each of the 8 spots is created simultaneously in each ring by 7 short pulses lasting a fraction of a second (200 msec) at a rate of 5 pulses per second. Treatment time lasts 3 seconds for both rings. The stroma is heated to 60°C causing shrinking of the cornea collagen in a circular manner, thus steepening the central cornea (Figure 16-3). Each spot is approximately 0.6 mm at the epithelial level. Figure 16-4 shows a postoperative photo 1 week after LTK. The 6 mm ring is laid down first quickly followed by the 7 mm ring, which needs to be created in approximately 60 seconds. The spots in the second ring are just radial to and contiguous to the spots in the 6 mm ring. The combined spots resemble snowmen. The epithelial portion of these spots is actually coagulated epithelium, which can be, and usually is, removed immediately after the laser treatment. Between each pair of laser thermal spots, induced by collagen shrinking, are deep stromal stress lines forming an octagonal pattern. The lesions tend to fade but not disappear. Figure 16-5 shows appearance of LTK lesions at approximately 1 month after treatment.

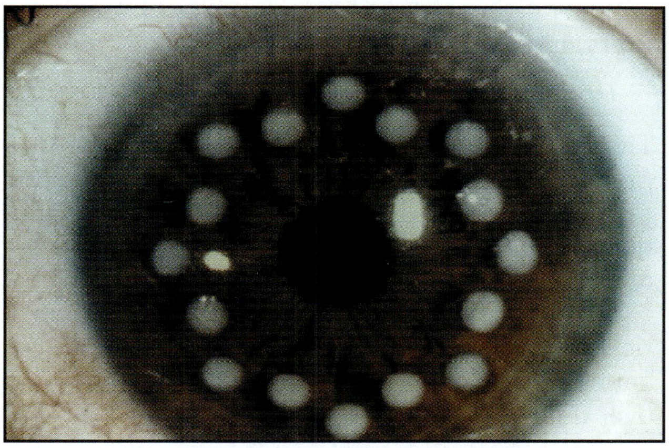

Figure 16-4. A postoperative photo 1 week after LTK. The 6 mm ring is laid down first quickly followed by the 7 mm ring, which needs to be created in approximately 60 seconds. The spots in the second ring are just radial to and contiguous to the spots in the 6mm ring. The combined spots resemble snowmen.

Laser power in millijoules (mj) is selected according to the amount of correction desired. There is some variation because there are 3 nomograms, 6, 12, or 24 months. In the 6-month nomogram the powers run from 226 mj to 258 mj. The 12 and 24-month nomograms give more overcorrection that lasts much longer. At present, many users have abandoned these nomograms.

The non-contact aspect of the procedure is of course a very important feature of the technique and is viewed as very patient friendly. Many potential laser refractive patients frequently voice a strong anxiety over the prospect of an instrument touching their eyes.

Pretreatment Drop Protocol

The preoperative anesthetic drop protocol (the patient sitting at the laser) was originally 1 drop of anesthetic every 3 minutes times 2 then a third drop after 5 minutes. The anesthetic drops were followed by speculum placement, a corneal wipe with a moist weck cell and a 5-minute wait. The wait was intended to allow for uniform corneal drying thus eliminating the tear film, which is regarded as an impediment to predictable laser absorption. Eventually the drying time concept was dropped and the drop repetition rate was altered to one drop of anesthetic every minute times 3 and no corneal wipe.

Postoperative Management

The postoperative course requires no restrictions or precautions because there is no corneal instability induced. There was no major propensity for infection or other complications to threaten the recovery or outcome.

Postoperative LTK patients generally do not experience a loss of best corrected vision. Any induced ammetropia, induced astigmatism, usually improves over time but not always.

Results from Published Studies

Koch, Kohnen et al[13] reported on the US FDA Phase IIa clinical trials for the Hyperion System. In this study, one eye of each of 28 patients was tested with a mean age 54.6 years and a mean preoperative spherical equivalent of +2.21 D (range +0.50 to +3.88 D). This experimental group received treatment with either one ring of LTK (8 spots) at a 6 mm optical zone or two rings (8 spots each, rotated by 22.5 degrees, so that the laser spots are staggered) at the 6- and 7-mm optical zones. At 2 years after surgery, uncorrected distance visual acuity was improved by 1 or more lines of Snellen visual acuity in 19 (73%) of 26 of the treated eyes. The mean lines gained was 2.5 ± 2.2/3.3 ± 2.7 for 1- and 2-ring treatment groups, respectively. The mean change in spherical equivalent of the subjective manifest refraction was -0.53 ± 0.33 D ± 1.48 ± 0.58 D for 1- and 2-ring treatment groups. Regression between 1 and 2 years was 0.01 D and 0.16 D, respectively. In the 1-ring treatment group (18 eyes), 13 eyes (72%) had refractive corrections (range, -0.38 to -1.13 D), and 5 eyes (29%) were unchanged (within +0.25 D) relative to their preoperative measurements. In the 2-ring treatment group, all 8 eyes (100%) had reductions in their hyperopia (range of corrections, -0.38 to -2.25 D). None of the eyes lost two or more lines of spectacle-corrected distance visual acuity. There were no sight-threatening complications. In general, 2-ring treatment group gained a greater number of Snellen lines, but the group also experienced greater regression

In another study, Alio et al[14] treated 57 sighted eyes of 42 hyperopic patients. All patients were followed for 15 months after surgery. The preoperative spectacle-corrected visual acuity returned to baseline levels from 2 to 6 weeks after treatment. Regression of effect was evident in all eyes, and after 15 months the regression was total in 18 eyes (31.5%). At the end of the study, 41 eyes (71.9%) had an uncorrected visual acuity of 20/40 or better. Thirty-two eyes (58.8%) were within ± 1.00 D of the intended refraction. The authors concluded that patient age and central pachymetry values were significantly correlated with regression (ANOVA, p less than .005). The authors concluded that the technique works best up to +3.00 D in older individuals with central corneal thickness less than 525 microns.

My Personal Experience (Peter Kansas, MD)

Fortified by favorable experience over the years in RK, ALK, PRK, LASIK and clear lensectomy, I ventured into what proved to be uncertain waters of LTK. Sunrise Technologies had carried out a series of experiments using its Corneal Shaping System (CSS). CSS corrects simple hyperopia by using a Ho:YAG non-contact laser performing thermal keratoplasty to steepen the cornea.[13,15-18] I followed the evolution of Sunrise until in 1996 the Sunrise CSS was in use at over 40 clinics worldwide. Sunrise eventually came out with an updated version of CSS called the Sunrise Hyperion LTK System. Hyperion LTK has many laudable characteristics that make it potentially a very desirable technique. It was thought to be safe with a short learning curve; the procedure requires no new surgical skills, there is little pain, and most enticing of all, it is a non-contact procedure. This was in contrast to two other devices developed in a similar time frame, which required a probe contacting the cornea: the Holmium-YAG by Summit Technologies[19] and the Holmium 25 Plus by Technomed (Germany).[20]

These theoretic advantages did not outweigh the disadvantages of the Hyperion System. Unlike myopic corrective procedures, where the patient experiences an immediate and dramatic improvement in vision, the LTK patient may experience worse vision due to the necessary over correction. A matter of months must pass before there is improved vision. Ideally the regression would end up near or at emmetropia. During the regression phase, the patients require extensive support and handholding. Some may need temporary myopic correction to be able to function normally. Patients also require longer and more frequent visits to the office than patients of excimer laser surgery.

In spite of explicit and emphatic preoperative explanations about what to expect during the postoperative course, patients for the most part did not react well to their surgically induced myopia. The LTK surgeon must acclimate to this negative reaction. The author was a little surprised and was not truly appreciative as to how consistently the patients would respond in this manner. Early enthusiasm and eagerness gradually eroded into patient frustration and disappointment. Lastly, it goes without saying that unhappy patients talk more than happy ones. In our practice, it gradually became apparent that the LTK patients were not referring others. In an effort to improve outcomes, it was decided to modify the protocol and revise the recommended nomograms in an attempt to minimize initial over correction. Some success was being recognized through these modifications when Sunrise ceased operations for financial reasons.

Complications

Refractive

One of the drawbacks of this procedure is the postoperative course: overcorrection followed by excessive regression. Overcorrections as much as 1.00 to 2.00 D were typical even at the lower attempted corrections of 1.00 D. Overcorrection subsides in the course of 3 or 4 weeks but in the meantime vision is problematic and distinctly disappointing.

In about 30% of patients there is an accompanying induced against the rule astigmatism. The reason for this unwanted meridianol change has never been scientifically elucidated. Speculation says that because the horizontal meridians are exposed the most and become dried out the fastest, they respond more than vertical meridians and are influenced more by the lid margins and their accompanying lacrimal tear strip. Although the over correction recedes in the subsequent 6 to 8 weeks, the astigmatism does not disappear. It may slowly diminish in 50% of cases, but never completely.

Epithelial Lesions

Even though the 16 spots represent disruptions to the corneal surface, these heal overnight and are rarely a problem. The deeper white stromal portion of the spots last several months and tend to fade over the next year.

Corneal Edema

An additional frequent reaction in 10% of patients is the development of corneal edema with Descemet's folds by the next morning. Although these recede over the subsequent 2 to 3 days, initially, they cause profound visual disturbance. The blurred vision frequently incites some anxiety.

Stromal Stress Lines

Deep stress lines develop between the LTK spots but gradually fade over a period of some weeks. They have no impact on vision and present no problem. These are similar to those seen with conductive keratoplasty (CK).

Pain

The procedure is painless and for most patients triggers little response or sensation. If pressed, a patient will admit to experiencing a vague sensation but never rising to the level of discomfort. In US clinical trials of the LTK procedure, patient complaints of postoperative discomfort were usually minimal, lasting about 24 hours or less.[21]

The Future of LTK

Overcorrection and regression presented LTK advocates with a huge challenge: how to modify this surgical technique to improve the results. At first, surgeons reduced the power as recommended by the nomograms to improve outcomes or at least reduce the initial over correction. The maximum power was reduced to the lowest setting—ie, 226 mj. Surgeons also no longer treated patients with more than 2.00 D [Hyperion was FDA approved for 2.50 D]. Although reducing the energy delivered helped, overcorrection still occurred. The protocol was further modified to single ring applications, a 6-mm ring with 8 spots. Overcorrection was decreased, but excessive regression continued to occur. The initial visions were tightly bracketed in a 20/40 or better grouping. This was more acceptable, but after 4 to 6 weeks, regression had erased some of the improvement in 70% to 75% of eyes.

For those who agreed, enhancements were performed. A second set of 8 spots was placed at the 6 mm ring level 22.5 degrees off the initial setting (this was default software adjustment), thus ending up with 16 spots at the 6 mm optical zone. This group of patients did the best. They did not endure distressing over corrections and this approach seemed encouraging.

The Hyperion is currently being modified to interface with wavefront technology. With the Hartmann-Shack wavefront sensor, surgeons can measure the refractive system of the eye before, during, and after LTK to determine the appropriate LTK nomogram and know when the peak of treatment has been reached to stop surgery immediately. In addition, LTK energy as low as 144 mj per pulse coupled with an increased number of pulses is being studied as a way to reduce regression. It is hoped that the Hyperion will be further modified to provide more versatility for selecting individual spots and locations so that individual meridians can be treated.

Conclusion

The Holmium-YAG laser as configured within the Hyperion system represented a significant effort in research and development in an effort to perform laser thermokeratoplasty in a safe and predictable manner. Unfortunately, issues of predictability, requirements for corneal drying, overcorrection, and regression have made this approach with this specific technology problematic. It remains to be seen whether modifications in equipment, nomograms, and techniques will make this procedure succeed in the refractive marketplace.

References

1. Lans LJ. Experimentelle Untersuchungen über die Entstehung von Astigmatismus durch nuicht-perforierende Corneawuden. *Graefes Arch Clin Exp Ophthalmol*. 1898;45: 117-152.
2. Rowsey JJ, Doss JD. Preliminary report of Los Alamos keratoplasty techniques. *Ophthalmology*. 1981 Aug;88(8): 755-60.
3. Peyman GA, Larson B, Raichand M, et al. Modification of rabbit corneal curvature with use of carbon dioxide laser burns. *Ophthalmic Surg*. 1980;11:325-329.
4. Neuman AC, Fyodorov S, Sanders DR. Radial thermokeratoplasty for the correction of hyperopia. *Refract Corneal Surg*. 1990;6:404-411.
5. Bende T, Seiler T, Matallana T. Regression of hyperopic correction with the Ho:YAG laser is dependent on coagulation depth. *Invest Ophthalmol Vis Sci*. 1991;32:995.
6. Kanoda AN, Sorokin AS. Laser correction of hypermetropic refraction. In: Fyodorov SN, ed. *Microsurgery of the Eye: Main Aspects*. Moscow, MIR Publishers; 1987;147-154.
7. Seiler T, Matallana M, Bende T. Laser thermokeratoplasty by means of a pulsed Holmium-YAG laser for hyperopic correction. *Refract Corneal Surg*. 1990;6:328-333.
8. Horn G, Spears KG, Lopez O, et al. New refractive method for laser thermal keratoplasty with the Co:MgF2 laser. *J Cataract Refract Surg*. 1990;16: 611-616.
9. Seiler T. Ho-YAG laser thermokeratoplasty for hyperopia. *Ophthalmol Clinics North Amer*. 1992;5:773-780.
10. Ren Q, Melgar TM, Parel JM, et al. New system for noncontact laser photothermal keratoplasty (LPTK). Proc SPIE. 1993;1877:57-60.
11. Majmudar P. *In emedicine*. Available at: http://www.emedicine. com/oph/topic660.htm. Accessed August 6, 2003.
12. Koch DD. Histological changes and wound healing response following noncontact Holmium-YAG laser thermal keratoplasty. *Trans Am Ophthalmol Soc*. 1996;94:745-802.
13. Koch DD, Kohnen T, McDonnell PJ, et al. Hyperopia correction by noncontact holmium:YAG laser thermal keratoplasty: US phase IIA clinical study with 2-year follow-up. *Ophthalmology*. 1997 Nov;104(11):1938-47.
14. Alio JL, Ismail MM, Sanchez Pego JL. Correction of hyperopia with non-contact Ho:YAG laser thermal keratoplasty. *J Refract Surg*. 1997 Jan-Feb;13(1):17-22.
15. Koch DD, et al. Instrastromal Procedure: The use of the noncontact Holmium:YAG laser for correction of hyperopia-Sunrise technologies experience. In: Sher NA, ed. *Surgery for Hyperopia and Presbyopia*. Baltimore, Md: Williams and Wilkins; 1997;135-144.
16. Kohnen T, Koch DD, McDonnell PJ, Menefee RF, Berry MJ. Noncontact holmium:YAG laser thermal keratoplasty to correct hyperopia: 18-month follow-up. *Ophthalmologica*. 1997;211(5):274-82.
17. Villareal RV, Koch DD, Kohnen T, et al. Hyperopia correction by non-contact holmium:YAG laser thermal keratoplasty: 5 pulse treatments with 1-year follow-up. *J Refract Surg*. 1996.
18. Azzolini M, Vinciguerra P, Epstein D, et al. Laser thermokeratoplasty for the correction of hyperopia: a comparison of two different application patterns. *Invest Ophthalmol Vis Sci*. 1995;36:S716.
19. Thompson, V. Holmium: YAG laser thermokeratoplasty: the Summit system, In: Sher NA, ed. *Surgery for Hyperopia and Presbyopia*. Baltimore, Md: Williams and Wilkins; 1997;157-162.
20. Eggink CA, Meurs P, Barduk Y. Holmium laser thermal keratoplasty for hyperopia and astigmatism photorefractive keratectomy. *J Refract Surg*. 2000;16:317-322.
21. FDA Approves Sunrise Technologies Hyperion LTK System. Available at http://www.prk.com/SunriseTech PressRelease. html. Accessed August 6, 2003.

Chapter Seventeen

Conductive Keratoplasty for Treating Hyperopia and Presbyopia

Jonathan Davidorf, MD and Daniel S. Durrie, MD

Introduction

The most common surgical techniques for treating refractive error today are laser ablation in the form of laser-assisted in-situ keratomileusis (LASIK) or photorefractive keratectomy (PRK). Outcomes following LASIK treatment of myopia have been especially good, with generally excellent visual results and a low incidence of complications. LASIK treatment for hyperopia, however, has been less successful and much less widely adapted by refractive surgeons. Relative to myopic LASIK, hyperopic LASIK results need improvement in accuracy, visual outcomes, optical aberrations, safety, and stability.[1-10]

To correct hyperopia and hyperopic astigmatism, the central cornea must be steepened. To accomplish this, the excimer laser is used to ablate the corneal periphery in a ring-shaped pattern under a LASIK flap. The best results have been obtained with large (9.0 mm) ablation zones made possible through a large diameter flap that creates a sufficiently large stromal bed. However, flaps of any size can be problematic. Thin, irregular, or buttonhole flaps, wrinkles, dislocations, and interface debris can occur and affect the outcome. Furthermore, a hyperopic ablation must be perfectly centered. Different excimer lasers, beam profiles, transition zone diameters, nomograms, and epithelial healing also affect results.

Conductive keratoplasty (CK) (Refractec, Inc., Irvine, Calif), is an entirely different approach to hyperopia correction. With CK, the cornea is reshaped through a non-ablative, non-incisional, collagen shrinkage procedure that inherently avoids flap problems and complications because a flap is not used for the procedure. The precise use of an excimer laser is also unnecessary because CK is a "laserless" procedure. CK's mechanism of action is through the application of high-frequency (radiofrequency) energy that the cornea converts to heat in a controlled fashion. Treatment is applied outside of the visual axis at 8 to 32 treatment spots (Figure 17-1). A full circle of treatment spots acts like a belt tightening the cornea in the periphery so that the central cornea steepens, thereby correcting hyperopic refractive error (Figure 17-2).

Historical Review

The intention of thermokeratoplasty (TK) techniques is to change corneal curvature through the application of heat, which shrinks corneal collagen. Although Lans attempted to shrink corneal collagen in rabbit eyes through thermal burns in the 19th century, it was not until the 1970s that various pathological conditions in humans, such as keratoconus and persistent corneal hydrops, were successfully treated

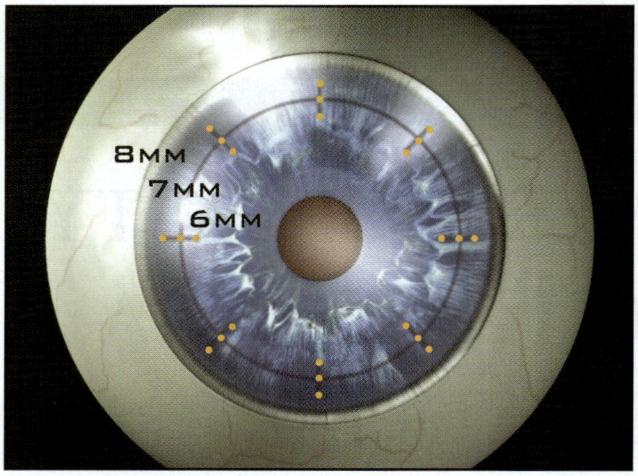

Figure 17-1. The optical zone marks made by the marker to guide the surgeon in placement of the treatment spots. A circular mark is made on the 7 mm optical zone with the CK marker. An inner hatch mark lies on the 6 mm and an outer hatch mark on the 8 mm optical zone. (Reprinted with permission from Agarwal A. *Presbyopia: A Surgical Textbook*. Thorofare, NJ: SLACK Incorporated; 2002.)

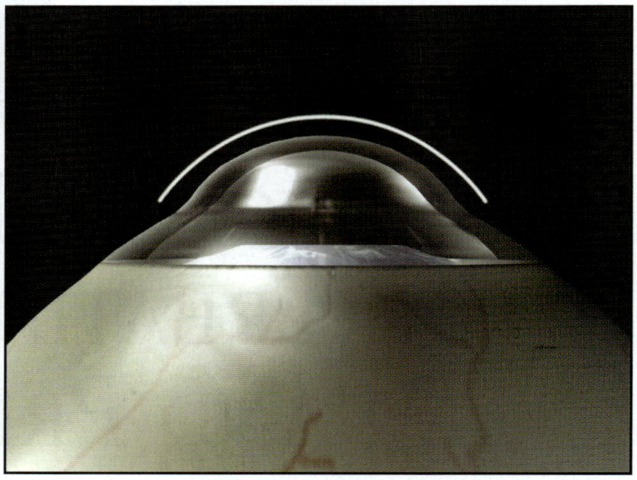

Figure 17-2. The conductive keratoplasty technique cinches the peripheral cornea which increases the curvature of the central cornea. (Reprinted with permission from Agarwal A. *Presbyopia: A Surgical Textbook*. Thorofare, NJ: SLACK Incorporated; 2002.)

with heated probes.[12,13] Although initially successful, corneal curvature returned to preoperative status and the complication rate was unacceptable.[14-16] The Russian surgeon Fyodorov was the first to use TK to change corneal refraction in 1981. Using a retractable probe tip, he and other investigators applied controlled thermal burns to treat spherical hyperopia and hyperopic astigmatism. The tip was heated to 600°C, and corneal penetration depth was reported to be 95%.[17-19] Although hyperopic corrections of up to 8.0 D were achieved, later studies showed lack of predictability and marked regression.[20,21] Also in the early 1980s, Rowsey and colleagues developed the Los Alamos TK probe. This instrument heated stromal collagen by means of radiofrequency waves, rather than by direct thermal conduction from a heated instrument. However, the topographical effect with this probe was short lived, and testing was terminated.[22-24]

Following the report by Seiler and associates of stable corneal steepening achieved in blind eyes with a pulsed Holmium-YAG laser used in the contact mode,[25] Sunrise Technologies of Fremont, California began to develop a non-contact method of Holmium-YAG laser treatment for hyperopia. The clinical studies with 2-year follow-up were published in 1996 and 1997.[26-27] The US Food and Drug Administration (FDA) approved the Hyperion LTK device in June, 2000, based on a study cohort of 612 eyes, with 80% available for analysis at 12 months and 12% at 24 months postoperatively.[28] Current physician labeling information for the approved Sunrise Hyperion LTK system limits the use of the device for treatment of patients 40 years of age or older, with a manifest refractive spherical equivalent (MRSE) of +0.75 D to +2.50 D at the spectacle plane and cylinder ≤0.75 D. The FDA submission data were never published.

The present Sunrise Hyperion LTK noncontact system provides 3 algorithms for pulse energy versus age of the patient. Less laser energy is indicated for older patients to achieve the same effect. The first algorithm provides the most refractive effect at 2 years postoperatively, but is associated with the most overcorrection initially. The second and third algorithms have less long-term effect, but also less initial overcorrection. In general, LTK has grown out of favor with many refractive surgeons because of lack of predictability and stability.

In the 1990s, Dr. Antonio Mendez studied radiofrequency as an alternative to procedures that applied heat directly to the corneal surface.[11] His success in denaturing collagen and steepening of the cornea led to the development of CK, performed with the ViewPoint CK System (Refractec).

In April 2002, the FDA granted approval of the ViewPoint CK System for the treatment of mild to moderate (0.75 D to 3.00 D) previously untreated, spherical hyperopia in persons 40 years old or older. Other potential uses of the CK technique, such as the

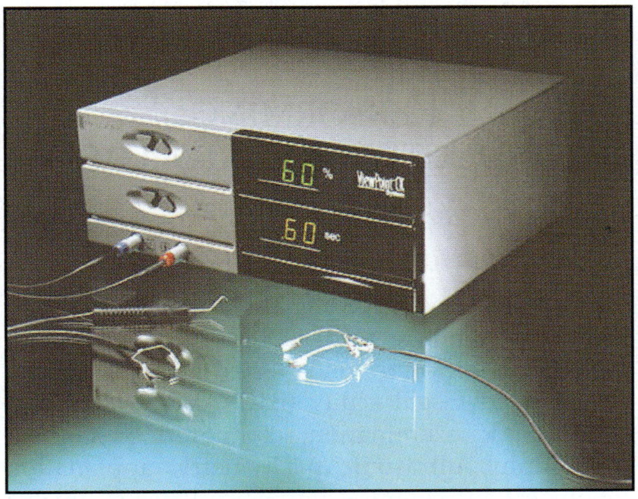

Figure 17-3. The ViewPoint CK system from Refractec, Inc. consists of a portable console, a corneal marker, choice of lid specula, a handpiece that holds the Keratoplast Tip, and a foot pedal. (Reprinted with permission from Agarwal A. *Presbyopia: A Surgical Textbook*. Thorofare, NJ: SLACK Incorporated; 2002.)

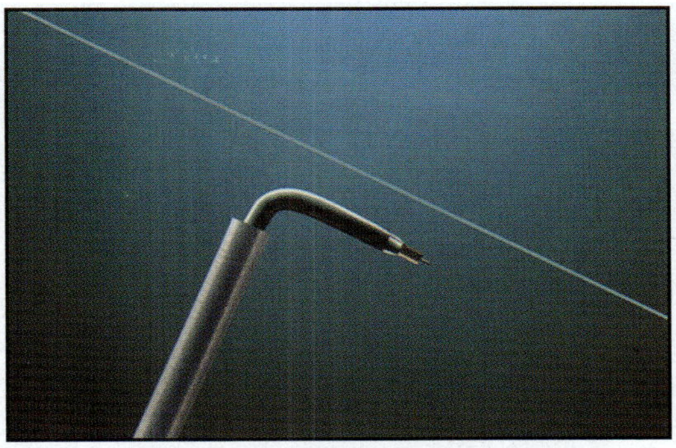

Figure 17-4. The Keratoplast Tip, (shown next to a 7-0 suture). The tip is 450 µm long and 90 µm wide and is used to deliver radiofrequency energy into the corneal stroma at 8 to 32 treatment points. A cuff on the probe assures correct depth of penetration. (Reprinted with permission from Agarwal A. *Presbyopia: A Surgical Textbook*. Thorofare, NJ: SLACK Incorporated; 2002.)

treatment of astigmatism, correction of hyperopia induced by previous refractive procedures, enhancing outcomes of cataract surgery, and the treatment of presbyopia through blended vision surgery, are under investigation.

The ViewPoint CK system (Figure 17-3) consists of a portable console, corneal marker, choice of lid specula (Lancaster, Barraquer, or Cook) that acts as the electrical return path for the radiofrequency energy delivered by the tip, a handpiece (probe) that holds the 450 µm long and 90 µm wide stainless steel tip (Keratoplast tip) (Figure 17-4), and a foot pedal. An insulated stop at the base of the probe controls the depth of penetration of the Keratoplast tip. Energy is delivered into the cornea by activation of the foot pedal.

Effect of Heat on Corneal Collagen

Although corneal collagen has great tensile strength and thermal stability, exposure to elevated temperatures for specific time periods transforms its native helical structure into a randomly coiled structure during the denaturation process. This is accompanied by contraction (shrinkage) of the collagen and changes in the mechanical behavior of the tissue.[29-31] In hyperopia treatment procedures, the desired mechanical change is peripheral corneal flattening and the resulting central corneal steepening.

Collagen denaturation depends not only on the temperature to which it is subjected, but also to the duration of exposure to the elevated temperature.[31] Minimal heating does not contract tissue enough to produce lasting refractive change. Intermediate denaturation is more permanent because wound healing may not completely replace the denatured collagen with new collagen. And finally, heating to the gelatin state (irreversible denaturation) leads to replacement with new collagen, which would not support a predictable refractive change and might cause scarring and damage to the endothelium. According to one study, some wound healing changes after thermal procedures are desirable, while others may contribute to postoperative regression and other unknown effects.[32]

CK uses the optimal combination of radiofrequency energy characteristics, including current, waveform, frequency, and duration of exposure, to raise the temperature of corneal collagen long enough to cause localized shrinkage of collagen fibers. The default CK treatment parameters are 0.6 W for 0.6 seconds at 350 kHz. Treatment application at these default parameters causes the surrounding tissue to undergo a temperature increase. As the heated tissue dehydrates, its resistance to radiofrequency current increases. Because current seeks the path of least resistance, the current path moves up the shaft of the Keratoplast tip.

Tissue heating progresses from bottom (deep in the stroma) to top (corneal surface), and creates a

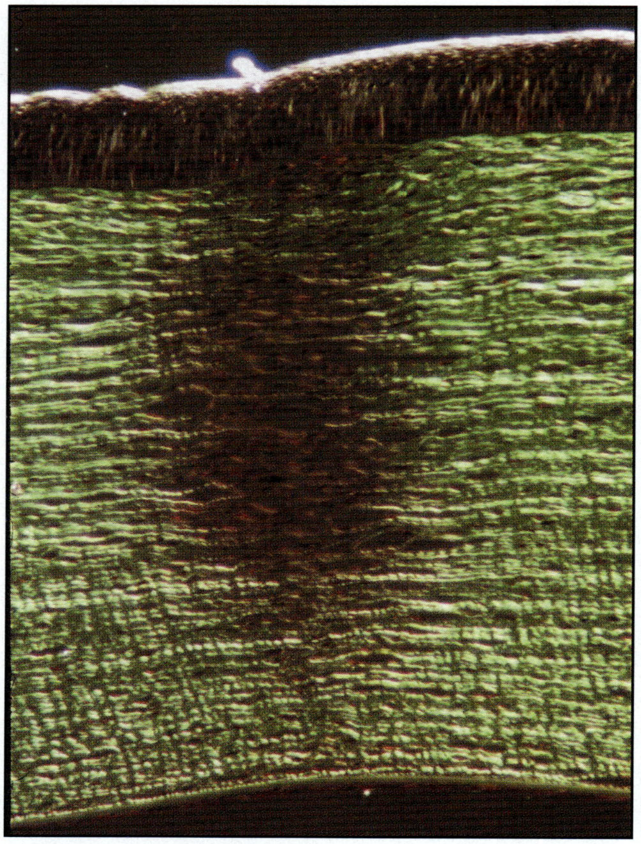

Figure 17-5. A polarized light micrograph of a histological section from a pig cornea, approximately 650 µm thick, seven days after CK treatment. The CK-treated spot (dark region) shows a cylindrical footprint 509 µm deep, which is approximately 80% of this cornea. (Reprinted with permission from Agarwal A. *Presbyopia: A Surgical Textbook*. Thorofare, NJ: SLACK Incorporated; 2002.)

thermal lesion that is uniformly cylindrical. The Keratoplast tip only delivers radiofrequency energy and heats up only in response to the increase in tissue temperature. The tip acts as a heat sink (takes heat away) rather than as a heat source (supplies heat). Histology studies on a pig cornea show that the cylindrical thermal lesion (footprint) formed as a result of CK treatment extends to approximately 80% of the depth of the stroma (Figure 17-5).

In contrast with CK, the noncontact LTK technique generates the greatest amount of heat at the surface of the cornea. Heat energy diffuses radially and axially into the tissue. The result is corneal denaturation decreasing from top to bottom, forming a cone-shaped zone of collagen shrinkage[32] of a depth that appears to be more shallow than that of a CK-treated spot. The shape of the footprint or lesion is believed to be critical to stability. Thus the instability associated with LTK treatment may be due to its conically shaped lesion, which does not reach the depth needed to produce a stable treatment effect.

Performing Conductive Keratoplasty

Patient Selection and Preoperative Examinations

The examinations preceding a CK procedure should include a complete medical history, manifest and cycloplegic refraction, uncorrected and best spectacle-corrected visual acuity (BSCVA), slit lamp and funduscopic examination, computerized corneal topography, ultrasonic pachymetry, applanation tonometry, and central keratometry. Patients suitable for the CK procedure should have visual acuity correctable to at least 20/40 in both eyes and pachymetry readings of at least 560 mm at the 6 mm optical zone. They should not have intractable keratoconjunctivitis sicca or unstable, progressive hyperopia. Contact lens wearers should have a stable refraction. Hard lens wearers should discontinue lens use 3 weeks and soft contact lens wearers 2 weeks before the procedure.

The Surgical Procedure

CK is a simple procedure that can be performed in an office setting with topical anesthesia. The entire CK procedure usually takes less than 5 minutes from the time the speculum is inserted to the time the speculum is removed. Administer 1 drop of topical anesthetic 3 times at 5-minute intervals and monitor the patient appropriately for the degree of anesthesia. Do not dilate the eye to be treated. Anxious patients can be given 5.0 mg of Valium (Roche, Switzerland) preoperatively. Begin by consulting the nomogram and establishing a surgical plan based on the patient's refraction and intended correction (both eyes or monovision [blended vision]). If mild myopia is desired to treat presbyopia by inducing blended vision, design an overcorrection, usually to no more than -1.00 to -1.50 D in the non-dominant eye.

Inspect the Keratoplast tip under the microscope to ensure it is not damaged or bent prior to application. Position the patient under the operating microscope, insert the lid speculum, and ask the patient to fixate on the fixation light. Dampen the CK marker with gentian violet or rose bengal stain, center the marker's cross-hair over the pupil center, and apply light pressure on the marker to make a circular mark with 8 intersections on the cornea. If using gentian violet, irrigate with balanced salt solution (BSS) to remove excess ink. Dry the surface of the cornea thor-

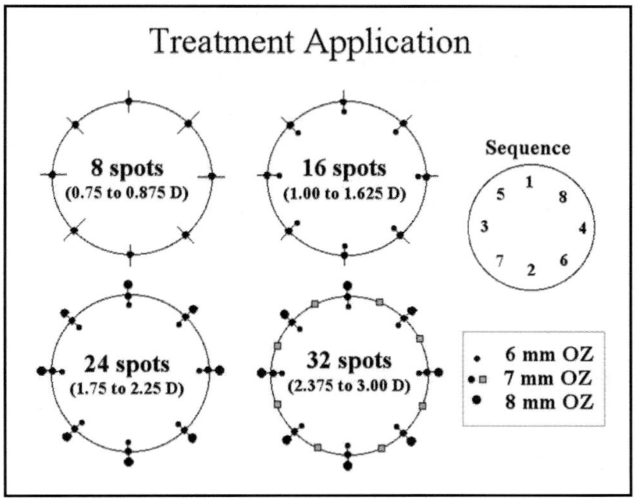

Figure 17-6. Conductive keratoplasty nomogram. Treatment is applied at the 6, 7, and 8 mm optical zones at 8 to 32 treatment spots, depending on the level of hyperopia to be treated.

oughly with a fiber-free sponge to avoid dissipation of applied energy by a wet or damp ocular surface. Marking the cornea properly is important for centration. Set the appropriate treatment parameters on the console, according to the nomogram and sequence of application (Figure 17-6). Apply treatment by inserting the Keratoplast tip into the stroma, perpendicular to surface, at the marked spots around the peripheral cornea. Apply an increasing number of spots for increasing levels of hyperopia, as indicated by the nomogram. Begin treatment at the 7-mm optical zone and continue to the 6-mm and 8-mm optical zones, if necessary. Apply light pressure until the tip penetrates the cornea down to the insulator stop, which prevents further penetration of the tip into corneal tissue. Place treatments in a cross-corneal manner as shown in sequence.

Depress the footpedal to apply the radiofrequency energy. A tone will sound as the energy is applied. The default setting for treatment is 350 kHz, 60% power (0.6 watt) for 0.6 seconds. At each treatment spot, keep the tip in place until the pre-programmed treatment time has been completed (the tone stops). Remove the tip of the delivery probe and repeat the procedure until the full series of spots has been treated according to the treatment plan. Clean the tip (as necessary) with a fiber-free sponge after each treatment spot to remove any tissue debris, taking care not to damage the tip.

As the current flows through the tissue immediately surrounding the probe tip, resistance to the current creates heat. Collagen in the area surrounding the tip shrinks uniformly and forms a column or cylinder. Following a full circle of treatment spots, the peripheral cornea flattens and the central corneal steepens. Postoperative medications include a broad-spectrum topical antibiotic, a topical nonsteroidal, a mild topical corticosteroid (ie, fluorometholone), and an oral analgesic, if needed.

Hyperopia Clinical Study

Patients and Methods

A 2-year, multicenter, prospective clinical trial (FDA phase III hyperopia trial) was conducted to evaluate the safety, efficacy, and stability of conductive keratoplasty when performed on eyes with +0.75 to +3.00 D of hyperopia and 0.75 D of cylinder or less. Some of the preliminary 1-year results were previously published.[33] Patients were selected according to the selection criteria described above (Patient Selection and Preoperative Examinations). Each procedure was performed by one of 12 surgeons at several centers according to methods previously described). The treatment goal was a full correction of spherical hyperopia (emmetropia). No retreatments were performed. A total of 400 eyes have been treated. Follow-up data on 98% of these eyes are available at 1 year and on 80% at 2 years.

Hyperopia Treatment Results

Efficacy

The mean age of enrolled patients was 55.3 ± 6.4 years (range = 40 to 74). The mean baseline cycloplegic spherical equivalent (SE) refraction was +1.86 ± 0.63 D, the median was +1.75 D, and the range was +0.75 to +4.00 D. Uncorrected distance visual acuity (UCVA) preoperatively was 20/40 or better in 26% of the eyes.

A summary of efficacy variables (visual acuity and predictability) is shown in Table 17-1. Twelve months postoperatively, UCVA was 20/20 or better in 174/320 (54%), 20/25 or better in 239/320 (75%), and 20/40 or better in 293/320 (92%) of the eyes. Results were similar at 24 months. The procedure was predictable. Mean MRSE values showed 199/320 (62%) within 0.50 D of intended correction and 284/320 (89%) within 1.00 D at 12 months.

Stability results are shown in Figure 17-7. In patients with consecutive follow-up visits, the MRSE changed ≤0.50 D in 283/383 (74%) between the 3- and 6-month visits, in 337/380 (89%) between the 6- and 9-month visits, in 335/381 (88%) between the 9-

Table 17-1

Summary Efficacy Variables: Hyperopia Study

Efficacy Variable	*3 Months*	*6 Months*	*12 Months*	*24 Months*
UCVA ≤20/20	40%	46%	54%	50%
UCVA ≤20/25	63%	65%	75%	75%
UCVA ≤20/40	85%	89%	92%	92%
MRSE ± 0.50 D	57%	61%	62%	54%
MRSE ± 1.00 D	82%	88%	89%	82%
MRSE ± 2.00 D	97%	98%	99%	98%

N=320 for all visits

UCVA = Uncorrected visual acuity; MRSE = Manifest refractive spherical equivalent

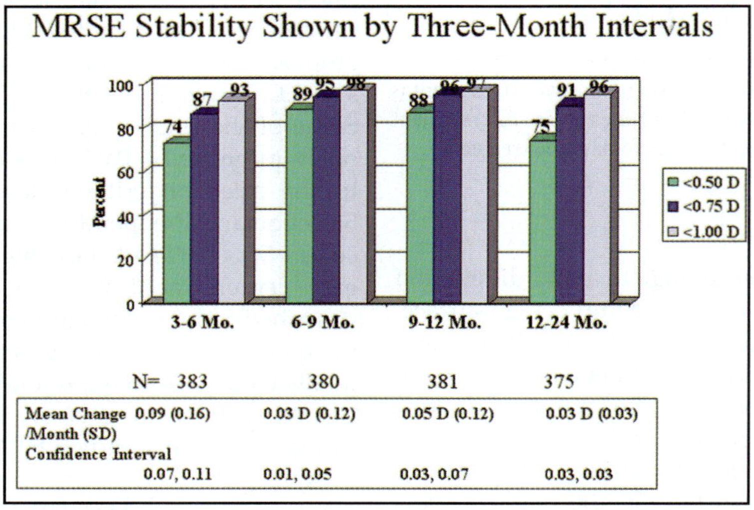

Figure 17-7. Stability Results: Hyperopia Study

and 12-month visits, and in 282/375 (75%) between the 12- and 24-month visits. The mean change in MRSE *per month* was 0.09 D, 0.03 D, 0.05 D, and 0.03 D, between months 3 to 6, 6 to 9, 9 to 12, and 12 to 24, respectively. Expressed as change per interval, the MRSE changed a mean of +0.25 ± 0.50 D between 3 and 6 months, +0.11 ± 0.41 D between 6 and 9 months, 0.13 ± 0.33 D between 9 and 12 months, and 0.28 ± 0.41 D between 12 and 24 months.

The mean MRSE over time shows an overcorrection of approximately 0.50 D at month 1, followed by slight regression over the following months. At 6 months the eyes were essentially emmetropic (mean MRSE = -0.03 D).

Corneal topography (Orbscan, Bausch & Lomb, Rochester, NY) shows postoperative central corneal steepening surrounded by mid-peripheral flattening (Figures 17-8A and B). The MRSE of this eye was +1.625 D before CK treatment and -0.375 D after CK. The lines of tension or striae that connect the treatment spots are responsible for the tightening of the peripheral cornea and the subsequent steepening of the central cornea.

Safety

Safety results are summarized in Table 17-2. Four of 392 eyes lost >2 lines of BSCVA at 3 months and none lost >2 lines at 12 months. Two lines were lost by 20/392 (5%) at 3 months and 9/391 (2%) at 12 months. However, the loss of 2 lines at 12 months left all 9 eyes with very functional vision. Preoperatively, all 9 of these eyes had 20/10 to 20/16 BSCVA. Postoperatively, 1/9 eyes had 20/16 BSCVA, 5/7 eyes had 20/20 and 3/9 eyes had 20/25. No eye had BSCVA worse than 20/40 at any follow-up visit. No eye that had 20/20 or better BSCVA preoperatively had worse than 20/25 BSCVA postoperatively. A total of 87% had no change from preop in cylinder at 12 months. One of 391 eyes (0.3%) had a cylinder increase of more than 2.00 D. A total of 7% had 1.00 D of induced cylinder and 4.8% had more than 1.00 D but less than 2.00 D of induced cylinder. Induced

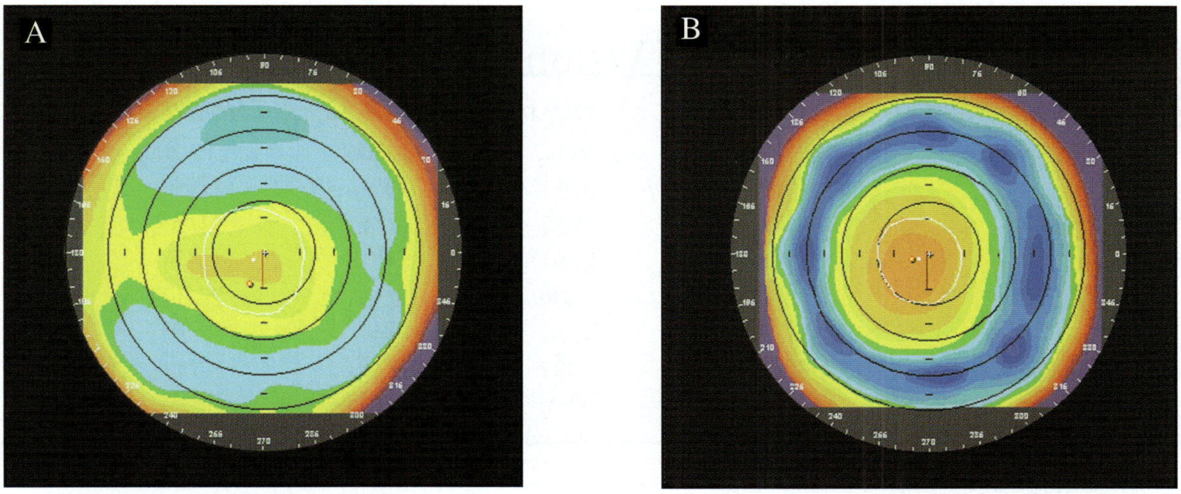

Figure 17-8A and B. Orbscan corneal topography before (left) and 12 months after (right) CK treatment with 16 spots. The MRSE was +1.625 D before CK treatment and -0.375 D after CK. (Courtesy of Daniel Durrie, MD. This figure was previously published in: *Ophthalmology* 2002;109:1978-89.)

Table 17-2

Summary of Safety Variables: Hyperopia Study

Safety Variable	*1 Month*	*3 Months*	*6 Months*	*9 Months*	*12 Months*	*24 Months*
2 Line Loss BSCVA	25/390 (6%)	20/392 (5%)	16/389 (4%)	13/386 (3%)	9/391* (2%)	6/376 (2%)
>2 Line Loss BSCVA	8/390 (2%)	4/392 (1%)	2/389 (0.5%)	2/386 (0.5%)	0/391 (0%)	1/376 (0.3%)
BSCVA Worse than 20/40	0/390 (0%)	0/392 (0%)	0/389 (0%)	0/386 (0%)	0/391 (0%)	0/376 (0%)
Increase >2.00 D Cylinder	13/390 (3%)	8/392 (2%)	3/389 (0.8%)	1/386 (0.3%)	1/391 (0.3%)	0/378 (0%)
BSCVA Worse than 20/25 if better than 20/20 preoperatively	14/390 (4%)	7/392 (2%)	3/389 (0.8%)	2/386 (0.5%)	0/391 (0%)	1/376 (0.3%)

BSCVA = Best spectacle-corrected visual acuity
*Preoperatively, these eyes had 20/10 to 20/16 BSCVA. Postoperatively, 1/9 eyes had 20/16 BSCVA, 5/9 had 20/20, and 3/9 eyes had 20/25. Thus all eyes with 2-line losses had functional vision.

cylinder decreased in frequency and magnitude over time.

Cylinder when present was usually regular and had no effect on BSCVA.

No intraoperative complications or adverse events occurred during any of the surgeries. There were also no treatment-related adverse events, such as peripheral corneal defect, corneal edema later than 1 week postoperatively, recurrent corneal erosion at 1 month or later, double or ghosting images at any time, foreign body sensation at 1 month or later, and pain at 1 month or later. No haze was seen in 384/390 (98%) of the eyes at 1 month postoperatively, in 97% at 6 months, and in 100% at 12 months. There were no occurrences of an uncontrolled intraocular pressure (IOP) increase of >5 mmHg above baseline.

Specular microscopy studies showed no statistically significant change in endothelial cell density from preoperative cell density counts to postoperative counts. Mesopic contrast sensitivity, both with and without glare, showed no difference between

Table 17-3

Patient Evaluation of Vision Quality: Hyperopia Study

Improvement	*Month 1*	*Month 6*	*Month 12*	*Month 24*
Extreme/Marked	210/321 (65%)	249/337 (74%)	258/343 (75%)	217/309 (70%)
Moderate	62/321 (19%)	52/337 (15%)	56/343 (16%)	51/309 (17%)
Slight	33/321 (10%)	19/330 (6%)	19/343 (6%)	26/309 (8%)
None	16/321 (5%)	12/337 (4%)	10/343 (3%)	17/309 (5%)

Table 17-4

Patient Satisfaction: Hyperopia Study

Patient Response	*Month 1*	*Month 6*	*Month 12*	*Month 24*
Very Satisfied/Satisfied	247/324 (76%)	279/338 (83%)	287/343 (84%)	241/310 (78%)
Neutral	52/324 (16%)	31/338 (9%)	26/343 (8%)	42/310 (14%)
Dissatisfied	15/324 (5%)	18/338 (5%)	22/343 (6%)	18/310 (6%)
Very Dissatisfied	10/324 (3%)	10/338 (3%)	8/343 (2%)	9/310 (3%)

the preoperative and the 6 month postoperative values.

Patient Satisfaction

Extreme, marked, or moderate improvement in postoperative vision was noted by a total of 372/321 (85%) of patients at one month and by 314/343 (91%) at 12 months (Table 17-3). Ten patients (3%) thought they had no improvement at 12 months. Patients who were very satisfied or satisfied with the results of their surgery numbered 84% at one month and 78% at 24 months (Table 17-4).

PRESBYOPIA TREATMENT THROUGH BLENDED VISION

Seventy-six million Americans are in the "baby-boomer" category (46 to 56 years old) and are or will soon become presbyopic. Many of these people are distressed by their declining near vision and need for spectacles, but would not consider LASIK surgery because of the perceived risks. These presbyopes represent a distinct population for a modified monovision CK treatment that is known as blended vision. The goal is to induce a mild myopia in 1 eye through an overcorrection designed by the surgeon.

Blended vision is believed to be a result of the multifocal corneal effect produced by CK treatment (Figure 17-9). In the multicenter clinical trial, most eyes were emmetropic at one year, yet the average patient had more than a 6-line improvement in near vision. These effects can be attributed to the corneal surface changes after the procedure. Small surface leukomas that do not require debridement appear at the treatment spots after CK at the 6, 7, and 8 mm optical zones. These leukomas gradually fade and are not cosmetically visible. Figure 17-10A shows a highly magnified slit lamp view of a CK lesion at 7 days after surgery. However, the striae between the spots are believed to be permanent and to be responsible for the multifocal effect (Figure 17-10B). This multifocality may reduce the effects of anisometropia, making CK-created blended vision more tolerable than LASIK- or contact lens-created monovision.

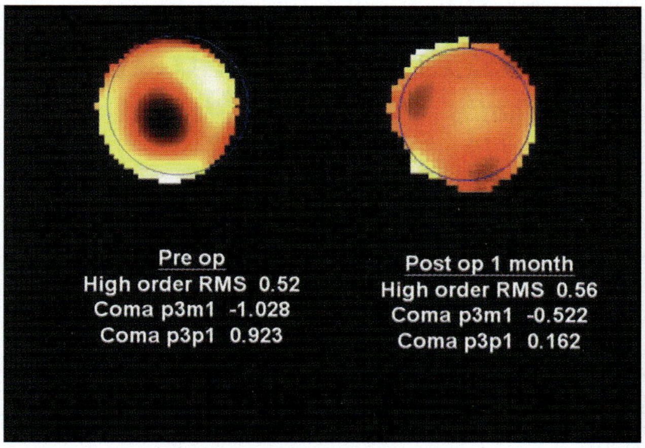

Figure 17-9. Multifocal cornea after CK Treatment. Caption: Corneal topography and wavefront images of a cornea after CK treatment show alternating rings of flat and steeper areas (ie, a flat central cornea surrounded by a ring of higher elevation which is then surrounded by a ring of flatness). These results resemble the effect that follows implantation of the Array multifocal intraocular lens (Allergan, Inc., Irvine, Calif) (courtesy of Ioannis Pallikaris, MD).

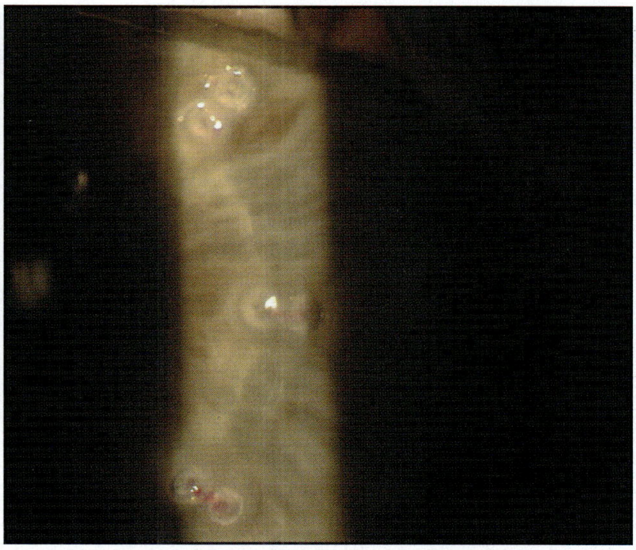

Figure 17-10A. Highly magnified view of CK lesion.

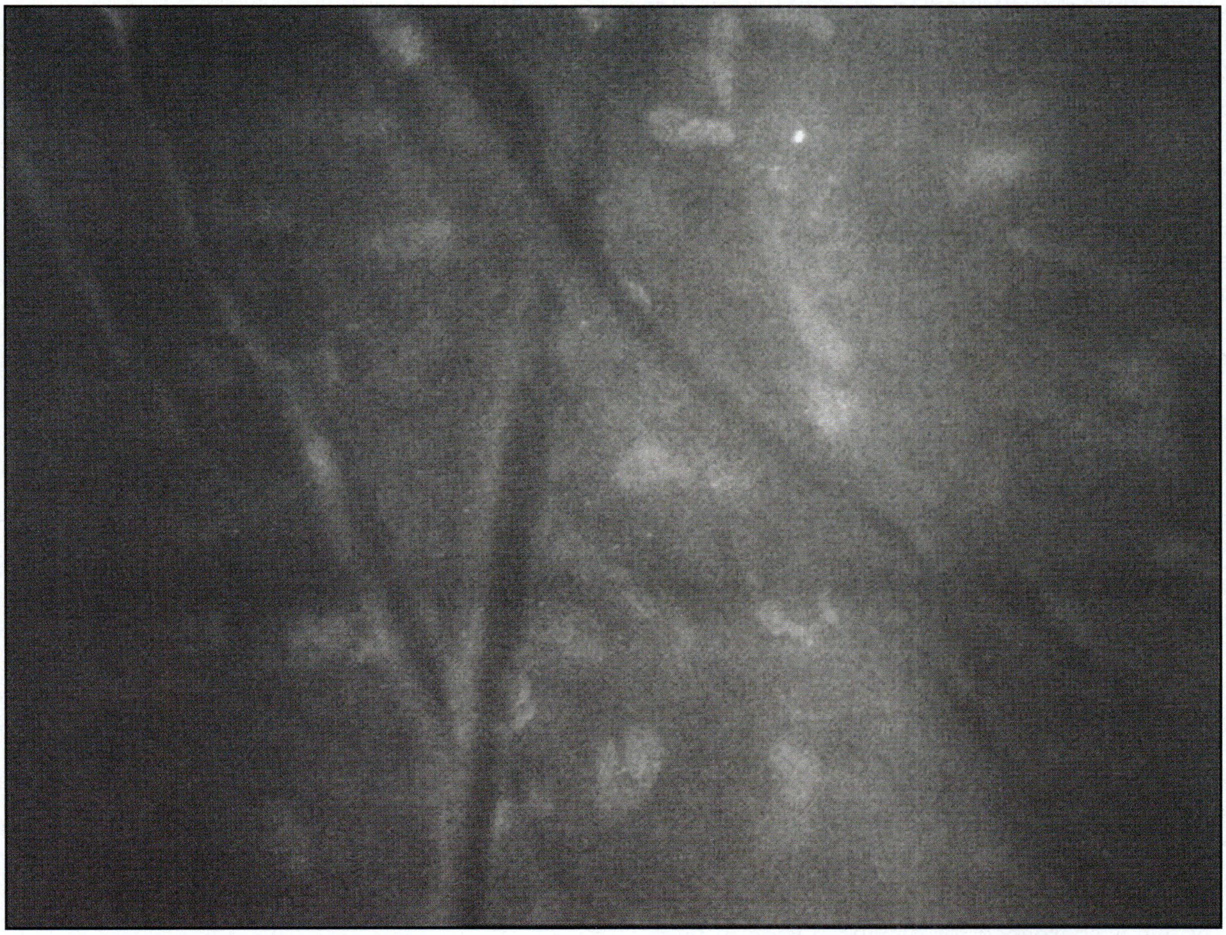

Figure 17-10B. Striae between lesions seen by confocal microscopy. (Courtesy of Drs. Sabry, McDonald, Klyce, and Refractec Inc.)

Table 17-5

Safety Results—All Treated Eyes: Presbyopia Study

	1 Month N=160	3 Months N=112	6 Months N=83
Loss of 2 Lines BCVA	2%	1%	1%
Loss of > 2 Lines BCVA	2%	0%	0%
BCVA Worse than 20/40	0%	0%	0%
Increase > 2.0 D Cylinder	0%	0%	0%
BSCVA worse than 20/25 postoperatively if 20/20 or better preoperatively	0%	0%	0%

Patient Selection

Good candidates for blended vision are 45 years old or older, have usually had very good uncorrected distance vision all of their lives, and strongly dislike their reading glasses. A thorough explanation of the nature of the patient's refractive error and nature of the procedure is particularly important for this older and well-informed patient population. To set appropriate patient expectations, the surgeon must explain that: 1) both hyperopia and presbyopia are progressive conditions, 2) the need for reading glasses will increase as patient ages, but that the benefits from the procedure will not be lost. The patient must also have appropriate short-term expectations because the refraction may be unstable at 1 week to 1 month.

Treat the full refractive error when planning the treatment. The recommended target refraction is -1.00 to -1.25 D in the non-dominant eye of a spherical hyperope (≤0.75 D cylinder). In lower hyperopes, target midway between cycloplegic and manifest refraction. Most well-selected patients will initially only need one eye corrected with the application of 16 spots. Avoid patients with high target anisometropia or strong ocular dominance.

Presbyopia Clinical Study

Patients and Methods

An FDA phase III clinical study is being conducted at 5 sites to evaluate the effectiveness and safety of treating presbyopia with CK. The non-dominant eye is overcorrected to produce a mild to moderate myopia, about -1.00 D to -1.50 D. Vision in the dominant eye is sharpened for distance vision, if necessary.

Patient selection factors were similar to those described for treatment of hyperopia. A total of 176 eyes of 143 patients were treated. One hundred forty-three eyes were treated to improve near vision and 33 eyes (fellow eyes) were treated to improve distance vision. The mean age of patients was 53.1 years ± 4.8, with a range of 44 to 71 years. The mean range of treatment was 1.86 D ± 0.655 D, with a range of +0.75 to +3.00 D. Data on 162/176 eyes (92%) was available at 1 month postoperatively and on 44/176 (25%) at 9 months postoperatively.

Results

Binocular distance and near UCVA results are shown in Figure 17-11. The percentage of eyes with 20/20 and J2 or better binocular UCVA increased from 7% preoperatively to 70% at 6 months postoperatively. Also at 6 months, 86% had 20/25 or better distance with J3 or better near, compared with 13% preoperatively, 92% had 20/32 or better distance and J5 or better near, compared with 35% preoperatively, and 98% had 20/40 or better distance and J7 or better near, compared with 59% preoperatively.

Accuracy results were good for the eyes treated to improve near vision. At 6 months, 66% had an MRSE within 0.50 D and 89% were within 1.00 D of intended correction. Regarding stability, 85%, 89%, and 95% changed 0.50 D or less between 1 and 3 months, 3 and 6 months, and 6 and 9 months, respectively. This was a change of 0.07 D per month in the first 1 to 3 months, 0.06 D per month between months 3 and 6, and 0.04 D per month between months 6 and 9.

Some increase in cylinder was seen at 1 month (26% with 1.00 to 1.50 D increase) but diminished to only 4/83 eyes (5%) having 1.25 D of induced cylinder at 6 months and 3/44 (7%) at 9 months. A summary of safety results is shown in Table 17-5.

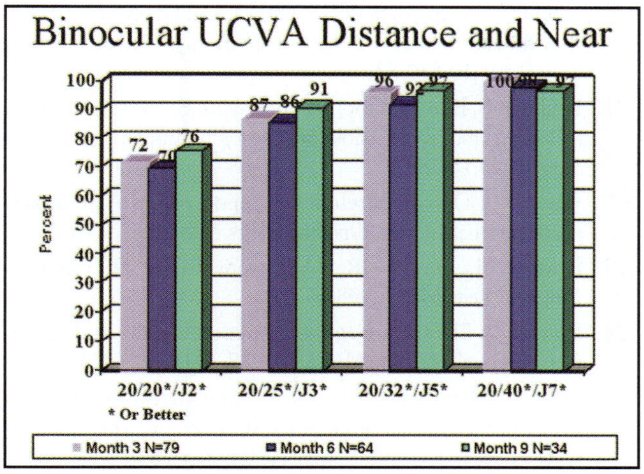

Figure 17-11. Binocular distance and near UCVA: Presbyopia study.

At 9 months postoperatively, 82% of patients were very satisfied/satisfied with the outcome, 13% were neutral, and 5% were dissatisfied.

Summary

CK is a new technique for changing corneal curvature that is approved for use in the United States for correcting low to moderate spherical hyperopia. Ongoing studies for presbyopia treatment through blended vision show promising results. The CK technique uses optimal temperature and time exposures of radiofrequency energy to denature corneal collagen in selected treatment spots. Following a full circle of treatment spots, the peripheral cornea flattens and the central cornea steepens.

During CK treatment, corneal tissue is exposed to the same temperature at the bottom of the probe as at the top of the probe (corneal surface). This is in contrast to non-contact holmium LTK, which has a significant axial gradient and produces the highest temperatures at the corneal surface. The footprint after CK is cylindrical and extends deep into the stroma to approximately 80% depth, which is likely to contribute to permanence of effect. This is in contrast to the conical stromal footprint made with the Sunrise LTK technique.

The multicenter hyperopia clinical study showed the procedure to be very safe; preoperative BSCVA was maintained and penetration of the CK treatment to 80% of the corneal depth did not reduce endothelial cell counts. The study also demonstrated the efficacy of CK in steepening the central cornea to correct low to moderate hyperopia, as well as predictability and stability of the procedure. At 1 year, UCVA was 20/25 or better in 75% of eyes and MRSE was within 0.50 D in 62%. Treated eyes were approximately 0.50 D myopic at month 1 and effectively emmetropic at 6 months. At 24 months, there was only a 20% loss of initial effect. CK outcomes are similar to those seen after hyperopic LASIK without the flap-related complications.

The multicenter presbyopia study showed that CK can be very effective for inducing blended vision in presbyopic eyes. The procedures appears to produce a multifocal cornea that allows for distance and near vision. At 6 months, 70% had binocular UCVA 20/20 or better together with J2 or better and 92% had 20/32 or better along with J5 or better. Safety results were exceptional; the incidence of all safety variables was 1% or less at 3 months and later. At the last visit, 82% of patients were satisfied or very satisfied with the procedure.

Compared with excimer laser treatments, CK does not invade the central cornea, compromise the integrity or structure of the cornea, or require creation of the flap. It is also technically easier to perform than hyperopic LASIK.

The small portable CK unit is much less expensive than other collagen shrinkage technologies. Because the tip can be placed anywhere on the cornea, CK may be useful for treating astigmatism after LASIK or cataract surgery, replacing incisional enhancement procedures, such as astigmatic keratectomy or limbal relaxing incisions. Treatment can be performed at the slit-lamp in a standard examination room instead of a surgical suite. The procedure does not weaken the eye as in the case of incisional enhancement procedures. CK is also a safe means of adjusting LASIK outcomes without the need to lift or recut the flap.

The CK non-laser procedure appears very promising for treating a number of refractive conditions, easily, effectively, and safely.

References

1. Anschutz T. Laser correction of hyperopia and presbyopia. *Intl Ophthalmol Clin*. 1994;10:S277-S280.
2. Argento CJ, Cosentino MJ. Laser in situ keratomileusis for hyperopia. *J Cataract Refract Surg*. 1998;24:1050-8.
3. Ditzen K, Huschka H, Pieger S. Laser in situ keratomileusis for hyperopia. *J Cataract Refract Surg*. 1998;24:42-7.
4. Williams DK. One year results of laser vision correction for low to moderate hyperopia. *Ophthalmology*. 2000;107:72-75.
5. Zadok D, Maskaleris G, Montes, et al. Hyperopic laser in situ keratomileusis with the Nidek EC-5000 excimer laser. *Ophthalmology*. 2000;107:1132-7.

6. Rashad KM. Laser in situ keratomileusis for the correction of hyperopia from +1.25 to 5.00 diopters with the Keracor 117C laser. *J Refract Surg.* 2001;17:123-8.
7. Tabbara KF, El-Sheikh HF, Islam SM. Laser in situ keratomileusis for the correction of hyperopia from +0.50 to 11.50 diopters with the Technolas Keracor 117C laser. *J Refract Surg.* 2001;17:113-2.
8. Pineda-Fernandez A, Rueda L, Huang D, Nur J, Jaramillo J. Laser in situ keratomileusis for hyperopia and hyperopic astigmatism with the Nidek EC-5000 excimer laser. *J Refract Surg.* 2001;17:670-675.
9. Cobo-Soriano R, Llovet F, Gonzalez-Lopez F, Domingo B, Gomez-Sanz F, Baviera J. Factors that influence outcomes of hyperopic laser in situ keratomileusis. *Cataract Refract Surg.* 2002;28:1530-8.
10. Ditzen K, Fiedler J, Pieger S. Laser in situ keratomileusis for hyperopia and hyperopic astigmatism using the Meditec MEL 70 spot scanner. *J Refract Surg.* 2002; 18:430-4.
11. Mendez A, Mendez Noble A. Conductive keratoplasty for the correction of hyperopia. In: Sher N, ed. *Surgery for Hyperopia and Presbyopia.* Baltimore, Md: Williams and Wilkins; 1997;163-171.
12. Gassett AR, Kaufman HE. Thermokeratoplasty in the treatment of keratoconus. *Am J Ophthalmol.* 1975;79:226-232.
13. Aquavella J, Buxton J, Shaw E. Thermokeratoplasty in the treatment of persistent corneal hydrops. *Archives Ophthalmol.* 1977;95:81-84.
14. Aquavella JV, Smith RS, Shaw EL. Alterations in corneal morphology following thermokeratoplasty. *Arch Ophthalmol.* 1976;94:2082-2085.
15. Arentsen J, Rodriquez M, Laibson P. Histopathological changes after thermokeratoplasty for keratoconus. *Invest Ophthalmol Vis Sci.* 1977;16:32-38.
16. Fogle JA, Kenyon KR, Stark WJ. Damage to the epithelial basement membrane by thermokeratoplasty. *Am J Ophthalmol.* 1977;83:392-401.
17. Caster AI. The Fyodorov technique of hyperopia correction by thermal coagulation: a preliminary report. *J Refract Surg.* 1988;4:105-108.
18. Neumann A, Sanders D, Salz J. Radial thermokeratoplasty for hyperopia. *J Refract Corneal Surg.* 1989;5:50-54.
19. Neumann A, Fyodorov S, Sanders D. Radial thermokeratoplasty for the correction of hyperopia. *J Refract Corneal Surg.* 1990;6:404-412.
20. Neumann A, Sanders D, Raanan M, DeLuca M. Hyperopic thermokeratoplasty: clinical evaluation. *J Cataract Refract Surg.* 1991;17:830-838.
21. Feldman S, Ellis W, Frucht-Pery J, et al. Regression of effect following radial thermokeratoplasty in humans. *J Refract Surg.* 1995;18:288-91.
22. Rowsey JJ, Doss JD. Preliminary report of Los Alamos keratoplasty techniques. *Ophthalmology.* 1981;88:755-760.
23. Rowsey JJ, Gaylor JR, Dahlstrom R, et al. Contact. *Intraocul Lens Med J.* 1980;6:1-12.
24. Rowsey JJ. Electrosurgical keratoplasty: Update and retraction. *Invest Ophthalmol Vis Sci.* 1987;28 (suppl):224.
25. Seiler T, Matallana M, Bende T. Laser thermokeratoplasty by means of a pulsed holmium:YAG laser for hyperopic correction. *Refract Corneal Surg.* 1990;6:355-359.
26. Koch DD, Abarca A, Villareal R, et al. Hyperopia correction by non-contact holmium:YAG laser thermokeratoplasty; clinical study with two-year follow-up. *Ophthalmology.* 1996;103:731-40.
27. Koch D, Kohnen T, McDonnell P, et al. Hyperopia correction by noncontact holmium:YAG laser thermal keratoplasty. U.S. Phase IIA Clinical Study with 2-year follow-up. *Ophthalmology.* 1997; 104:1938-47.
28. Hyperion LTK System Device Labeling, PMA P990078. Fremont, Calif: Sunrise Technologies; May 2000.
29. Pearce J, Thomsen S. Rate process analysis of thermal damage. In: Welch AJ, van Gemert MJC, eds. *Optical-Thermal Response of Laser-Irradiated Tissue.* New York: Plenum Press: 1995; 561-605.
30. Chen SS, Humphrey JD. Heat-induced changes in the mechanics of a collagenous tissue: pseudoelastic behavior at 37° C. *Journal Biomechanics.* 1998;31:211-216.
31. Chang J, Soderberg PG, Denham D, et al. Temperature induced corneal shrinkage. In: Parel JM (ed). *Ophthalmic Technologies VI. Proc SPIE.* 1996;2673:70-76.
32. Koch DD, Kohnen T, Anderson JA, et al. Histologic changes and wound healing response following 10-pulse noncontact holmium:YAG laser thermal keratoplasty. *J Refract Surg.* 1996;12:623-34.
33. McDonald MB, Hersh PS, Manche EE, Maloney RK, Davidorf J, Sabry M. Conductive keratoplasty for the correction of low to moderate hyperopia: US clinical trial 1-year results on 355 eyes. *Ophthalmology.* 2002;109:1978-89. Discussion 1989-90.

Chapter Eighteen

Keratophakia: Corneal Implants

Stephen C. Kaufman, MD, PhD and Herbert E. Kaufman, MD

Introduction

Keratophakia involves the use of a lenticule or other device that is surgically placed within the cornea to alter the refractive state of the eye. These corneal implants are an intriguing means of correcting hyperopia. Devices composed of different compounds have been used to alter the refractive properties of the cornea, either by changing the anterior corneal curvature or increasing the refractive index of the cornea. Some of these implants have been designed for placement within a stromal pocket, while other implants are designed for placement under a lamellar dissection, like that produced by the microkeratomes used in laser-assisted in-situ keratomileusis (LASIK). Another type of implant has been designed for placement anterior to Bowman's membrane. The common advantages of these techniques are: 1) no intraocular surgery is involved, 2) the devices can be removed and, 3) the surgical procedures are relatively straightforward. Thus, the "additive" nature of corneal implants offers the promise of correcting spherical and astigmatic refractive errors in a simple, reversible way that does not require intraocular manipulation.

History and Background

Any review of corneal implants must focus upon 3 key aspects: the biocompatible nature of the material, the surgical technique required for placement, and the predictability of the induced refractive change. These properties and others are listed in Table 18-1.

If alloplastic keratophakia is to succeed, the implanted biomaterial must possess certain qualities. The implant must change the refractive state of the eye. The anterior corneal surface is the primary point of refractive power of the eye. To alter the refractive state of the eye, either the anterior corneal radius must be altered or a change in refractive index must be introduced.

Next, any implant must permit the free flow of water and nutrients from the anterior chamber to the anterior corneal surface (Figure 18-1), or the implant must reside in the posterior cornea and possess a small diameter that will allow the nutrients to "flow around" a non-permeable implant. Maurice described the nutritional requirements of the cornea in his 1969 writings.[1] Likewise, oxygen must reach the posterior cornea. The material must remain clear and stable under physiologic conditions. Finally, the implant must alter the refractive state of the eye in a predictable manner.

Table 18-1

Ideal Properties of Biomaterials Used for Keratophakia

- Permit the passage of oxygen, water, nutrients, and lactic acid
- Optically clear
- Stable under physiologic conditions
- Nontoxic/biocompatible
- Predictably alter the refractive state of the eye
- Easy surgical placement
- Reversibility of implant procedure

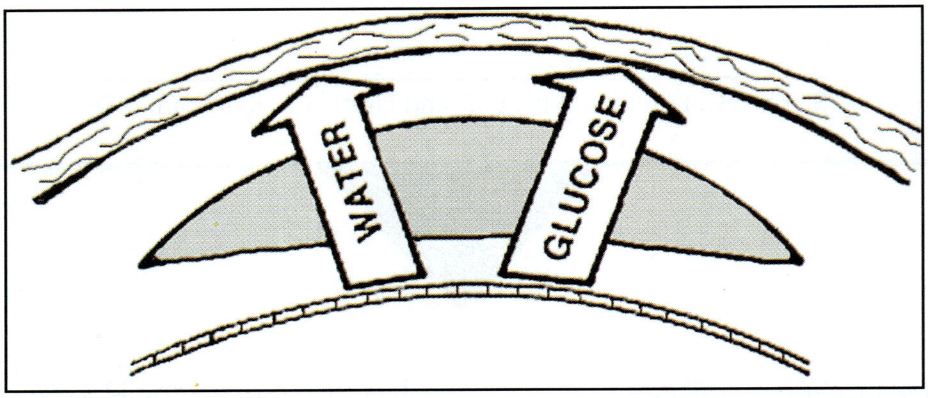

Figure 18-1. Intracorneal implants must permit the free flow of water and nutrients from the anterior chamber to the anterior corneal surface, or the implant must reside in the posterior cornea and possess a small diameter, which will allow the nutrients to "flow around" a non-permeable implant.

Alloplastic Keratophakia

Refractive keratophakia was described by Barraquer in 1949 but technological limitations made the technique inaccurate and not generally usable.[2] Barraquer sought to alter the anterior curvature of the cornea to provide a stable and predictable change in refraction. He understood that the primary refractive effect was produced at the interface of the air and the pre-corneal tear film. Thus, very small changes in the radius of curvature of the cornea resulted in a relatively large change in refractive state of the cornea. The basic principles described by Barraquer were employed by later generations of refractive surgeons in a variety of procedures, ranging from radial keratotomy (RK) to corneal implants and keratophakia.

Barraquer's initial alloplastic implants were composed of flint glass and plexiglass.[3] When these alloplastic materials failed, he redirected his efforts toward the production of autologous corneal tissue as an implant material. Intracorneal implants of multiple design and composition have been studied. Many synthetic biomaterials have been proposed for lenticule composition (Table 18-2), which will be discussed.

Epikeratophakia

Further studies by Kaufman and Gasset investigated the use of a methacrylate lens as a keratoprosthesis.[4,5] These initial experiments led to the procedure of epikeratophakia, which alters the refractive power of the cornea by sewing a tissue lens, pre-lathed to the desired curvature, onto the anterior corneal surface (Figure 18-2). The goal of epikeratophakia was to provide a safe, straightforward surgical procedure that produced a permanent refractive correction.

The Epikeratophakia Procedure

The procedure involves the use of a donor lenticule, which is ground to the desired curvature from the endothelial side of the "button." The central epithelium of the host cornea is removed. A shallow, peripheral trephination is performed, which is followed by

Table 18-2

Biomaterials for Keratophakia

Material	*Advantages*	*Disadvantages*
Glass	Clear, stable	Impermeable to water and nutrients.
PMMA	Clear, stable	Impermeable to water and nutrients.
Polysulfone	Clear, long-term survival in some patients	Impermeable to water and nutrients. Must be placed in posterior cornea. Lens associated deposits reported. Possible UV degradation
Hydrogel	Clear, stable, Long-term survival, Permeable to water and nutrients. Can be placed under lamellar keratectomy (easy placement)	Difficult to manipulate thin lenses. Can decenter under lamellar keratectomy. Water content can affect refractive state of lens by altering size/thickness of lens

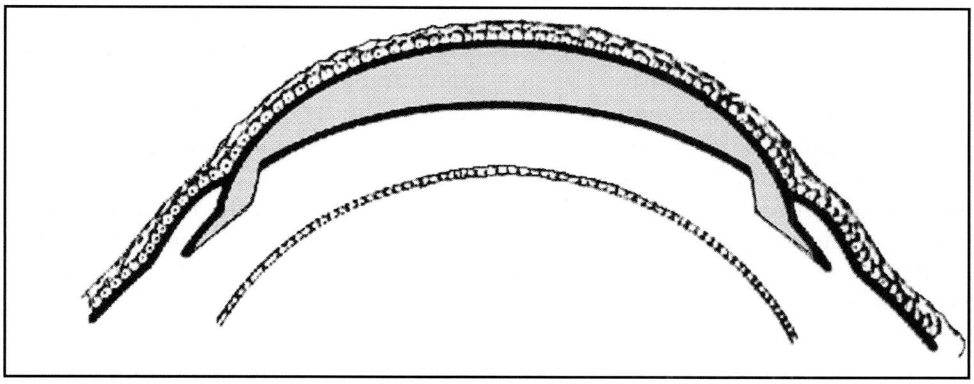

Figure 18-2. Epikeratophakia alters the refractive power of the cornea by sewing a tissue lens, pre-lathed to the desired curvature, onto the anterior corneal surface. Adapted from Brightbill FS, ed. *Corneal Surgery*. Mosby, St. Louis; 1993.

a short undermining dissection at the peripheral edge. Next, the stromal side of the donor lenticule is placed on the bare surface of the host's Bowman's membrane. The wing of the lenticule is then tucked into the peripheral edge of the previously undermined region of the host cornea. Sutures are then used to anchor the tissue lenticule into place. Contraindications to this surgery include: poorly controlled blepharitis, significant dry eyes, exposure keratitis, or a central corneal scar.

Evaluation of Epikeratophakia

Although this procedure is straightforward in its description, it requires a precision ground lenticule and skill in applying the corneal sutures. The procedure was designed for use in 4 basic areas: aphakic patients who could not tolerate an intraocular lens (IOL), pediatric patients who could not tolerate a contact lens (CTL), CTL-intolerant patients with high myopia, and keratoconus patients who can not wear a CTL. Major studies were performed to evaluate the procedure of epikeratophakia in each of these applied areas.

In 1987, a large group of investigators published a series of studies for epikeratophakia in children, individuals with high myopia, patients with keratoconus, and for adults with aphakia.[6-9] One hundred and fifty-four surgeons performed 519 epikeratophakia procedures for the correction of aphakia in adults. Seventy-five percent of the study eyes were within 3.00 D of emmetropia, while 95% of 259 eyes demonstrated an improvement of the uncorrected visual acuity. Preoperative mean astigmatism was 2.10 D and the postoperative astigmatism was 2.70 D. Four percent of the onlays were removed due

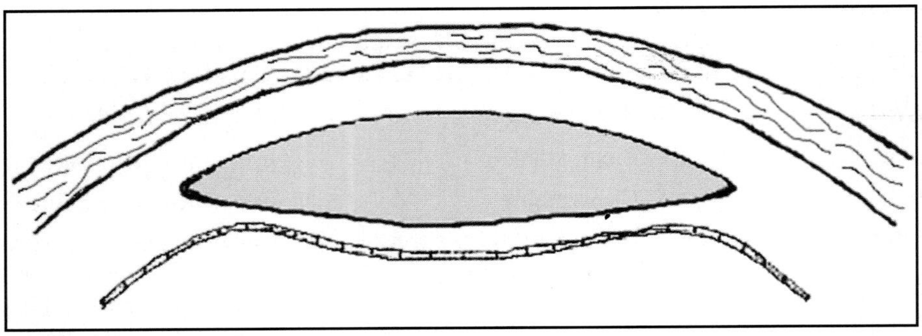

Figure 18-3. Polysulfone implants have a higher index of refraction than that of the cornea, thus, it is not necessary to alter the anterior corneal curvature. Because of the impermeable nature of the polysulfone material, these lenses must be placed deep within the stroma of the cornea.

to failure to re-epithelialize, refractive errors, or a torn lenticule.

In the next study, 97 surgeons performed 335 epikeratophakia procedures for aphakia in children under 8 years of age. Surgical success was achieved in 89% of patients and 73% of the eyes were within 3.00 D of emmetropia. An investigation of epikeratophakia for myopia was undertaken by 116 surgeons, performed 352 procedures. Seventy-five percent of the eyes were within 30% of emmetropia and all but 1 patient improved their best-corrected visual acuity (BCVA). The mean preoperative astigmatism was 1.40 D and the postoperative astigmatism was 2.60 D. A total of 10% of the lenses were removed due to refractive errors or failure to re-epithelialize. The preliminary results of the nationwide study of epikeratophakia for keratoconus involved a small number of patients but stated that epikeratophakia was as efficacious at penetrating keratoplasty for the treatment of keratoconus.

While epikeratophakia was successful as a refractive procedure, was reversible, and did not involve the risk of an intraocular procedure; epikeratophakia did require a prolonged healing time for vision to stabilize and the refractive outcome was not as predictable as one would like. However, newer technologies and materials may make it a viable option in the future.

"Buried" Corneal Silicone Prosthesis

As early as 1965 Dohlman, Brown, Miller and coworkers had studied the use of silicone rubber as a possible fluid barrier on the posterior corneal surface.[10-13] The theoretical value of such a device was appealing for patients with endothelial dystrophies and decompensation resulting in corneal edema. In their major paper, the investigators described 2 types of silicone implants. One was a mushroom-shaped buried implant (Brown–Dohlman implant, Dow Corning Corp, Midland, Mich). The second was a silastic-type membrane for attachment to the posterior corneal surface as an artificial endothelium. The authors described their implants as "buried prosthesis."

The index of the refraction of the implants was 1.48. The thickness of the mushroom-shaped implant was 1.65 mm while that of the thinner silicone-type membrane was 0.23 mm. The diameter of the primary cylinder of the mushroom-shaped implant was 2 mm and the diameter of the silicone-type implant was 8 mm. In their 8 series of experiments, the authors described the use of the mushroom-shaped implant within a bovine corneal lenticule and the membrane-type implant placed under a plano contact lens or worn directly on the surface of the cornea. The authors ultimately discussed the possible use of these implants on the posterior surface of the cornea. However, to the best of our knowledge, further experiments were never published. Because silicone will not transmit nutrients from the aqueous humor through the material, anterior corneal tissue would ultimately necrose. These silicone implants were actually intended as a therapeutic device but are discussed in this chapter in the historical context of their use as an implantable alloplastic lenticule.

Polysulfone Intracorneal Implants

Although other impermeable materials had failed when implanted within the cornea, Choyce implanted polysulfone corneal inlays within the corneas of patients in 1980. Choyce described the outcome of his initial study and stated that the implants were well tolerated and able to correct significant levels of refractive error.[14]

Polysulfone lenses have a refractive index of 1.633. This higher index of refraction eliminates the need to alter the anterior corneal curvature (Figure 18-3). Thus, these lenses can be placed in the posterior corneal stroma where they have little or no effect on the anterior corneal curvature. In fact, because of the impermeable nature of the polysulfone material, these lenses must be placed deep within the stroma of the cornea.

Polysulfone Lens Implantation

An eyelid speculum is inserted. The center of the cornea was marked with the tip of a 23-gauge needle, the border of the proposed lamellar pocket was outlined with a 6-mm RK optical zone marker. A penetrating corneal incision, approximately 6 mm in length, was performed central to the superior limbus using a diamond knife. The blade of the diamond knife was set to 100% of the measured superior corneal thickness. An intrastromal corneal pocket was constructed using a #66 Beaver blade. The polysulfone lens was irrigated with a balance salt solution (BSS) and subsequently cleaned with a cellulose sponge moistened in BSS. The lens was inserted into the stromal pocket with a smooth Kelman-McPherson forceps. The corneal wound was then closed with 4 to 5 interrupted, 10-0 nylon sutures.

In Vivo Studies of Polysulfone Lenticules

In 1985, Choyce published a paper describing the outcomes of 40 patients who had polysulfone lenses implanted within the cornea.[15] Some of these patients had retained their lenses for up to 50 months. Although no complications were noted, he did recognize that the non-permeable polysulfone lenses required implantation deep within the corneal stroma. It was hypothesized that the deeply implanted lenses permitted water and glucose from the aqueous to flow around the lens and supply the anterior corneal stroma and epithelium with water and nutrients. That same year, Lindstrom and coworkers described their independent examinations of a limited number of Choyce's early patients.[16] The majority of Choyce's claims were verified; however, concerns involving clinically observed changes within the cornea were expressed. Chiefly among these were: necrosis or thinning of the anterior stroma from reduced water and glucose levels, precise placement of the polysulfone lens within the cornea, the stability of the polysulfone material and whether accurate clinical assessment of the intraocular pressures and endothelial cell density could be assessed after polysulfone lens implantation.

Other concerns involving the use of polysulfone corneal inlays were expressed and later in 1985 Dr. Kirkness and Dr. Steele expressed this in a letter to the editor of *The LANCET*.[17] The letter read, "We have reported adverse reactions to polysulfone in two patients, (three eyes), who were referred to us. We have since had the opportunity to examine 10 of the 40 eyes in Mr. Choyce's original series (some at his direct invitation) and none of them is without pathological changes."[17]

Climenhaga and co-workers devised a unique study concerning corneal changes associated with polysulfone lenses of different diameters implanted at different depths within the cornea.[18] The depth of the corneal implant was determined by using an ultrasonic pachymeter to measure the thickness of the cornea prior to insertion of the polysulfone lens. After the lens was inserted, the ultrasonic pachymeter was again used to measure the thickness of the cornea over the polysulfone lens. The thickness of the anterior lamella could be determined because the ultrasound waves were reflected off the anterior surface of the polysulfone lens. Then the ratio of the two numbers permitted the determination of the depth of the polysulfone lens within the cornea.

The diameter of the inserted lenses ranged from 4 to 7 mm. The author's initial results indicated that central opacities developed within the corneas of the more superficially placed and larger diameter intracorneal lenses, but after 6 months, differences between corneas with lenses at different depths were not deemed significant. Twenty months after implantation, 100% of the 7-mm lenses had produced anterior corneal opacification, while only 66% of the 4-mm lenses were associated with corneal opacification. Interestingly, the measured depth of the lens was not directly correlated with the appearance of opacities.

In their conclusion, the authors wrote that their attempts to circumvent the hindrance of nutrients to the anterior cornea by the polysulfone lens within a deep corneal placement—in the hopes that nutrients would diffuse around the lateral edges of the lens to prevent metabolic changes—failed. Additionally, while the 4-mm diameter lenses stayed clearer longer, they worried that lenses smaller than 5 mm might produce significant nighttime glare.

Later, Deg, and Binder performed a subsequent study in 1987 concerning the behavior of polysulfone intracorneal implants in a baboon model.[19] The lenses were implanted deep within the corneal stroma and ranged in diameter from 3.975 to 6 mm. The first series of 6 subjects all failed within 6 days to 6 months. Anterior corneal melting, epithelial haze, stromal haze, neovascularization, anterior erosion, anterior corneal necrosis, and interface opacification were all described in various subjects in this first series. The second series contained 3 subjects who received lenses between 3.975 mm and 4.978 mm. Similar to the first series of subjects, 2 of 3 subjects in this study experienced failure. However, one subject did maintain corneal clarity up to 27 months after surgery.

Compared to other studies, this study experienced a statistically higher failure rate. It was proposed that this was due to the possibility of retained toxic material within their polysulfone implants. The authors concluded that the design of the implant used in their study was not compatible with normal corneal nutrition and was therefore not an acceptable implant.

In a later study, Rodrigues and co-workers described lipid deposits posterior to the intracorneal lenses.[20] Although deposits had been noted in other studies, these investigators documented the presence of lipid in a position that was posterior to the polysulfone lenses. This seemed paradoxical initially, because nutrients from the aqueous would initially reach this posterior surface. However, it was noted that this type of lens blocked oxygen diffusion and the metabolic stress of the decreased oxygen tension may have caused production of lipids by stromal keratocytes. Conversely it was also hypothesized that the lipids may have been produced by the posterior stromal keratocytes in response to the polysulfone foreign body reaction.

In a 1997 published letter, Choyce summarized his feelings concerning polysulfone implants by saying that "the bottom line, as far as I'm concerned, is that polysulfone corneal inlays do work and can be tolerated for many years, up to 15 so far, but they need to be equipped with microperforation surrounding a central 3-mm diameter zone."[21]

Thus, the work of Choyce and McCarey highlight the potential for polysulfone intracorneal implants, and although this material is an impermeable barrier within the cornea, it may be tolerated by virtue of its high refractive index and discrete placement within the cornea or possibly with microperforations to allow nutrient flow through the lens.

Hydrogel Implants

The first hydrogel material that was used in corneal surgery was glyceryl methacrylate. The material was initially used by Dohlman and associates in 1967 and, although the material was not used in a refractive manner, it did demonstrate the potential biocompatibility of this material.[22]

Most hydrogel material currently being investigated is hydroxy-ethyl methacrylate (HEMA). Mester first used this HEMA hydrogel lens in 1976 in an experimental keratophakia study and this was followed by extensive studies by McCarey, Andrews, Binder, Werblin, Kaufman, and others.[23-27]

Hydrogel material has pore channels throughout the matrix of its substance. The polymer chain makeup of the hydrogel material has hydrophilic sites, which attract water, and the more water that is associated with the material, the greater spreading that will occur between polymer chains. Thus, the number of hydrophilic sites within the material affects the pore size and thus the diffusion through the lens.[28]

The ability of these lenses to permit the passage of water and nutrients is essential, because these lenses must be placed in the anterior half of the cornea. Their refractive index is very similar to that of the cornea and they change the refractive state of the eye by altering the anterior corneal curvature (Figure 18-4).

In 1985 Watsky and co-workers published an algorithm to predict the refractive alteration in the cornea after insertion of an intracorneal space-occupying material.[29] These basic calculations permit the prediction of the final refraction of an eye after insertion of an anteriorly placed intracorneal lens.

Surgical Implantation of Hydrogel Lenses

Three techniques have generally been used to implant hydrogel lenses. The first technique involves construction of a stromal pocket, as was described in the placement of the polysulfone lens. However, because the hydrogel lens must alter the anterior corneal curvature, Bowman's membrane must be incised to permit an alteration in the anterior corneal curvature. The second surgical technique involves the use of a microkeratome to produce a lamellar keratectomy. Initially, when this procedure was used, the keratectomy produced a "free cap." This disk of anterior corneal tissue was placed over the hydrogel lens and sutured into place. This technique was soon abandoned after microkeratome technology improved and a lamellar flap could be reliably produced with a hinge. The hinge provided additional stability and although sutures were still used to anchor the graft, they were typically removed after only a few weeks. Newer techniques may eliminate the need for sutures altogether.

Results After Hydrogel Keratophakia

Sendele and co-workers were the first to report the implantation of hydrogel lenses in humans.[30] Multiple studies have demonstrated successful long-term results with hydrogel intracorneal lenses in primates and human subjects.[31-34] Furthermore, studies have revealed that removal of the lens returned the eye to its original refractive state.[32]

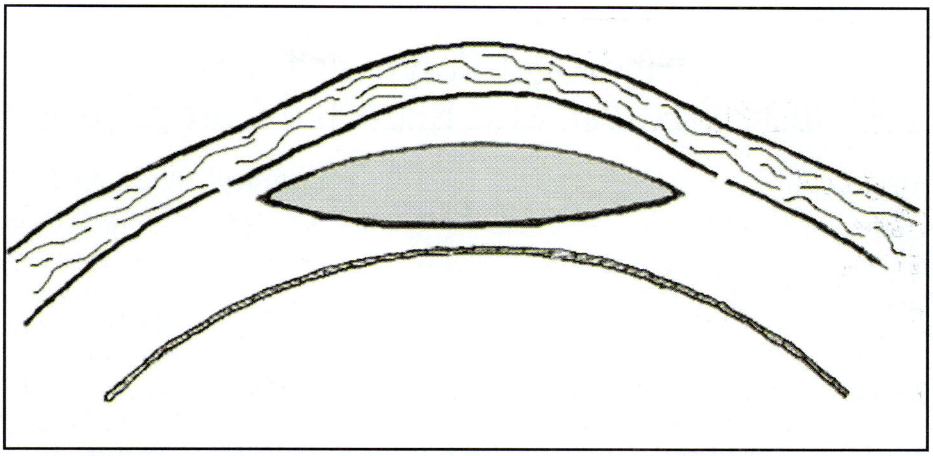

Figure 18-4. Hydrogel intracorneal implants change the refractive state of the eye by altering the anterior corneal curvature.

One of the primary goals of any refractive surgery is to consistently and accurately eliminate preoperative refractive error. Although the biocompatibility of the lens has been proven, there are studies that demonstrate an unpredictable refractive outcome after the surgery.

An early hydrogel study from Binder demonstrated variability in the final refractive outcome that appeared to be somewhat unrelated to the predicted power that would be produced by the hydrogel implant.[35] These errors were attributed to two factors: 1) difficulties in measuring the refractive error in the baboon model preoperatively and, 2) some possible irregular astigmatism that was present in the implant preoperatively.

A further study of hydrogel implants by Werblin also demonstrated an undercorrection of the preoperative refraction in a human model.[36] The authors were uncertain whether the residual refractive error was the result of the keratomileusis flap, other factors induced by the surgical procedure, changes in the hydration of the hydrogel material, or some other lens-related factor. Despite the undercorrections experienced, the lenses were well tolerated for 18 months in these human subjects.

Hydrogel Lens Design and Manufacturing Issues

Early hydrogel lens studies demonstrated the importance of quality control in the manufacturing process of these implants. There are numerous examples of intracorneal and intraocular implants that have produced postoperative complications due to lens design or contamination of the material during the manufacturing process or the packaging process. Beekhuis and his co-workers discussed the importance of implant design and specifically concentrated their analysis on the construction of the edge of the lens. They determined that it was important to gently taper the edge of the lens to produce a fine wedge-shaped periphery rather than to produce a lens with an abruptly cut edge.[37] This type of lens construction aided in the biocompatibility of the lens, the improved conformation of the keratomileusis flap to the anterior surface of the lens, and decreased light scattering produced by the lens edge. Table 18-3 discusses some of the types and characteristics of the various hydrogel polymers available.

A study by Werblin discussed the results of 63 surgical cases of hydrogel lens implantation with a 30-month to 8-year follow-up. This study was significant for associating postoperative complications with lens contamination during the manufacturing process and contamination originating from materials within the lenses container.[38] Additionally, a study by Zavala and co-workers demonstrated that polymer types and chemical additives may play a role in encapsulation of the hydrogel implant.[39] Encapsulation is an undesirable event that appears as a "marbleization" at the interface of the lens with the cornea. This area of encapsulation appears as fibrosis and haze on examination.

In 1984, a study was performed with hydrogel lenses. Virtually all the corneas showed sign of opacification, vascularization, and chronic inflammation in a rabbit model.[40] Because of these results, it was unclear whether the cause was related directly to the hydrogel material, the surgical method or simply the fact that the rabbit's eye does not react in the same manner as a human or a primate eye. The authors concluded that due to the immune response of the rabbit and because the rabbit possesses thinner

Table 18-3

Hydrogel Polymer Types+, Characteristics,+ and Reported Complications*

Hydrogel Type	Polymer+	Hydration+	Surface Charge+	Reported Complications*
Lidofilcon A	Methyl methacrylate & N-vinyl pyrrolidone	70 %	Neutral	Deposits, Lens extrusion, Lens encapsulation, Epithelial downgrowth, Corneal ulceration
Lidofilcon B	Methyl methacrylate & N-vinyl pyrrolidone	79 %	Neutral	Deposits, Lens extrusion, Corneal ulceration
Perfilcon A	2-hydroxyethyl methacrylate, N-vinyl pyrrolidone, & methacrylic acid	71 %	No data	No data
Bufilcon A	2-hydroxyethyl methacrylate, diacetone acrylamide, & acrylic acid	55 %	Negative	No data
Polymacon	Poly (hydroxyethyl methacrylate)	38.6 %	Neutral	No data

Adapted from: +Zavala EY, Nayak SK, Deg JK, et al. Human keratocyte interactions with hydrogel materials. *CLAO J.* 1986;12(1):55 and *McDonald MB, McCarey BE, Storie B, et al. Assessment of the long-term corneal response to hydrogel intrastromal lenses implanted in monkey eyes for up to five years. *J Cataract Refract Surg.* 1993;19:217.

corneas, it is difficult to use as a suitable animal model in keratophakia studies. This illustrates the need to evaluate the model used in any nonhuman corneal implant investigation.

Collagen Type IV Intracorneal Implants

Like the other materials discussed, collagen type IV has been used as an intracorneal implant. A significant study of this material involved human placental derived collagen type 4 in a dog model. Dupont and co-workers described the implantation of these lenses in 8 canine subjects. Although the study was of a short duration, no inflammation was noted from the collagen and no encapsulation or fibrotic activity was identified on microscopy. It was noted that there was one case of anterior corneal necrosis, that occurred without any alteration in clarity of the implant or cornea.[41] Primate implantation was also performed with clarity of the lenticules and good tolerance but slow dissolution, sometimes after a year , began in the absence of any apparent corneal abnormality. Other types of collagen have been studied (Table 18-4). Further studies with collagen materials are underway.

Current Trends in Keratophakia

Previous surgical procedures laid the foundation for our understanding of altering the refractive state of the cornea. New instrument technologies and materials insure continued research into this promising area of refractive surgery. A discussion of current research can be divided by the material of the implant and the location of the implant within the cornea.

Collagen I Coated Perfluoropolyether Lenticules

In 2000, a study by Evanes, Xie, and co-workers described the use of a synthetic polymer lenticule for epikeratophakia. The lens is clear (Figure 18-5) and designed for placement anterior to Bowman's membrane after epithelial debridement, as was described with epikeratophakia. But, an alternative procedure, which involved construction of an anterior stromal pocket for the placement of the lens, was also described.[42] Four-millimeter diameter lenticules of perfluoropolyether (PFPE) were constructed with a central thickness of 80 µm, which tapered to 70 µm

Table 18-4

Collagen Biomaterials for Keratophakia

Material	*Advantages*	*Disadvantages*
Pure Collagen (Collagen type I, III, or IV)	Relatively clear, non synthetic	Susceptible to enzymatic degradation, May not be completely transparent
Synthetic-Coated Collagen [Collagen type I Coated Perfluoropolyether Lenticules (PFPE), and other coatings]	Transparent, good optics, possibly more stable and resistant to enzymatic degradation	Requires addition of synthetic coating during manufacturing process, some coatings cause decreased epithelial adhesion

Adapted from: Thompson KP, Daniel J. Synthetic epikeratophakia. In: Elander R, Rich LF, Robin JB, eds. *Principles and Practice of Refractive Surgery*. Philadelphia, PA: WB Saunders Co; 1997: 406.

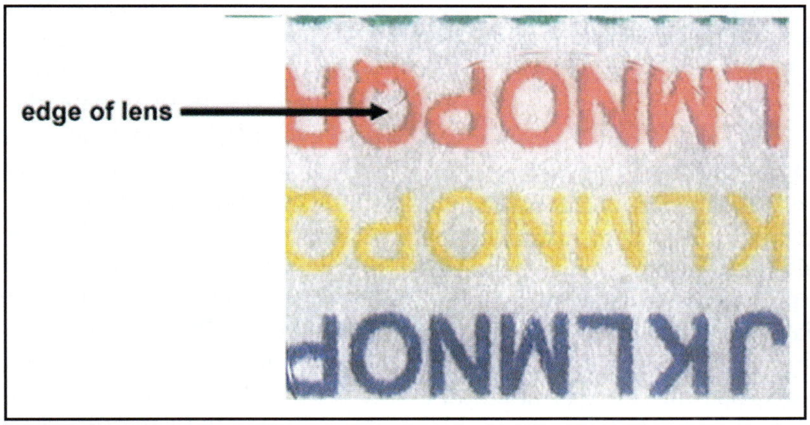

Figure 18-5. The clear nature of the collagen I coated perfluoropolyether lenticules (PFPE) can be seen in the photograph. (Photo courtesy of the Cooperative Research Centre for Eye Research and Technology [CRCERT].)

and terminated in a squared edge. The lenses had a water content of 52%.

Surgical Procedure

The lenses were implanted in 4 feline subjects by using a beaver blade to remove the corneal epithelium in a 4-mm diameter area. A 150 μm deep circular keratectomy was performed in the debrided area with a 2-mm diameter trephine. The stroma within this 2-mm region was removed. Next, a 1-mm wide stromal pocket was produced extending from the keratectomy site. The superior region of this keratectomy was extended superiorly 5 mm in an arcuate fashion. A 5-mm keratectomy was then performed at the superior margin of the previously made pocket. This was used to deliver a 4-mm diameter lenticule, which was tucked into the previously made circular stromal pocket.

Study Results

Evans noted complete growth of the epithelium over the debrided area within 5 to 9 days. The cats were maintained for 34 to 39 days post surgery. The authors determined that the PFPE lenticules were transparent and bio-stable. The lenses were determined to be permeable to a nutrient flow by measurement of glucose, inulin, and human serum albumin measurements. An additional study has been performed by placing the lens on Bowman's membrane after debridement of the epithelium. Postoperatively, epithelial re-growth covered the lenticule in 5 to 11 days. The feline subjects were followed for either 4 or 8 weeks. Complications included post-surgical inflammation in 1 subject and a small focal epithelial detachment in 2 subjects. All subjects' eyes implanted with the PFPE lens developed "fine crystalline deposits" around the periphery of the lenticule. Upon histological examination the deposits appeared to be lipid in nature. Overall, the authors considered this preliminary study a success.[43]

One year later the Cooperative Research Centre for Eye Research and Technology (CRCERT) further

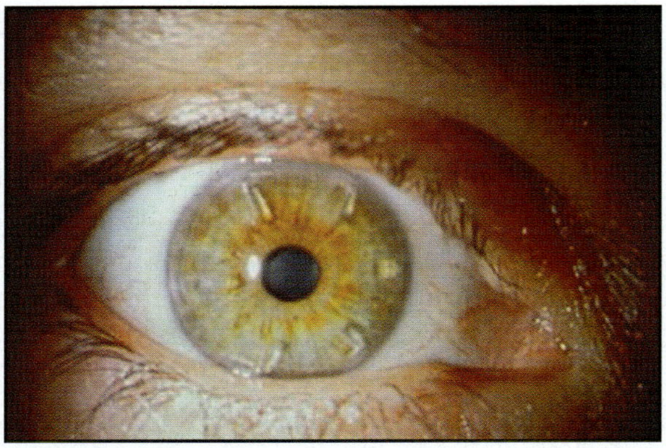

Figure 18-6. Intrastromal corneal segments (ICS) for hyperopia are PMMA segments that are placed deep within the corneal stroma in a radial orientation. The segments correct hyperopia by flattening the peripheral cornea, while steepening the central cornea. (Photo courtesy of Addition Technology.)

examined the use of the PFPE lens.[44] The lenses are composed of PFPE, which is a class of fluoropolymer with index of refraction of 1.344. They examined the biostability, permeability, transparency, and the biocompatibility of the polymer lens. Their study found that corneal epithelial cells coated and adhered to the lens surface best when the pore size of the polymer ranged between 50 and 300 μm. Furthermore, they developed a "coral-like" surface of fused globular submicron sized particles on the lenticule, which is believed to promote adhesion of epithelial cells. Further research with this implant is underway.

Intrastromal Corneal Segments for Hyperopia

Like the intracorneal ring segments (ICRS) designed to treat myopia, Addition Technology (Fremont, Calif) has designed a corneal implant to treat hyperopia. These PMMA corneal inserts are small segments that are placed deep within the corneal stroma in a radial orientation (Figure 18-6).

Each intrastromal corneal segment (ICS) is 1.8 mm in length and placed in the peripheral cornea; therefore, the central optical zone is not invaded. The segments produce their effect by flattening the corneal periphery while steepening the central cornea. The degree of refractive correction can be increased by increasing the number of the segments implanted and by using segments of greater thickness.

ICS Study Results

The initial clinical trials of the ICS were performed in Mexico, by Chayet.[45] The study involved the implantation of 6 radially placed segments in each of 16 eyes. The mean preoperative cycloplegic refraction was +2.29 (range: +0.75 to +4.50). After 18 months, 69% of the patients were 20/20 or better and 94% of the patients were better than 20/50. None of the patients were reported with more than 0.50 D of induced cylinder. Complications were experienced in 6 of the 16 patients who had segments removed due to shallow placement or epithelial ingrowth.

A second European hyperopia study was performed with the ICS.[46] This secondary investigation utilized different numbers of segments implanted in each eye and different size segments were implanted in different arms of the study. The flexible protocol employed either 0.5 or 0.8 mm wide by 1.8-mm length segments. Additionally, by varying the segment thickness, the degree of correction can be altered. Segment thickness ranged from 0.35 mm to 0.50 mm, in 0.05 increments. Either 6 or 8 segments were implanted at 2/3 corneal depth. The study involved 34 eyes of 34 patients. The mean preoperative cycloplegic spherical refraction was +1.97 D preop cycloplegic (range: +0.50 to +4.75). Resulting visual acuities after 1 year were 20/20 in 29% to 47% of the eyes and 100% of the subjects were better than 20/40. Fourteen percent to 100% of the eyes were within 1.00 D of emmetropia. The better results were obtained by the groups with the wider (0.8 mm) implant or with 8, rather than 6, implants (Table 18-5). Seven of 34 patients had more than 1.00 D of induced astigmatism postoperatively. Further investigations with these devices are planned.

PermaVision Intracorneal Hydrogel Lens

The PermaVision intracorneal lens is manufactured by Anamed (Lake Forest, Calif) and is designed to correct up to 6.00 D of hyperopia. This new hydrogel lens has received the CE mark in Europe, has begun FDA trials, and has already successfully completed long-term animal studies in rabbits and swine. The hydrogel lens material has successfully passed testing concerning sterility, stability under physiologic conditions, and optical clarity.

This proprietary hydrogel material has the trade name "Nutrapore." Anamed's studies of the basic properties of the material indicate that it has a refractive index of 1.374. The transmission of light through the lens is dependent upon the wavelength measured; however, over the visible spectrum, the transmission ranges between 96.8% and 99.8%. The water content and glucose transmission of the Nutrapore material is 78.9% and 433 μg/hr/cm^2 respectively (Table 18-6).

Surgical Implantation

Due to advances in automated microkeratome technology and hinged flap lamellar dissections, surgical

Table 18-5

Spherical Equivalent of Postoperative Manifest Refraction Results

Study Arm	*N*	*Mean (D)*	*Std. Dev.(D)*	*Minimum (D)*	*Maximum (D)*
1 (M12)	16	-0.891	0.816	-2.500	1.000
2 (M6)	7	-1.321	0.494	-1.750	-0.500
3 (M6)	6	-2.458	1.219	-4.750	-1.250

Data Provided by Addition Technology from the European ICS Hyperopia Study.

Table 18-6

Permeability of Nutrapore and Lidofilcon-A Hydrogel Materials (ug/hr/cm2)

Lens Material	*Glucose Transmission*	*Fluorescein Transmission*	*Water Transmission*
Nutrapore	433	161	40
Lidofilcon-A	201	91	1

Information provided by: Anamed, November, 2002

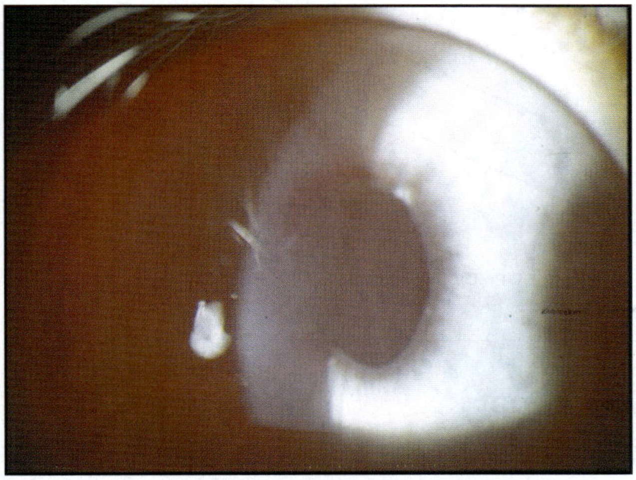

Figure 18-7. PermaVision intracorneal implants are designed for placement under a LASIK-type corneal lamellar "flap." This photo illustrates the clear nature of the PermaVision lens within the cornea, two years after implantation. (Photo by SC Kaufman, MD, PhD.)

techniques have become significantly more reliable and easier to perform. Therefore, like the previously described technique for implanting a hydrogel lens, this lens is placed underneath a "flap"; however, there is no need to suture this flap in place. It is believed that this will reduce astigmatism and corneal irregularity while improving the refractive predictability of this new lens. Anamed has developed a new delivery system for the implant, which resembles a modified Patton spatula, so that it can be placed in the corneal pocket with minimal manipulation.

In Vivo Studies of the PermaVision Lens

Results of the animal studies are presented first, followed by the results of the human trials.

Eight Nutrapore lenses were implanted in 1 eye of 8 swine. The treated eyes were examined immediately postoperatively and monthly for 1 year. The edges of two lenses were noted to have been folded at their periphery. This finding was thought to be due to the crude delivery system used for the lenses in this initial study. The reported results demonstrated that the lens material remained clear in all subjects the 1-year period. Regions of stromal haze were noted in two animals. The haze persisted in one animal over the 1-year period. Intraocular pressure (IOP) measurements did not reveal any significant differences between test and control subjects.[47]

Four lenses were placed in the eyes of New Zealand white rabbits in a long-term biocompatibility study. The eyes underwent regular slit lamp and confocal microscopy examination. After over 2 years, the lenses remained clear and in place (Figure 18-7). No anterior corneal thinning was seen nor was any fibrosis or inflammation associated with the PermaVision lenses.[48]

Table 18-7

PermaVision Intracorneal Lens

Clinical Summary-All Patients

			Preoperative		*Postoperative*	
Period	*N*	*Age*	*Manifest*	*MRSE*	*Manifest*	*MRSE*
1 week	109	45.1	+3.74 x -0.45	+3.51	-0.26 x -0.57	-0.57
1 month	101	44.4	+3.63 x -0.44	+3.41	+0.17 x -0.56	-0.10
3 months	82	44.2	+3.61 x -0.43	+3.40	+0.43 x -0.66	+0.09
6 months	50	44.2	+3.61 x -0.49	+3.58	+0.70 x -0.67	+0.36
9 months	24	45.1	+3.71 x -0.58	+3.43	+0.54 x -0.44	+0.30
12 months	15	44.2	+3.36 x -0.50	+3.12	+0.18 x -0.53	+0.06
24 months	2	51.5	+2.87 x -0.75	+2.50	+0.25 x -0.25	+0.125

Information provided by Anamed.

Table 18-8

Attempted Vs. Achieved Outcomes With PermaVision Lens Implants

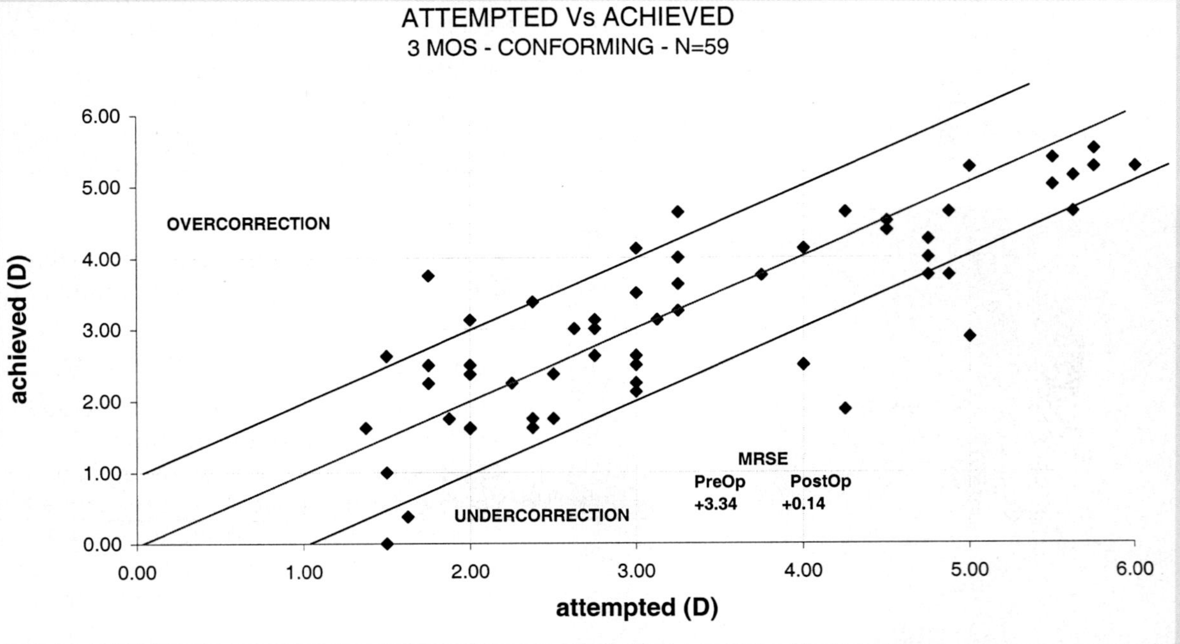

Human studies with the PermaVision lens were begun in 1997 and 109 eyes have been treated to date.[49] The patients had a mean preoperative cycloplegic, spherical error of +3.53 D. Postoperative follow-up ranges from 1 week to greater than 24 months. The mean postoperative cycloplegic, spherical error was +0.36 D across all treatment groups. Tables 18-7 and 18-8 summarize the study results. Complications included a torn lenticule, an inverted lenticule, and slight haze associated with the implant. The haze was minor but noticeable at the slit lamp. The fibrosis, which caused the haze, was postulated to be related to material from the stainless-steel lens delivery device. The delivery device was changed to titanium and no further incidents of lenticule-associated haze have been reported.[50]

Conclusion

Results of preliminary studies suggest that keratophakia is feasible. Current implants appear to be well tolerated, with no evidence of corneal necrosis in long-term studies. Multiple materials may prove effective; however, it is clear that any successful biomaterial must possess the characteristics listed in Table 18-1. Newer technologies and biomaterials will undoubtedly improve the refractive results and ease of implantation of the lenses or other devices. In the future, it may be possible to perform this safe refractive procedure without dependence upon complex lasers. Research will continue in this reversible form of refractive surgery.

References

1. Maurice DM. Nutritional aspects of corneal grafts and prostheses. In: Rycroft PV, ed. *Corneo-Plastic Surg: Proceedings of the 2nd International Corneo-Plastic Conference*. New York: Perganon Press; 1969;197-207.
2. Barraquer JI. Queratopoastia refractiva, estudios e informaciones. *Oftalmologicas*. 1949; 2:1-21.
3. Barraquer JI. Modification of refraction by means of intracorneal inclusions. *Int Ophthalmol Clin*. 1966; 6:53-78.
4. Kaufman HE, Gasset AR. Clinical experience with the epikeratoprosthesis. *Tr Am Acad Ophthalmol & Otolar*. 1969;73:1133-1140.
5. Kaufman HE, Gasset AR. Clinical experience with the epikeratoprosthesis. *Am J Ophthalmol*. 1969; 67(1):38-45.
6. McDonald MB, Kaufman HE, Aquavella JV, et al. The nationwide study of epikeratophakia for aphakia in adults. *Am J Ophthalmol*. 1997;100(3):358-365.
7. Morgan KS, McDonald MB, Hiles DA, et al. The nationwide study of epikeratophakia for aphakia in children. *Am J Ophthalmol*. 1997;100(3):366-374.
8. McDonald MB, Kaufman HE, Aquavella JV, et al. The nationwide study of epikeratophakia for myopia. *Am J Ophthalmol*. 1997;100(3):375-83.
9. McDonald MB, Safir A, Waring GO, et al. A preliminary comparative study of epikeratophakia or penetrating keratoplasty for keratoconus. *Am J Ophthalmol*. 1997;100(3): 467.
10. Brown SI, Dohlman CH. A buried corneal implant serving a barrier to fluid. *Arch Ophthalmol*. 1965;73:635.
11. Dohlman CH, Brown SI. Treatment of corneal edema with a buried implant. *Tr Am Acad Ophthalmol & Otolar*. 1965;70:267.
12. Dohlman CH, Brown SI, Martola E. Artificial corneal endothelium. *Arch Ophthalmol*. 1966;75:453.
13. Dohlman CH, Brown SI, Martola E. Replacement of endothelium with alloplastic material. *Tr Am Acad Ophthalmol & Otolar*. 1967;71:851.
14. Choyce DP. Semi-rigid corneal inlays used in the management of albinism, aniridia and emmetropia. *Ophthalmology*. 1982; 89(supplement):55.
15. Choyce DP. Polysulfone corneal inlays to correct refractive errors. *Cataract*. 1985;7:6-11.
16. Lindstrom RL, Lindstrom CW, Lane SS, et al. Polysulfone intracorneal lenses. *J Refract Surg*. 1985;1:207-16.
17. Kirkness CM, Steele AD. Polysulfone corneal inlays. *The LANCET*. April 1985;811.
18. Climenhaga H, Macdonald JM, McCarey BE, Warring GO. Effect of diameter and depth on the response to solid polysulfone intracorneal lenses and caps. *Arch Ophthalmol*. 1988;106:818-824.
19. Deg JK, Binder PS. Histopathology and clinical behavior of polysulfone intracorneal implants in the baboon model. *Ophthalmol*. 1988;95(4):506-515.
20. Rodrigues MM, McCarey, BE, Warring GO, et al. Lipid deposits posterior to impermeable intracorneal lenses in rhesus monkeys: clinical, histochemical, and ultrastructural studies. *Refract and Corneal Surg*. 1990;6:32-36.
21. Choyce DP. Additional thoughts on polysulfone corneal inlays. *J Cataract Refract Surg*. 1997;23:8-9.
22. Dohlman CH, Refojo MF, Rose, J. Synthetic polymers in corneal surgery. *Arch Ophthalmol*. 1967;77:252-257.
23. Mester U, Heimig D, Dardenne MU. Measurement and calculation of refraction in experimental keratophakia with hydrophilic lenses. *Ophthalmic Res*. 1976;8:111-116.
24. McCarey BE, Andrews DM. Refractive keratoplasty with intrastromal hydrogel lenticular implants. *Invest Ophthalmol Vis Sci*. 1981;21:107-115.
25. Werblin TP, Blaydes JE, Fryczkowski AW, et al. Stability of hydrogel intracorneal implants in non-human primates. *CLAO J*. 1983;9(2):157-161.
26. Binder PS, Deg JK, Zavala EY. Hydrogel keratophakia in non-human primates. *Current Eye Research*. 1982;1:535-542.
27. Koenig SB, Hamano T, Yamaguchi T, et al. Refractive keratoplasty with hydrogel implants in primates. *Ophthalmol Surg*. 1984;15(3):225-229.
28. McCarey BE. Current status of refractive surgery with synthetic intracorneal lenses: Barraquer lecture. *Refract Corneal Surg*. 1990;6:40-46.
29. Watsky MA, McCarey BE, Beekhuis WH. Predicting refractive alterations with hydrogel keratophakia. *Invest Ophthalmol Vis Sci*. 1985;26:240-243.
30. Sendele DD, Abelson MB, Kenyon KR, et al. Intracorneal lens implantation. *Arch Ophthalmol*. 1983;101:940-944.
31. McCarey BE, McDonald MB, van Rij G, et al. Refractive results of hyperopic hydrogel intracorneal lenses in primate eyes. *Arch Ophthalmol*. 1989;107:724-730.
32. McCarey BE, Storie BR, van Rij G, et al. Refractive predictability of myopic hydrogel intracorneal lenses in nonhuman primate eyes. *Arch Ophthalmol*. 1990;108:1310-1315.
33. McDonald MB, McCarey BE, Storie B, et al. Assessment of the long-term corneal response to hydrogel intrastromal lenses implanted in monkey eyes for up to five years. *J Cataract Refract Surg*. 1993;19:213-222.
34. Stinert RF, Storie B, Smith P, et al. Hydrogel intracorneal lenses in aphakic eyes. *Arch Ophthalmol*. 1976;14:135-141.
35. Binder PS, Zavala EY, Deg JK, et al. Hydrophilic lenses for refractive keratoplasty. *CLAO J*. 1984;10:105-111.
36. Werblin TP, Patel AS, Barraquer JI. Initial human experience with perma-lens myopic hydrogel intracorneal lens implants. *Refract Corneal Surg*. 1992;8:23-26.

37. Beekhuis WH, McCarey BE, Waring GO, et al. Hydrogel keratophakia: a microkeratome dissection in the monkey model. *Br J Ophthalmol.* 1986;70:192-198.
38. Werblin, TP, Peiffer RL, Binder PS, et al. Eight years of experience with perma-lens intracorneal lenses in non-human primates. *Refract Corneal Surg.* 1992;8:12-22.
39. Zavala EY, Nayak SK, Deg JK, et al. Human keratocyte interactions with hydrogel materials. *CLAO J.* 1986; 12(1):54-58.
40. Ohrloff C, Duffin RM, Apple DJ, et al. Opacification, vascularization and chronic inflammation produced by hydrogel corneal lamellar implants. *Am J Ophthalmol.* 1984; 98:422-425.
41. Dupont D, Gravagna P, Albinet P, et al. Biocompatibility of human collagen type IV intracorneal implants. *Cornea.* 1989;8(4):251-258.
42. Evanes MDM, Xie RZ, Fabri M, et al. Epithelialization of a synthetic polymer in the feline cornea: a preliminary study. *Invest Ophthalmol Vis Sci.* 2000;41(7):1674-1680.
43. Evanes MDM, Xie RZ, Fabri M, et al. Epithelialization of a synthetic polymer in the feline cornea: a preliminary study. *Invest Ophthalmol Vis Sci.* 2002;43(10):3196-3201.
44. Evans MDM, McLean KM, Hughes TC, et al. A review of the development of a synthetic corneal onlay for refractive correction. *Biomaterials*. 2001;22:3319-3328.
45. Information Provided by Addition Technology (Fremont, Calif).
46. Clinch T. Compilation of Addition Technology European hyperopia data. Provided by Addition Technology.
47. Anamed material, November 2002.
48. Kaufman SC. Long-term biocompatibility of the PermaVision hydrogel lens. Paper presented at: *Assoc. of Cataract and Refract Surg.* June 2002.
49. Kaufman HE. *The PermaVision Lens for hyperopia.* Presented at the AAO Subspecialty Day. October 2002.
50. Information provided by Anamed (Lake Forest, Calif).

Section Five

IMPLANTS

Chapter Nineteen

Refractive Lensectomy for Hyperopia

Trevor Woodhams, MD

Introduction

It is interesting to note that the original intended use for the intraocular lens (IOL) was to correct ametropia, albeit myopia rather than hyperopia. We are, of course, all familiar with the story of the development of the IOL since its inception in the 1949. Its use in the course of cataract surgery to preclude the high degree of induced hyperopia was one of the seminal medical achievements of 20th-century medicine, all the more remarkable in the face of its invention, adoption, improvement, and finally general acceptance despite the formidable attempts by some in the ophthalmology academic establishment to suppress and/or seize control of the technology. If a Nobel Prize for medicine were ever richly deserved by an individual for his selfless and courageous acts, it would surely be to Dr. Harold Ridley of England.

It may be useful at this point to review the visual effects of inducing high degrees of hyperopia in wearing spectacles with a typical aphakic +8.00 to +12.00 D lens so as to better appreciate his accomplishment.

Magnification

Because the correcting lens sits on average about 12 to 14 mm from the corneal plane, significant magnification of the apparent image is created on the order of 25% to 35% from an otherwise emmetropic eye. This makes the scene perceived visually as being the same degree of distance closer to the observer. The necessary accompanying lateral expansion of the image occupying the eye's central view "pushes" the otherwise full (approximately 150-degree) field out of the visible peripheral field. This "ring scotoma" effectively eliminates much peripheral vision, causing objects traversing the field of observation to suddenly "jump" into view. The optical effect on a patient more or less emmetropic or myopic was a visual effect not unlike looking through a very low-power telescope.[1]

Pincushion Effect

A second undesirable visual effect of a high plus spectacle lens is the variable magnification created by the thick lens. This causes a greater degree of relative magnification as an image approaches the visual axis of the correcting lens. This creates the effect of "pincushion" distortion, where straight lines curve along their midpoints towards the optical center of the thick plus lens.

Higher Order Aberrations

A more recent visual problem of the high plus spectacle lens is a phenomenon that has only recently begun to occupy the attention of ophthalmologists: higher order optical aberrations (previously known as irregular astigmatism). The most common if not most bothersome of these in an otherwise "normal" eye is spherical aberration. This phenomenon is due to the increasingly acute angle of incidence that paraxial rays of light meet at the refracting surface of a lens. In effect, this causes the increasingly peripheral parts of an image plane to be refracted in an even higher "plus" fashion so that the peripheral parts of an image come to focus more anterior to the retina than centrally. While aspherical, prolate lenses have been used for years in photography to offset this phenomenon, their introduction into aphakic spectacles only occurred at about the same time as the introduction of the IOL into medical practice (ie, the 1970s).

Small Incision Lensectomy

Because the natural, or native, lens has a diameter considerably larger than even a fully dilated pupil, lensectomy has historically been associated with the need to create a corneal-scleral wound of about 12 to 14 mm, about 150 to 180 degrees of a typical limbus. Dr. Troutman had pioneered utilization of the operating microscope for corneal transplants. It took the advent of phacoemulsification, however, to realize the full advantages of microsurgery in the removal of the human lens. Its inventor, Dr. Charles Kelman, has related the story of its development in fascinatingly human and political detail elsewhere.[2] Suffice to say that he, too, faced the opposition and attempted repression of new technology that threatened the status quo.

Up to that time, the surgeon attempting to remove the intact nucleus of a lens from the eye faced the same problem as the furniture mover dealing with the need to remove a grand piano from a room with a normal-sized entrance: how does one extract a substantially large object through a smaller window or door without destroying the enclosing walls? The answer, of course, is to dissemble it first. With the ultrasonic breakup and fluid-based evacuation of lens material afforded by a typical limbal, 2- to 3-mm phaco wound, cataract surgery went from requiring a week of uninterrupted flat-on-the-back recuperation (with its consequent risks of bed rest complications in the usually elderly patient) to a 15-minute, ambulatory center procedure under local anesthesia.

Much of the advantage of the small incision afforded by phacoemulsification in the days of its early rapid run-up in acceptance (the late 1970s) was obviated by the necessity to extend the corneal/scleral wound in order to insert a typically 6- to 7-mm IOL. Such early attempts at dealing with this problem (eg, "folding," elliptical, and truncated IOLs) encountered various practical and optical problems. The solution was fairly intuitive: an IOL made of a soft or flexible transparent material that could be temporarily deformed by folding for insertion through a small incision. Early materials included silicone, hydrogel, and temperature-sensitive acrylic. These have been steadily and relentlessly improved over the years in terms of surface and edge smoothness, biocompatibility, and stability of haptic support, either in the ciliary sulcus or within the preserved capsular bag itself.[3]

The overwhelming triumph of the successful union of phaco technology with foldable IOLs has led in turn, to a considerably more favorable risk/benefit ratio in the consideration of cataract-based lens surgery that encouraged ever earlier surgical intervention. Despite Medicare and privately funded Health Insurance programs' continued erosion of cataract surgery fees, the irresistible advantages to both physician and patient made the continued expansion of lensectomy/IOL implantation inevitable.

IOL Calculation for Optimizing Emmetropia

The induced high hyperopia of lensectomy in cataract surgery (or for purely refractive reasons) has been discussed previously. While replacement of the cataractous natural lens with a synthetic IOL offered distinct advantages over aphakia in visual rehabilitation, early implant surgeons were faced with the challenge of determining preoperatively how to calculate the ideal dioptric IOL power in order to optimize the achievement of postoperative emmetropia. All formulas sufficient to do this require precise measurement of intraocular axial length for the visual axis of the intended eye. Additionally, accurate measurement of the cornea's refractive surface has been recognized from the start as mandatory in successful IOL implantation for postoperative refractive optimization. Early formulas such as the Collanbrander and Fydorov were based on theoretical models of the eye taking into account the third most important variable, anterior chamber depth.

Unfortunately, preoperative measurement of the central anterior chamber depth does not reflect the actual postoperative anatomy. The distance measured from the corneal surface at its intersection with the visual axis to the corresponding point on the anterior capsule of the natural lens will change as a result of the surgery itself. Due to a differing index of refraction, the typical silicone, PMMA, or acrylic IOL has a central thickness about 25% that of an equivalent power natural lens. This causes a posterior displacement of the IOL/iris diaphragm after surgery that alters the optical inter-relationship of these 3 main variables used in IOL calculation. Furthermore, the ratio of anterior chamber depth to axial length is not consistent. Large series of eyes studied by optical biometry have shown that there are various "subtypes" of ocular anatomy consisting of uncharacteristically deep anterior chambers in short-diameter eyes as well as unexpectedly deep or shallow chambers in otherwise normal eyes that more classically approximate the "ideal" Gullstrand model eye's 23 mm.

These physiologic variations were often the explanation for the "3-diopter surprise" that frequently plagued early cataract implant surgeons. This consisted of an intolerably large disparity between the planned postoperative refraction and what actually occurred. A significant step forward, then, was the development and widespread adoption of the theoretical models of predictive optical outcomes in lensectomy/IOL implantation. Theoretical-based formulas used multi-variable regression analysis of large databases of actual refractive outcomes to greatly refine the predictive property of an IOL formula. The original Sanders-Retzlaff-Kraff formula was soon joined by that of Hoffer,[4] Holladay, and Haigis. These later formulas have continued to be refined, taking into account a greater array of variables and the increased "outlier effect" of unusually short or long eyes.

The effect of these increasingly precise formulas has been matched by technological improvement in the measuring devices themselves. Axial length biometry was once compromised by the imperceptible indentation of the cornea utilizing contact, or applanation ultrasound probes. Contact axial length biometry has largely been rendered obsolete by the use of improved methodology that eliminates the need for actual physical contact between the measuring probe and the eye itself. Water-bath immersion ultrasound was actually the original procedure for ultrasound biometry. The cumbersome nature of the early set-up has largely been replaced by the relative ease of a compact Praeger shell whose ocular surface contour and shape requires less than 10 cc of saline. This permits a single, well-trained operator to perform highly accurate biometry. In recent years, Zeiss-Humphrey has eliminated the water bath entirely as well as the need for supine positioning of the patient with its IOL master. This compact device employs laser partial coherence interferometry rather than ultrasound, thus allowing the patient to be seated with face positioned on a chin rest, a comfortable position already familiar from past exposure to the bio-microscope, or "slit lamp."[5] This type of biometry is brief, uncomplicated, and can be performed by any reasonably trained technician. Measurement of the anterior chamber, however, still requires optical biometry although this is built into the IOL master device.

Patient Selection and Education

Even before the relative merits of lensectomy versus keratorefractive surgery can be discussed, it is essential that a patient understand the physiology of farsightedness to the best of his or her ability. Unfortunately, having only one lay word in English for both presbyopia and hyperopia creates ambiguity and lays the ground for misunderstanding and disappointment later, even if the surgery is otherwise completely successful in the professional and technical sense. For this reason, we find that considerably extensive patient education is mandatory even before the surgeon meets the patient.

The first order of analysis is, of course, to ascertain that a prospective refractive surgery patient is truly hyperopic. This is not really as trivial an issue as it may appear at first. The overwhelming triumph of LASIK worldwide as a refractive procedure has been based on its success in treating nearsightedness, not farsightedness. This is not as unremarkable as it may seem. After all, the incidence of myopia in America is estimated at only 25% of the general population while at least the presbyopic form of farsightedness has (or will have) an incidence of 100% should the patient live long enough for the inevitable diminution of accommodation. Yet almost every single myope in developed countries wears or at least owns (in low degrees of nearsightedness) a pair of spectacles or contact lenses (CTLs).

This is not necessarily the case, however, with either hyperopia or presbyopia. A young hyperopic patient is often unaware of "having a vision problem" at all unless other related symptoms (such as headache or esotropia) bring him to the attention of the optometrist or ophthalmologist. Even anisometropic amblyopia can easily be missed by nonprofessional observation until well after patching therapy would have been effective. The typical hyperope presenting for consideration of refractive surgery of any type is rarely a young person unless the degree of hyperopia is quite high. This is of course quite different from the myope who knows from an early age that he cannot function in the outdoor world without some kind of prosthetic help.

The degree of myopia in a patient who describes his condition ruefully as being "legally blind" seems to start at levels of dioptric correction that would be invisible to a young hyperope!

Age, then, is a major factor (if not *the* major factor) in the consideration of refractive lensectomy. The accommodative capability of the natural lens is such that its near-total loss must be very carefully weighed against any anticipated advantages in post-lensectomy, uncorrected distance vision. Unless a potential patient is physically wearing a high plus pair of spectacles on presentation to the clinic for evaluation, claims of CTL intolerance need to be viewed with a certain degree of suspicion. A young potential patient (for our purposes under 40) is unlikely to truly appreciate the impact of a near blur sufficient to make even simple everyday tasks (such as application of makeup or shaving) impossible without assistance from such devices as illuminated concave mirrors or magnifying lenses. I have not yet encountered even one very young hyperope (under 30), who I felt would be genuinely better off with lensectomy. While an argument could be made in such unusual cases as a monocular, hyperopic anisometrope, I feel this should await a more structured and formal clinical trial. This conservatism will not be appreciated by a very young hyperope; it is not at all unusual for this patient to suppose the experience of his myopic friend (who had laser-assisted in-situ keratomileusis [LASIK]) will be identical to the likely outcome of his own situation.

Another reason that the inexorable success of LASIK has depended on myopia, rather than hyperopia is the simple reason that LASIK seems to "work better" in flattening a cornea than in steepening it. The latter requires much better centration and seems more prone to induce cylinder (and other forms of astigmatism). While the FDA has approved treatment of hyperopia for most excimer lasers up to +6.00 D, many surgeons voluntarily limit the upper ceiling to about +3.00 or +4.00 D.

For these reasons, we find it mandatory to educate the "farsighted" patient as to the true underlying nature of his visual problem(s) to a degree that he or she no longer uses the word "farsighted" at all, but rather the proper medical terminology of "hyperopia" and "presbyopia." It might profitably be added at this point that this also has the advantage of eliminating the familiar time-wasting conversation: if a hyperopic patient's friend is nearsighted (can see up close but not far off), then the opposite should be the case for him whereas he can't see either distance or near very well! Why is that, doc?

Anybody suspected of having a hyperopic component to their visual problem should have both a manifest and cycloplegic refraction. It is not unknown to encounter a patient with less than 20/20 distance acuity whose manifest Rx is slightly myopic, but whose Rx without accommodation is somewhat plus. This "spasm of accommodation" can paradoxically occur even in the presbyopic age group. It should go without saying that surgery on such a patient of any kind is asking for trouble.

It is not unusual to have a hyperopic patient in the presbyopic age group insist that there is no problem with distance vision even when acuity is measured under physiologic conditions as 20/40 or worse. Fortunately, a suitable plus trial lens held in front of the eye while the patient focuses on the eye chart is usually sufficient to disabuse the patient of this notion. Consideration of age is of paramount importance, though, in determining the actual impact of hyperopia on visual function.

The typical lensectomy candidate in the case of hyperopia, however, is much more straightforward. This patient is usually full-time spectacle dependent for both distance and near. In the case of the prepresbyopic (ie, young) patient, the lens Rx is often over +5.00 D, and occasionally as high as +10.00 D, with or without significant cylinder. The issue of preservation of accommodation in the young patient is dealt with elsewhere in this chapter. Much of the final decision, though, as to the propriety of lensectomy, can be resolved subjectively in discussion with the patient. Success with CTL wear can often be the deciding feature. While it can always be argued that yet another fitting may yield better CTL tolerance than the last, this does not necessarily cut off consideration of an intraocular procedure with its attendant risks. A rule of thumb we use at our clinic is quite simple: did the patient arrive for consultation and examination wearing plus contacts, or are they wearing thick glasses?

It is my experience that even with ample education, it is quite difficult for the average patient to truly appreciate the implications of being able to only "fix" the hyperopic component of a compound hyperopic/presbyopic situation. For this reason, we find it mandatory to actually demonstrate it rather than relying on conversation and pictures. Using one eye at a time, we have the patient hold a near card at whatever distance the patient finds best while gazing at the far acuity chart. The near card contains 2 different size fonts in the form of an actual paragraph; the sizes on our cards are 8 points and 18 points respectively. (This is not the place to deal with the generally outdated system commonly in use of using Jaeger-denominated size print.) A plus lens appropriate to the degree of hyperopia is held in front of the subject's eye (after first reconfirming for the patient the uncorrected visual acuity [UCVA] without the lens). The improvement is of course quite dramatic to the patient. Attention is then redirected to the near card first without and then with the same power lens. Usually the patient can discern the fact that there is indeed a significant improvement, often facilitating recognition of the larger-print paragraph, but not enough to allow reading of the smaller text. This needs to be imprinted in the patient's memory for future reference.

Monovision and multi-focal lenses as possible solutions to the challenge of loss of accommodation will be dealt with later in the chapter. It may well prove necessary, though, to wait for truly accommodating IOLs for this problem to be reliably solved.

Last of all, it must be admitted that even the case of the "perfect" lensectomy outcome of a hyperopia case is inferior to the visual performance of a naturally occurring emmetrope. This is because the natural lens seems exquisitely designed (whether by design, evolution, or other cause). Putting aside for the moment the fact that only the natural lens is capable of true accommodation, there are many "design features" of a natural lens that are only now coming to be appreciated by clinical visual science.

A good example of the superiority of the natural lens to even a perfectly implanted pseudophakos is the onion-layer architecture of the natural lens. As subsequent, less dense outer layers are grown by this sealed-off structure (of ectodermal origin) the index of refraction becomes progressively higher in the inner, nuclear parts. This mitigates the otherwise sharply demarcated refractive surface encountered in spectacles and IOLs with its attendant reflections and Purkinje images.

One of the most recently appreciated of these naturally occurring lens functions is the realization (from LASIK) of the importance of asphericity, the most commonly encountered of the higher-order optical aberrations. The natural lens is quite prolate, most of this occurring on its posterior surface. In combination with the natural prolate shape of the cornea, a significant amount of peripheral distortion is avoided in normal vision, especially under mesopic and scotopic conditions. The optical advantage of this prolate asphericity is substantially reduced when a plano-convex or even bi-convex pseudophakos is substituted. Recently, Pharmacia (New York, NY) has introduced a prolate IOL design (Tecnis Z-9000) that hopefully will be the harbinger of future more sophisticated IOL design.[6]

Complications of Refractive Lensectomy

Because most ophthalmic surgeons receive ample experience in cataract surgery during their residencies, the basics of phacoemulsification and IOL implantation are usually not new surgical skills that need further training to acquire. This is also the case then for the surgical complications attendant to routine cataract surgery. These include in descending order of severity: endophthalmitis, hemorrhage (choroidal or iris-root), corneal decompensation associated with endothelial trauma, iris prolapse associated with post-operative wound dehiscence, rupture of the posterior capsule with or without vitreous prolapse into the anterior chamber, and cystoid macular edema (CME).[7]

In addition, because refractive lensectomy has as its aim the optical goal of emmetropia, a final refraction severe enough to require spectacle correction must also be considered an undesirable side-effect. This should be quantified for purposes of formal outcome analysis. Not only is minus or plus sphere as a refractive outcome missing the mark, but the inducing of unwanted cylinder (or other types of astigmatism) must also be considered as a non-vision-threatening complication. Simple measurement of uncorrected spectacle visual acuity (USCVA) is probably not sufficient to judge the quality of outcome.

The Risk/Benefit Ratios of Lensectomy Versus Keratorefractive Hyperopia Surgery

We have discussed the work-up, education, and "training" of the prospective refractive surgery patient. At this point, sufficient data has been gathered for the surgeon to start to make a case for lensectomy, should that be agreed by patient and doctor as a reasonable or even preferable alternative to a keratorefractive procedure.

In a patient over the age of 65, or who has been diagnosed with a cataract, the decision can be rather straightforward. Such people are usually aware of cataract and lens implant surgery or even know friends or relatives who have undergone such surgery successfully. At this age, it is not unexpected to be diagnosed with at least some nuclear sclerosis and to elicit a positive response upon being questioned about halos and/or generally increasing difficulties with driving at night.

The argument could be made that keratorefractive procedures such as LASIK or any of the mid-peripheral corneal collagen shrinking procedures (eg, hyperopic thermal keratoplasty [HTK], laser thermal keratoplasty [LTK] or conductive keratoplasty [CK]) are "safer" than an intraocular procedure such as lensectomy. After all, there is almost no risk of actual loss of an eye as can occur with endophthalmitis associated with intraocular surgery. However, this must be balanced against the strong possibility of future lensectomy surgery anyway. This would then subject the patient to two, rather than just the one operation. Besides the matter of added expense, it is my experience that there will usually be a continued, albeit slow myopic shift of the eye's refraction that will prompt a patient to later seek an "enhancement." When told of the presence of an "early" cataract causing the progressive myopic blur which should not be treated with further keratorefractive surgery, even a very close patient rapport can be strained by discovering that later lensectomy will be able to take care of the developing vision problem. The author learned this the hard way when my inclination to conservatism left him on more than one occasion being asked "So why didn't we just remove the early cataract in the first place?" Why not indeed?

The issue of LASIK as an alternative for the surgical treatment of hyperopia is dealt with elsewhere in this volume. Suffice to say for the purpose of this chapter that while this is certainly a viable alternative in low and perhaps even moderate levels of hyperopia, there as yet does not exist any support for successful LASIK in the case of high (>+6.00 D) hyperopia.

The issue of third-party reimbursement, especially through government health insurance such as Medicare can also be a complicating factor, although not strictly speaking a medical concern. Nevertheless, the actual practice of Medicine does not operate hermetically sealed off from the outside real world, so this must be taken into account. Because the degree of lens opacity (or more properly lack of transparency) is not defined (or probably even definable) objectively, there is great temptation on the part of the patient and the surgeon to see the visual defects in terms of the cataract, rather than a purely refractive defect. A cataract is not a foreign presence from outside the eye, as is often thought by the public; rather, it should be more properly thought of as a process whereby there is progressive loss of visual functioning. This can culminate in measurable acuity loss to the degree that the patient can no longer perform normally.

In reality, though, this is more a function of the patient's lifestyle, expectations, and resources—all of which are notoriously subjective. It could reasonably be considered that the meaning of the word "cataract" has evolved from its origin as a synonym for "whitewater" with its attendant "white pupil" and sub-total visual incapacitation. Perhaps a more suitable term might be the more subtle "lens dysplasia." This would then include the entire age-related process of general degeneration of visual function from undesirable changes in the natural lens from age 40 on due to its progressive loss of flexibility and transparency. In effect, this could well comprise presbyopia and the gradual unveiling of the unwelcome effects of latent or manifest hyperopia. Could myopia itself eventually be considered a "lens dysplasia?" Time will tell.

In the total absence of any significant lens sclerosis or discoloration, there are still noteworthy reasons to prefer lensectomy to keratorefractive procedures. Chief among these is the induced spherical (and other) aberrations that can even reduce best spectacle-corrected visual acuity (BSCVA). Dr. Perry Binder and I have both reported this phenomenon (before the days when wavefront analysis would have been able to pinpoint the nature of the aberrations). A rule of thumb (never submitted for prospective analysis) is that the cornea does not seem to function optimally as a primary refractive surface with curvature over about +49.00 D.

Many hyperopic eyes' corneas are already steeper than average, presumably due to the as yet poorly understood "emmetropization principle of Sorsby."[8] This means that even with a lack of strict 1:1 correlation between corneal and refractive post-keratorefractive steepening, many hyperopic eyes would be pushed into the pseudo-keratoconus ranges of +50.00 D curvatures. This would be even more so in the case of highly hyperopic eyes beyond the range of facile accommodative compensation (ie, +4.00 D and up).

From a purely safety perspective, it is unarguable that HTK is the preferred modality for at least modest degrees of hyperopia. Unfortunately, this method of increasing the cornea's curvature through the judicious application of collagen-shrinking heat in the mid periphery has been plagued with shortcomings. These challenges have limited its adoption by the world-wide ophthalmic community despite its enviable safety track record. Chief among these has been instability, specifically the progressive tendency for regression, often to preoperative levels. This should perhaps not be unexpected given the body's propensity to heal. Within the professional lifetime of most practicing ophthalmogists, we have seen many forms of HTK: radio frequency induction, Fyodorov's needle cautery, the Sunrise Holmium LTK, and most recently CK. Only the most recent of these has not been shown to suffer from the same regression effect mentioned. Many are convinced this is only because not enough time has elapsed to confirm its instability. The stability of IOL-dependent hyperopic adjustment remains unchallenged; however, given the many years of cataract-based correction outcomes.

Other than the previously mentioned and very real possibility (fortunately quite rare) of loss of an eye to endophthalmitis, the major risks of refractive lensectomy for hyperopia are: later retinal detachment, choroidal expulsive hemorrhage (or its less-malignant cousin, sub-choroidal transudative expulsion), CME,[10] and corneal decompensation due to either excessive surgical trauma or to preoperative pathology (eg, Fuchs' endothelial dystrophy).

It is probably important to separate hyperopic from myopic lensectomy (whether associated with cataract or not) for analysis of risk assessment of these. While retinal detachment has long been recognized as a late complication of lensectomy, this appears to be more related to the particular anatomic defect in the myopic eye itself, rather than to some defect in the surgery itself. It appears that the abnormally enlarged diameter of the myopic eye with subsequent stretched thinning of the retina predisposes to localized thinning and frank tears with possible detachment from fluid penetration through these compromised retinal areas into the subretinal space. While further data is definitely needed to support the hypothesis, it appears that the smaller sized hyperopic eye with its thicker sclera and lack of retinal stretching is not nearly as disposed to this complication.

Because patients presenting for refractive surgery—whether keratorefractive or lensectomy—tend to be younger and healthier than the elderly, it is reasonable to discount the already rare incidence of choroidal problems during surgery. These are generally associated with older, more frail patients, often in association with hypertensive pathology. The risk of CME, of course, is nothing to take lightly, as will be discussed further in the section on management of the capsule. Still, its incidence has seen a gradual but steady decrease with improvements in anesthesia and minimally invasive surgical techniques. In the presence of diabetes or other vascular problems, however, the patient must be adequately counseled. Corneal decompensation as a complication of lensectomy has seen a similar strongly decreased incidence as young surgeons are increasingly well-trained in microsurgical techniques, utilizing protective viscoelastic materials and non-steroidal anti inflammatory agents (NSAIDs) and preoperative screening by specular microscopy for suspected endothelial problems.

Management of the Capsule

Standard lensectomy, whether for cataract or ametropia, recognizes the desirability of preserving an intact posterior capsule. This of course is for its obvious suitability as a support platform for the IOL. As of this writing, intracapsular fixation is deemed preferable to ciliary sulcus placement by reason of its isolation of the synthetic IOL material from direct contact with (and possible degranulation of) the pigmented posterior iris layer. Proper centration is also more readily obtained within the capsular bag; this becomes of even greater importance in the high plus pseudophakos where decentration can produce undesirable prismatic optical effects.

The argument against opening of the posterior capsule as a primary procedure at the conclusion of the lensectomy was decided almost two decades ago. There is a tendency for a capsular tear to extend itself in an uncontrolled fashion, rendering primary capsulotomy to be generally unmanageable in establishing the proper size of opening to allow unimpeded passage of all image-bearing rays of light. This can create many problems such as decentration or even loss of the IOL into the vitreous. Even movement of the IOL laterally in the direction of least tension can seriously degrade optical performance. Primary capsulotomy has also been shown to be associated with an increased risk of CME and its attendant risk of visual loss either short or long term.[11]

Much of contemporary IOL technology seems directed at efforts to prevent later capsular clouding whether from fibrosis or subcapsular cellular migration from the equatorial recesses of the capsule. While such strategies as squared edge design do indeed seem to be capable of creating some sort of barrier effect, there is reason to doubt that ultimately this may truly be the best solution to the problem of opacification. The post-lensectomy capsule is prone to contraction. This of course is manifested by the typical white/gray clouding seen easily in retro-illumination at slit-lamp biomicroscopy. Before this opacification becomes visible, wrinkling and striation of the capsule can be noted. Even a smooth capsule, however, can be seen to lose its luster and shiny surface with time resulting in an appearance not unlike that of a "dirty window." With the advent of low-contrast vision testing and modulation transfer function (MTF) measurement and analysis, it appears more likely that there is a degree of subtle degradation of visual function occurring long before a patient may present with complaints. While this may be tolerable in the case of previous presence of cataract, it should not be expected to be so well accepted in the case of younger and more active patients who are accustomed to a better quality of vision. Intolerance of the imperfections of spectacles or CTLs may well be a clue to patient suitability for refractive lensectomy.

The likelihood of post-lensectomy YAG laser capsulotomy, then, should be discussed prior to the original surgery. The risks associated with this, such as retinal detachment, do not seem to be as much of a concern as in the greater-diameter eye typical of myopic patients (previous to their lensectomy surgery). In any case, YAG-laser complications are fortunately quite rare. The question of who will bear the cost of this almost inevitable procedure should also be addressed before its actual necessity.

Special Challenges of Lensectomy in the Hyperopic Eye

The hyperopic eye tends almost uniformly to be a short eye with a shallow anterior chamber. While this is not universally the case, it is certainly often enough the case to require certain surgical precautions.

Chief among these is adequate protection of the corneal endothelium during intracameral surgical maneuvers. The more highly dense and dispersive viscoplastic materials can often be used to deepen the anterior chamber prior to introduction of instruments into the eye. These also, of course, serve to mitigate the possibility of impact by lens fragments and the IOL on the non-reproducing endothelial cell population, which is critical in maintaining corneal dehydration and clarity.

The very high plus power of an IOL sufficient to eliminate a patient's hyperopia is also often a source of difficulty. Most foldable and/or injectable IOLs are not available in powers over +30.00 D. Storz is greatly appreciated for its manufacture of PMMA (ie, rigid) IOLs in powers up to +40.00 D. These do require a much larger corneo-scleral wound with its tendency to induce unwanted post-operative cylinder.

Another way to deal with the lack of availability of appropriate high plus power IOLs is to resort to "piggyback" IOL insertion—ie, the use of two (or more) IOLs of more conventional powers in order to achieve emmetropia. This is possible because, as has been pointed out, the different index of refraction of IOL materials is such that a typical IOL center thickness is only about the corresponding thickness of a natural lens. Unfortunately, "piggy-backing" of IOLs has been plagued with problems. Perhaps the most basic one is the unfortunate fact that two IOLs do not function additively in power when placed face to face within the capsular bag. That is, a calculated +40.00 IOL cannot be achieved by insertion of two +20.00 IOLs. This is due to posterior displacement of the primary IOL upon insertion of the second IOL. This new dual IOL nodal point sits further posterior than the nodal point of a single high-power IOL. Dr. Holladay has added this feature to his very sophisticated IOL calculation computer application. Centration of both IOLs is also made more difficult with the possibility of disparity of optical centers along the visual axis. Nevertheless, there is an even more potentially vision-threatening complication in "piggy-back" IOLs in the form of interpseudophakos membrane formation. This appears to be a variation of the well-known proliferation of Elschnig's pearls and/or fibrosis that eventually cloud most posterior capsules after extracapsular-type lensectomy. Management of this problem has been quite taxing to even superb surgeons, so much so that interest in primary, planned "piggy-back" IOL implantation has faded greatly.

Some would argue that a "bioptics" approach (lens implant + keratorefractive procedure) is a safer, more predictable, and more accurate method of dealing with postoperative under- and overcorrections through the use of a staged or planned secondary keratorefractive procedure such as LASIK.[13] This of course can also be used to deal with unintended residual or induced cylinder. The implications of this will be addressed in the next section.

Astigmatism

Cylinder is the most common type of astigmatism. Indeed, most people (including no doubt many optometrists and ophthalmologists) use the two terms interchangeably. With the advent of sophisticated methods of computer enhanced corneal topography, however, it has become abundantly clear that there exists in reality much variation in even regular forms of astigmatism. What was once deemed "regular astigmatism" and was corrected by spherocylindrical lenses can now be seen to be only an idealized form of optical aberration.

Still, the binomial consideration of ametropia (with the addition of axis orientation in degrees) as a sphero-cylinder has had too much historical and practical usefulness to abandon just now. Furthermore, advances in IOL technology have tended to languish somewhat in the past decade in the face of declining reimbursement as an added disincentive to continued research and development by commercial medical industry.

Other than variations in manufacturing materials, the only real optical breakthrough in IOL technology has been the availability of the toric IOL from STAAR. Available in 2.00 and 3.50 D. cylinders, the toric STAAR IOL has greatly enhanced the ability of "lens replacement" surgery to offer optical benefits approaching emmetropia.[14]

Nevertheless, even with toric IOLs, small incision phacoemulsification, and third generation IOL formulas, the ability of lens implant surgery to approach the level of predictive accuracy of LASIK has not yet arrived. It is not uncommon to perform a flawless hyperopic (or myopic for that matter) lensectomy/ lens implant and be left with a disappointed patient. Even small degrees of cylinder or sphere can present unsatisfactory unaided visual impairment, especially under glare or low-light conditions.

Limbal relaxing incisions, developed by Dr. Stephen Hollis and popularized by Dr. Jim Gills,[15] are useful in low degrees (up to 2.00 D) of residual or induced compound cylinder (mixed astigmatism). These are inexpensive to perform, do not require a high level of precision for good results, and can even be performed in the exam lane under slit-lamp biomicroscopy.

Higher degrees of post-IOL cylinder, if not successfully addressed at the time of surgery through a toric IOL, can also be greatly reduced or even eliminated through PRK, LASEK, or LASIK once adequate wound-healing can be assured (typically 12 weeks in our practice). This involves an appreciation of the cost issues that are sometimes not practical in the absence of a practice-owned and operated excimer laser. It should go without saying that these need to have been discussed preoperatively to maintain the patient's good faith.

The Challenge of Accommodation

As was discussed in the section outlining my skepticism toward performing refractive lensectomy on a very young patient, the advantages of a naturally accommodative lens are not to be dismissed in a cavalier fashion (even in the face of relative high degrees of hyperopia). It is not unusual to encounter a patient with a latent, resting accommodative load of many diopters. In the absence of esophoria or frank esotropia (which is anyway typically identified in childhood), the fairly vague condition of aesthenopia or a premature discovery of the benefits of off-the-shelf readers is often the sole complaint.

Most everybody expects at some point in their life to be compelled to seek the help of magnifying lenses for near task help at some point in middle age, if only "drugstore readers." This is of course the case for the hyperope, albeit perhaps at an earlier age than his contemporaries. Once a hyperopic patient realizes that distance vision is now becoming a challenge, an appointment with the eye doctor becomes something that can no longer be put off! This often is the first occasion whereby a person discovers what hyperopia is. The "double duty" that accommodation has been serving (ie, for near tasks as well as compensation for distance focusing), then, is naturally conflated in the patient's perception of his condition. Consequently, the expectation of a successful surgical outcome is no less than a return to that level of visual performance before decreasing accommodation began to affect vision at any distance. The necessity of disabusing the patient of this (and its method) has already been described in the section on patient selection.

The "traditional" method of dealing with a lack of accommodation has been through some degree of planned monovision, whether attained through CTLs, keratorefractive surgery of refractive lensectomy. This is usually most successful when the dominant eye is assigned the role of distance vision. The degree of planned myopia in the other eye must ride a careful balance between magnification, depth of field, and toleration for anisometropia. LASIK actually holds the edge in monovision because of the increased depth of field afforded by the change of cornea architecture from prolate to oblate. It is my experience that unless there is a history of previous successful monovision from CTLs, there is not nearly the patient satisfaction that can be seen in postoperative myopic lensectomy. Presumably this is because of the myope's expectation of persistent unaided near vision as was the experience in his uncorrected preop state.

There is little argument that if a synthetic lens implant could successfully mimic accommodation, this would be preferable to monovision. Technology in IOLs, happily, is progressing at a rapid rate. Already there are IOL designs for use in refractive lensectomy that address the challenge of reproducing (or at least mimicking) accommodation. Currently, only multifocal IOLs are approved by the FDA for use in the United States. The Array lens by Advanced Medical Optics[16] (AMO) (Santa Clara, Calif) has enjoyed limited success in treating hyperopic patients, mostly in the eye with frank cataract, but to a certain degree in the pre-cataract or completely clear lens presbyope. While perhaps more a marketing maneuver than a designation of a truly original operation, presbyopic lens exchange (PRELEX, Indianapolis, Ind)[17] has been promoted as the first effective surgical alternative to simple monovision in the treatment of the presbyopic hyperope. This is indubitably the case. Nevertheless, acceptance has been limited by many reports of multiple halos around point sources of light nocturnally and by complaints consistent with a loss of contrast sensitivity. These are not entirely surprising considering that the pseudo-accommodation is provided by a concentric sequence of lenticular zones of differing focal power.

An entirely different approach to hyperopic/presbyopic restoration through pseudophakos implantation is provided by the AT-40 "Crystalens" (C & C) and Humanoptiks[18] IOLs. There will be a chapter of this text devoted to to the Crystalens. These take advantage of the fact that anterior displacement of the lens nodal point in an otherwise emmetropic eye creates a state of myopia by moving the near point of that eye closer. Reportedly, this is provided by both forward movement of the lens plane from contraction of the ciliary muscle (even in a presbyopic eye) along with increased posterior pressure on the IOL by the vitreous body. It is unclear at this point in the early experience of the IOL use whether the inevitable fibrosis and hardening of the capsule will permanently reduce this pseudo-accommodative effect. Likewise, it is not known whether YAG laser capsulotomy will effectively relieve this contraction-induced reduction of effect. In any case, the future trend in IOL technology is bright. Further refinements and improvements in optical design will undoubtedly provide greatly enhanced approximation of the smooth, seamless accommodation experienced in the youthful eye. It is not unreasonable to expect that at some point in the future, IOL technology will be able to even improve on Mother Nature with such features as telephoto and macro focusing effects.

Conclusion

Refractive lensectomy in the presbyopic hyperopic patient is rapidly finding a place for itself among our surgical armamentarium. Nevertheless, the definite difference in risk and benefit in comparison with keratorefractive surgery behooves the surgeon to explore the full range of implications (both surgically and optically) with the patient prior to intervention.[19] IOL planning formulas need to be further developed for greater accuracy. We can expect to see even greater advances in IOL technology in the near future to meet the needs of the surgical hyperope.

References

1. Applegate RA, Howland HC. Magnification and visual acuity in refractive surgery. *Arch Ophthalmol.* 1993;111: 1335-1342.
2. Kelman CD. *Through My Eyes: The Story of a Surgeon Who Dared To Take On the Medical World.* New York: Random House; 1985.
3. Holladay JT. Analysis of edge glare phenomena in intraocular lens edge designs. *J Cataract Refract Surg.* 1999;26:748-752.
4. Hoffer KT. The Hoffer Q formula. *J Cataract Refract Surg.* 1993; 19:700-712.
5. Lazzerini A. *Evaluation of IOL power calculation in cataract surgery. Refractive results obtained with partial coherence interferometry and ultrasound biometry.* Paper prestned at: ESCRS XX Congress; ; 2002; Nice.
6. Samalonis L. The 21st Century IOL. *Eyeworld.* Aug 2; 30.
7. Fink AM, Gore C, Rosen ES. Refractive lensectomy for hyperopia. *Ophthalmology.* 2000;107:1540-1548.
8. Stromberg. Refraction and axial length of human eyes. *Invest Ophthalmol.* 1936;14:281-285.
9. Nano H, Muzzin S. Non-contact holmium:YAG laser thermal keratoplasty for hyperopia. *J Cataract Refract Surg.* 1998;24:751-757.
10. Irvine AR, Bresky R, Crowder BM, et al. Macular Edema after cataract surgery. *Ann Ophthalmol.* 1971;3:1234-1240.
11. Srinivas K, Rao DO, et al. Cystoid macular edema after pediatric intraocular lens implantation: fluoroscein angioscopy results and literature review. *J Cataract Refract Surg.* 2001;27:432-436.

12. Shugar JK. Interpseudophakos Elschnig pearls associated with late hyperopic shift: a complication of piggyback posterior chamber intraocular lens implantation. *J Cataract Refract Surg*. 1999;25:863-867.
13. Davidorf JM, Zaldivar R, Oscherow S. Posterior chamber phakic intraocular lens for hyperopia of +4 to +11 diopters. *J Cataract Refract Surg*. 1998;14:306-311.
14. http://www.staar.com/toric/toricmed.htm
15. http://www.stlukeseye.com/professionals/lri_nomogram.htm
16. http://www.arraylens.com/cataracts/
17. http://www2.prelex.com/
18. http://www.humanoptiks.com
19. Koch DD. The cornea or the lens? Editorial. *J Cataract Refract Surg*. 2002;28:379.

Chapter Twenty

Lens Implants For Hyperopia in Adults and Children

Daljit Singh, MS, DSc

Introduction

Of all the refractive errors, with the exception of irregular astigmatism, early onset hyperopia has the most negative visually crippling effects. The reasons for this include poor visual acuity, strabismus, amblyopia, nystagmus, poor cosmesis of thick spectacles, and the resultant psychic impact on the patient. Unless the condition is detected and treated at an early age, visual damage with lifelong consequences is inevitable. However, there are enormous problems in early detection and management, due to the young age of the patient. With full cooperation of the family, a combined effort of the refractionist, strabismologist, orthoptist, and ophthalmic surgeon can help provide and maintain good vision. Low to medium refractive errors are easily managed with glasses. For higher errors, there is no agreement as to the lowest age when an excimer laser or a phakic lens type of intervention is in order, or where possibly a contact lens may be maintained. The absence of extensive clinical experience and the legal constraints in different parts of the world prevent the use of phakic lens implants in children.

Implantation of a phakic lens is an intraocular invasive procedure with a risk of serious early and late complications that may permanently damage the eye. If a phakic lens could be sequestrated and the surgeon could avoid any physical effect on adjacent intraocular structures, a larger margin of safety could be achieved. However, every design of phakic lens presses and erodes a uveal tissue. It occupies a space that keeps slowly shrinking over the years, increasing the need for regular lifetime follow-up. If cataracts develop (natural- or phakic lens-induced), explantation will be necessary. The phakic lens implant surgery involves a healthy eye, therefore to be done with the greatest caution, and the patient to be followed meticulously to detect and nip a budding problem.

Three types of phakic intraocular lenses are in use—posterior chamber lenses, angle-supported lenses, and iris-supported lenses. The choice of a lens depends upon its availability in a country (depending upon current regulations), the surgeon's training and experience, and the informed consent of the patient. Whatever the technique used, a life-long regular follow-up is necessary.

The iris-fixated lens, the Artisan Phakic Claw Lens (Ophtec Inc., Netherlands), is fixed to two points on the iris by means of claws, while the whole lens floats in the aqueous. In the author's experience, the lens is well tolerated by the iris tissue. It does not produce angle-related, posterior pigment epithelium, or crystalline lens-related problems (Figure 20-1).[1]

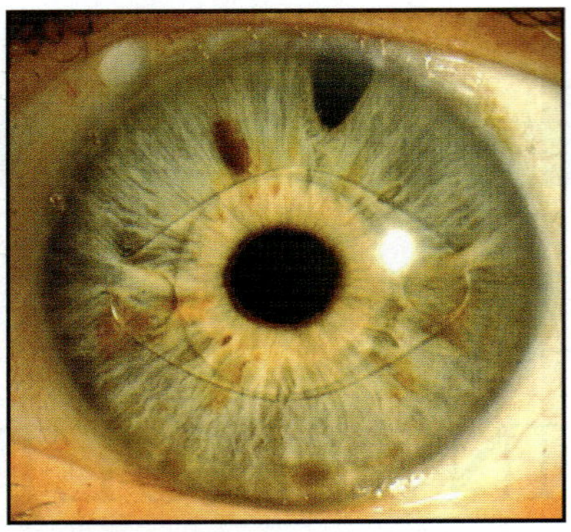

Figure 20-1. Iris-fixated lens 22 years postoperative, in an aphakic eye, showing excellent tolerance.

Historical

The early phakic lens studies were nearly drowned in the flood of laser refractive surgery by PRK and later by LASIK. Besides other simmering safety issues, there has been an increasing concern about the upper refractive limits for LASIK. This has created an impetus for the refractive surgeon to look at intraocular lenses (IOLs), or combined approaches such as bioptics.

Strampelli in 1953 was the first to implant phakic angle supported lenses.[2] Barraquer reported an angle supported PMMA lens in 1959.[3] In 1988 Baikoff presented their angle-supported lens for phakic eyes.[4] The first iris-fixated phakic lens was implanted in 1978 by Jan Worst as a blinding lens in a desperate patient who suffered from intractable diplopia.[5] Fechner implanted an iris-fixated lens in a myopic in 1986 and the author implanted one in a hyperopic in 1987. Fyodorov started posterior chamber phakic lenses in 1986.[5] Zaldivar, 1996, reported the use of foldable posterior chamber lenses in myopia and hyperopia.[6]

Anatomy and Pathophysiology

The tissues involved and the ocular spaces available for lens implantation have an important bearing on the early and late results.

A posterior chamber phakic lens has to occupy a triangular space of 65 µL that has zero depth at the pupillary margin. The configuration of the IOL is just the reverse, being thinnest at the periphery and thickest at the center, an unavoidable perfect anatomical mismatch. There is no way the lens can avoid touching, rubbing, or pressing the tissues around it—ie, ciliary epithelium, the posterior pigment epithelium of the iris, and the anterior surface of the crystalline lens. A lens design can reduce (not abolish) contact/pressure on one of them, at the cost of more pressure on the others. A less vaulted lens rubs against the crystalline lens (risk of cataract), while a high vault increases pressure on the ciliary epithelium and the posterior pigment epithelium of the iris (risk of blood-aqueous barrier breakdown and pigmentary glaucoma). The crystalline lens grows throughout life, increasing in volume from a mere 150 µL to 240 µL in 6 decades, mostly at the cost of the cramped posterior chamber. The resistance to the flow of aqueous in the presence of a phakic posterior chamber lens has to be overcome by a patent iridectomy.

The anterior chamber anatomy, although variable, has an average depth of 3.15 mm and a volume of 250 µL. The growth of crystalline lens reduces the volume by about 7.5% each decade, a matter of concern when an angle-supported or iris-fixated lens is contemplated.

The iris thickness is about 0.6 mm, being thicker in brown and black eyes. An iris-fixated phakic lens has to avoid rubbing the anterior surface of the iris during pupil movements. This is done by vaulting and having a concave posterior surface of the optic. A correctly fixed lens remains far away from the angle as well as the corneal endothelium. The crystalline lens does not come in the picture at all. However, the compression of the iris tissue in haptic (claw) is ever present. The pupils in the brown and black eyes are smaller and dilate less in the dark than the pupils in blue eyes.

The capillaries and blood vessels of the iris are anatomically designed to minimize blood aqueous barrier breakage, in comparison to the capillaries of the ciliary body that behave just the opposite. If an excessive amount of iris tissue is included in the claw of the iris-supported lens, the iris gets compressed between the crystalline lens and the phakic lens, resulting in synechiae formation and obstruction to the free flow of the aqueous.

The haptics of an angle-supported lens press against corneo-scleral trabeculae, Schlemm canal, the ciliary body in the angle recess, and sometimes the blood vessels and the nerves in the vicinity. Sizing is very important as well as vexatious, because there is no perfect size. A lens has to be somewhat oversized to stay in place. Therefore, it compresses the tissues. A short lens invariably rotates. The lens haptic may press the segmental supply of the iris, causing atrophy that manifests as progressive ovalization of the pupil. Uveitis-Glaucoma-Hyphema (UGH) syndrome and cystoid macular edema (CME) are other feared possibilities.

Micro-trauma and occasional macro-trauma in every day life has adverse effect on the tissues, provided the trauma force can reach IOL-tissue contact sites. Necrosis and shedding of cells and breakdown of blood-aqueous barrier occurs. The surgery itself is a considerable initial trauma, which may be even more severe when a lens is exchanged.

Criteria for Patient Selection

The aim of phakic lens implantation is either refractive correction or a part of prevention/treatment of amblyopia. The patients who need it most are young to very young unilateral or bilateral hyperopes. They are generally not suitable candidates, either because of regulatory restrictions, because the surgeon fears that surgery may introduce a damaging complication connected with high reactivity of a young eye, or due to underdeveloped or changing anatomy of the eye. The solid basis of amblyopia treatment, especially in unilateral hyperopia, is the correction of refractive error. In contrast to myopia, hyperopia does not increase with age, thus making the correction goal easier.

The ideal patient for a phakic refractive intraocular lens is one who does not like or tolerate hyperopic spectacles or contact lens (CTL) and does not wish a keratorefractive procedure. The other group of patients has high refractive errors, for which the surgeon usually suggests a phakic lens or a dual operation of phakic lens implant, followed, by a later laser refractive technique[7] so that an accurate refractive correction is achieved.

There are contraindications of IOL implantation including age, mental status, the ability to cooperate, and the intelligence of the patient; the patient must be able to refrain from rubbing the eyes. (The presence of amblyopia is not a contraindication.)

If other more objective indications exist, the surgeon must judge the severity of the condition and the preference of the patient before deciding if IOL implantation is the best route to take.

Contraindications of Phakic IOLs

Contraindications of phakic intraocular lens implantation:

- Early cataract
- Uveitis
- Posterior synechia
- Glaucoma or intraocular pressure more than 20 mmHg
- Diabetes mellitus
- Arthritis
- Anterior chamber depth less than 3 mm
- Corneal diameter less than 11 mm

Diabetes mellitus (DM) is a common disease. A strong family history of diabetes is a matter of concern. It adversely affects the posterior pigment epithelium of iris. A phakic lens in the posterior chamber is likely to shed pigment from the iris. This modality should be avoided if a patient is very likely to develop DM. Before implanting a phakic lens to correct hyperopia or myopia, the pros and cons of the various treatment modalities must be weighed. These include CTLs, keratorefractive surgery, cataract or clear lens extraction (CLE) with monofocal or multifocal IOLS, and phakic IOLS.

Laser refractive surgery has an advantage over phakic implants in that it does not require lifetime attention. It also reduces or removes existing astigmatism, while a phakic lens normally does not. However, the visual results after laser surgery do not match those of phakic lens implantation.

Preoperative Management

Examination

The following factors need consideration:

1. *Age of the patient*:
   A. Adults are generally non-problematic. One can advise phakic lens for young adults. Cataract extraction with a high power intraocular lens suffices the needs of the elderly.
   B. With children, a surgeon must refer to judgment as well as the prevailing practice patterns of the country or region. Phakic lens can be an effective treatment option for children when the parents are unable to manage contact lenses or thick spectacles.
2. *Nystagmus*: This is not a contraindication and has an advantage over spectacles.
3. *Corneal diameter*: Special angle-supported or posterior chamber lenses are not available for eyes with cornea smaller than 11 mm. However, iris-fixated lenses can be custom made by several companies in India as small as 5.5 mm width with an optic diameter of 3 mm. Horizontal white-to-white distance is a rough guide to select an angle-supported or a posteri-

or chamber lens. It does not always relate well to sulcus-to-sulcus distance.

4. *Depth of anterior chamber*: A good depth of anterior chamber reflects on the spaciousness of the posterior chamber, as well as on the ease of aqueous circulation. A depth of 3.0 mm or more is desirable. On the lower side a depth of 2.5 may be considered a risky extreme. Such patients are suitable either for laser refractive surgery or for cataract extraction with IOL implantation including piggyback lens implantation.
5. *Pupil size*: Pupils are smaller in brown and black eyes, compared to eyes with light-colored iris. The latter group needs lenses with bigger optics to avoid edge effects.
6. *Axial length of eye*: All hyperopic eyeballs are smaller than normal, yet the anterior segment dimensions may be normal. The smallest eye that we operated upon was 18.3 mm long.
7. *Refractive error*: The lenses are available from +1.00 D upward.The higher the refractive error, the thicker the optic of the phakic lens, a point to be kept in mind. Small optics lenses are thinner and provide a greater depth of field, but the edge effect has to be kept in mind.
8. *Corrected visual acuity*: The refractive surgery is in essence to preserve or gain visual acuity. An accurate visual acuity record of both the eyes and the recording of amblyopia, if present, are important.
9. *Intraocular pressure*: There should be no doubt about the absence of glaucoma.
10. *Fundus examination*: The condition of the optic disc, the macula and the periphery is noted. High hyperopes often complain of defective night vision, but the fundus is normal.

Preoperative Procedure

Nd:YAG laser peripheral iridotomy (LPI) is performed at one or, preferably, at two places a few weeks prior to posterior chamber lens implantation. If this facility is not available, a manual peripheral iridectomy is done at the time of surgery. LPI is more difficult in highly pigmented eyes.

Surgical Procedure

Preparation for Operation

1. Calculation of phakic IOL power from the results of refraction, the depth of the anterior chamber and the keratometric readings, with the help of the tables for different types of intraocular lens.
2. Conjunctival swab for culture and sensitivity.
3. Instillation of ofloxacin or ciprofloxacin eye drops 6 to 8 times on the preceding day and 4 to 6 times on the morning of the operation.
4. Pilocarpine 2% drops to contract the pupil, for iris-supported or angle-supported lenses. Phenylephrine 10% drops to dilate the pupil for posterior chamber lens. (*Care must be taken when using 10% Phenylephrine due to cardiovascular considerations.*)

Anesthesia

It is possible to implant a phakic lens after topical, intracameral, subconjunctival, peribulbar, or retrobulbar anesthesia. The author, however, prefers general anesthesia because it allows the surgeon to concentrate fully on the procedure. The operation takes about 5 to 7 minutes.

Surgical Preparation

1. Painting the skin around the eye with povidone-iodine 10%.
2. Washing the conjunctival sac with povidone-iodine 5%.
3. Passing a superior rectus suture and a suture through the lower lid.
4. Plastic adhesive drape and an eye speculum. The author uses none of these, because they seem to put pressure on the eye ball. The cilia are cut if they are likely to touch the operating instruments or the intraocular lens.The lid margin and the conjunctival sac are thoroughly washed with povidone-iodine 5%.

Implantation Steps

Iris-Fixated Lens

The steps of this procedure are described in greater detail, as iris-fixation is a more demanding procedure. A step-by-step procedure follows.

Step One

A trifacet adjustable depth diamond knife is used to make 0.3 mm deep grooves on the limbus, 1 mm wide on the sides and 4.25 mm to 6 mm (according to lens size) at the upper limbus. The side ports are opened in to the anterior chamber as 1 mm deep pockets in the clear cornea. The anterior chamber is filled firmly with viscoelastic material. The viscoelastic material should be injected after taking the cannula clearly in to the anterior chamber. Injecting

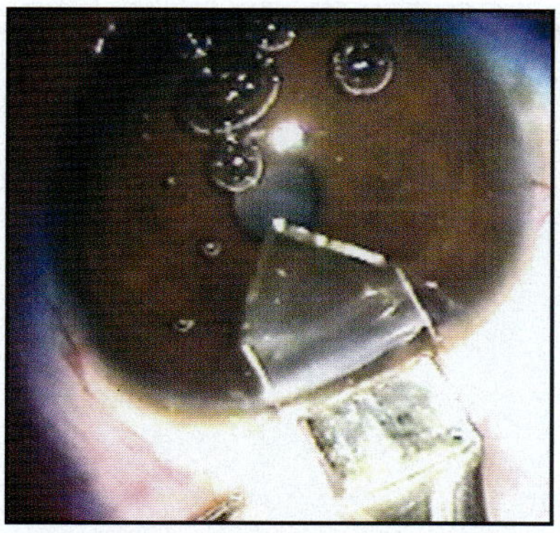

Figure 20-2. Pocket incision being made with a diamond knife. The knife is moved parallel to the iris. The anterior chamber is deepened by injecting viscoelastic from the side port before making the incision.

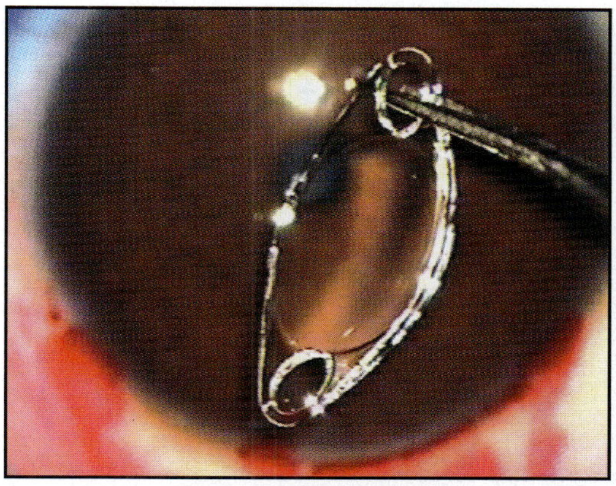

Figure 20-3. Phakic hyperopic iris fixation lens, showing a convex-concave configuration (Artisan Lens, Ophtec Inc., Netherlands).

merely inside the pocket can sometimes cause a disastrous separation of the Descemet membrane. The top incision is made with a 4.25-mm diamond knife and a 1.5-mm deep pocket is fashioned. A diamond knife makes the cleanest cut. The knife should be moved in the plane of the iris and never toward it (Figure 20-2).

Step Two

A peripheral iridectomy or iridotomy is performed either prior to lens implantation or at the end of the operation. To do an iridotomy or iridectomy, a utility forceps lifts the iris just inside the incision. The lifted iris is snipped by a scissors inside the anterior chamber. The iris is never pulled out of the incision line, as this can tear the iris root and cause bleeding.

Step Three

Lens implantation. The iris-fixated lens is vaulted and has a convex-concave optic (Figure 20-3). The author commonly uses a lens with eccentric claws, which need to face superiorly for proper fixation. Others use a lens with claws 180 degrees apart. Keeping the anterior chamber filled with viscoelastic, the intraocular lens is introduced and rotated to make it horizontal. The author likes to see the lens floating in the viscoelastic, so that when the lens holding forceps enters the anterior chamber, the upper edge of the intraocular lens moves in to the open jaws.

The Lens-Holding Forceps

Passing a fold of iris through the claw needs to be understood clearly. Each haptic of the iris supported lens has a springy flexible claw. The claw can be opened by anything stiff—a thin forceps, a hook, or a cannula. The iris can be introduced into the claw either by:

1. Carrying it along with the stiff instrument that opens the claw.
2. Gently pressing the claw on the iris. The iris holding forceps opens the claw in motion; the moment the two sides of the claw fall back, they immediately pinch the iris immediately underneath. The amount of the iris in the claw can be increased by feeding more iris or reduced by opening the claw backward (Figure 20-4).

During manipulations for claw fixation, the chamber has a tendency to collapse. Lack of control on the depth of the anterior chamber could upset the surgeon. If the iris follows the leaking viscoelastic material, the situation could become nightmarish. To overcome this problem the author has a few solutions.

The maintenance of the anterior chamber and the passage of the iris through the claw are done with a simple device. A small, stiff, 25-gauge cannula is attached to an irrigating handle, which in turn is connected through 6 inches long silicone tubing to a 2-ml syringe containing viscoelastic of surgeon's choice. The surgeon handles the instrument, while the assistant pushes the viscoelastic on command.

The viscoelastic is injected into the anterior chamber in small amounts, with the sole aim of simply keeping the iris-supported lens separated from the tissues. Overfilling tends to prolapse the iris and make lens fixation difficult.

When the Artisan lens is steadied in front of the pupil, the claw is fixated with an instrument through the side port. A shift in the position of the lens-hold-

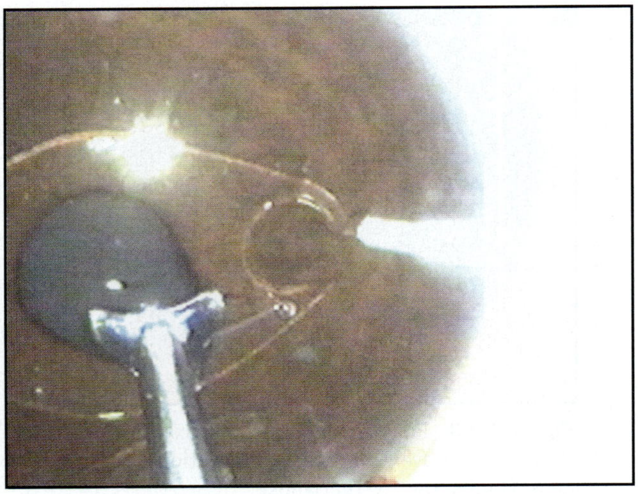

Figure 20-4. The Artisan lens is held with the forceps, while the iris is passed through the claw by a 25-gauge viscoelastic irrigating cannula.

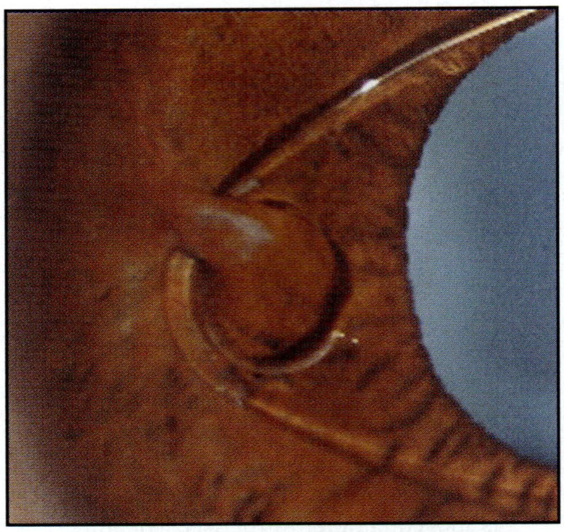

Figure 20-5. Sufficient iris in the claw for a proper fixation.

ing forceps will lead to a misplaced fixation. Fixation close to the angle of the anterior chamber and excessive iris enclavation can cause a tear in the iris root and bleeding. If that happens, wait for the bleeding to stop, fill the anterior chamber with viscoelastic, remove the iris from the claw by pushing the claw backwards, and refix the lens at correct place. Remember that there is crystalline lens under the iris that should not be hit when pushing the claw backwards.

A surgeon new to the procedure may make a small iris fixation on one side, then take out all instruments. He or she then refills the anterior chamber with a viscoelastic, reassesses the optic centration and the fixation of the first claw, and then makes the fixation of the second claw at the proper place. He or she then goes back to the first claw and completes the fixation.

The centration and fixation of an iris-fixated lens has to be done by the surgeon him or herself. The implanted lens should remain at the same position for the rest of the patient's life.

Another way to stabilize the implant is to use any horizontally or vertically acting plain lens holding forceps, to hold the lens haptic close to the claw, while another device (forceps or cannula or a hook) is used to pass the iris through the claw. Yet another way is to hold the lens with dolphin tail forceps while the iris is passed through the claw with the help of a hook passed through the same upper incision.

The iris should be moved in to the claw tangential to the pupillary margin. This preserves the circular appearance of the pupil. If the iris tissue gets pulled at a right angle to the pupil margin, an oval pupil results. The defect is especially noticeable when the pupil is contracted. It is an avoidable 1-time error and does not progress.

Tiny amounts of iris tissue in the claw of the lens can be responsible for dislocation months or years later. Too much iris tissue inside the claws, in a way, makes the lens optic press against the iris tissue, thereby reducing the freedom of the aqueous to move freely under the lens edges. It also encourages synechia formation between the iris and crystalline lens. In brown and black eyes a thicker fold of iris is necessary, because the collagen and elastic tissue are situated deep under the anterior pigmented stroma. In the light-colored eyes a relatively thin fold may actually be full iris thickness deep. Surgeons must pay careful attention to have neither too little nor too much iris in the claw (Figure 20-5).

Step Four

Clearing the anterior chamber of viscoelastic by irrigation with a wide-bore cannula helps remove the viscoelastic without much turbulence.

Step Five

Closing the incision line. Because the corneal pocket has a width of nearly 1.5 mm, the two walls of the upper pocket can be brought together effectively with the help of a medium-sized air bubble. The side pockets need no special attention.

Having no suture and no air bubble in the anterior chamber runs a risk of leakage or aspiration. A medium-sized air bubble is a great help. When the patient sits up, the air bubble helps to bring the two

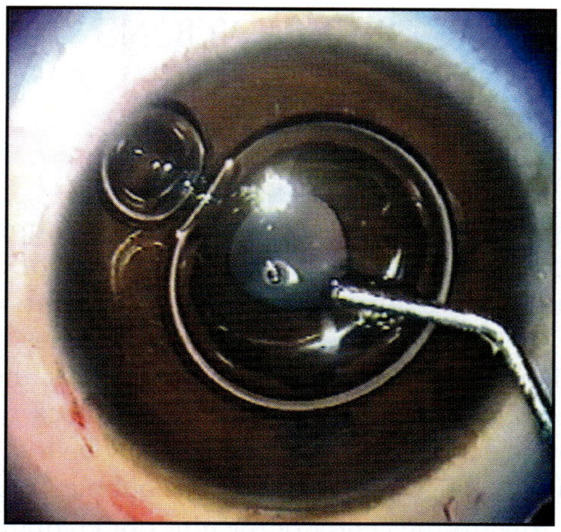

Figure 20-6. A medium size air bubble at the end of surgery ensures good apposition of the pocket incision. The cannula is being pressed on the cornea to judge the lifting force of the air bubble.

sides of the pocket incision together and gives further safety to the incision (Figure 20-6).

Step Six

Subconjunctival injection of 20 mgm of gentamycin and 2 mgm of dexamethasone.

Angle-Supported Lens

Step-by-step procedure:

1. A 6-mm corneo-scleral incision is made in the steepest meridian.
2. The anterior chamber is filled with viscoelastic.
3. A 5-mm silicone sheets glide is introduced in to the anterior chamber. A viscoelastic is injected over the glide.
4. The phakic IOL is held with a utility forceps and the inferior haptic is slipped into the anterior chamber.
5. The IOL is slid over the glide, until both ends of the inferior haptics are in contact with the angle. The glide is then pulled out gently.
6. The upper haptic is pushed in to the anterior chamber and under the posterior lip of the incision, using a double-tip nucleus manipulator.
7. The phakic IOL is rotated with a Sinskey hook, to the horizontal meridian, where white-to-white distance is measured.
8. A small peripheral iridectomy is performed.
9. If the pupil is not round, a Sinskey hook is used to pull the haptic away from the angle; then it is released.
10. Verify that the optic is centered, the pupil is round, and there is no iris traction by the foot plate.
11. Apply 2 to 3 bite running 10 zero nylon. Before the knot is tied, the viscoelastic is carefully washed out. Nylon is used to close any conjunctival flap made. After the incision is closed, it is important to perform gonioscopy to properly position haptic ends and check iris tuck. This important step is easy to forget.

Posterior Chamber Lens

A few days before lens implantation, a peripheral iridectomy is performed with Nd:YAG laser.

Before the surgery the pupil is fully dilated. The step-by-step procedure is:

1. One 0.6-mm side port is made. It is needed to inject viscoelastic material in the anterior chamber.
2. For a precrystalline lens, a 3.2-mm clear corneal incision is made on the steep meridian.
3. The lens is introduced with angled-suture forceps, or an injector and then positioned.
4. The lens is manipulated to center the optic on the pupil.
5. The viscoelastic material is removed from the anterior and posterior chambers with an aspiration syringe (23-gauge cannula) or by copious irrigation with saline.
6. The pupil is contracted with intraocular acetylcholine 1%, or pilocarpine 0.5% solution.
7. The incision is closed by hydrating the corneal incisions. A suture is rarely needed.

It is obvious from the 3 descriptions of lens implantation given above that the implantation of every phakic lens needs thorough knowledge of the procedure and an average degree of surgical skill.

Postoperative Management

Preventing a postoperative reaction is crucial:

1. Anti-inflammatory—Prednisone 40 mg daily for the first 3 days, 20 mg for the next 7 days, 10 mg for the next 15 days, and 5 mg daily for the next 15 days. It is important to take the standard precautions in administering oral corticosteroids. This is followed by indomethacin slow release 250 mg capsules once daily for the next 30 days. Then fluoromethalone 0.25% drops are prescribed, 6 times a day for 2 weeks, 5 times a day for the 2 weeks after, and so on reducing the amount of daily drops by 1 every 2 weeks. Non-steroidal agent ketorolac tromethamine 0.5% is added 6 weeks after the surgery. It is instilled 3 times a day and is continued for 4 to 6 months. The regime might appear excessive,

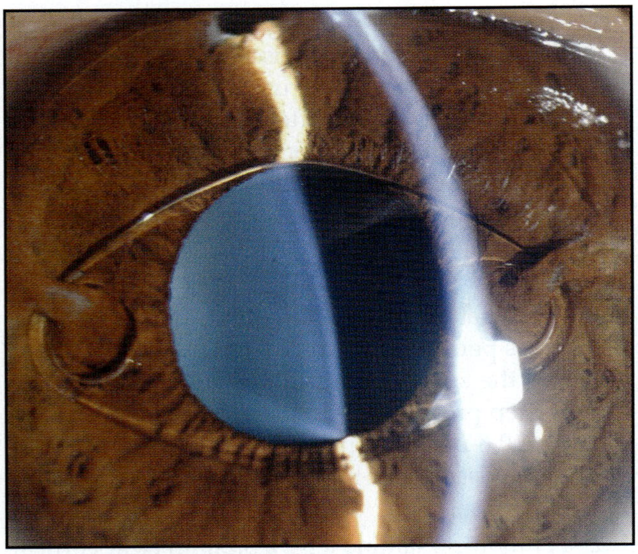

Figure 20-7. Phakic iris fixated lens for hyperopia, 4 years postoperative. The overall width of the lens is 7.25 mm, while the optic is 4.25 mm.

but the stakes are too high to take chances. The intraocular pressure (IOP) is monitored closely.

2. Dilation of the pupil—The pupil is kept moving by the instillation of homatropine 2% and phenylepherine 5% once or twice a day. At the slightest sign of posterior synechia, the treatment is intensified.
3. Refraction—The first postoperative refraction may be done after 1 or 2 days.
4. Follow-up—The patient is examined daily for 3 days. The next examinations are performed after 15 days, 1 month, 2 months, 3 months, 6 months, and then twice a year. At every visit, uncorrected and best-corrected visual acuity (BCVA) is recorded. The eye is examined under the slit lamp microscope, with the pupil fully dilated. IOP is measured. Six months postoperative and then twice a year thereafter, gonioscopy is done in angle support and posterior chamber lens cases. Endothelial cell counts are done in every case. Figure 20-7 shows a phakic iris fixated lens 4 years postoperative.
5. Warning to the patientùThe patient is advised to report immediately if there is pain, redness, or a fall in the sharpness of vision. He or she is advised to never rub the operated eye.

Complications

Early

Pupil Block Glaucoma

A pupil block is possible with an angle-supported lens if a peripheral iridectomy is not done or it does not function. If an iris-fixated lens patient with a large air bubble sits up, the bubble presses on the peripheral iridectomy as well as presses the lens optic against the iris, initiating pupil block glaucoma. Such a patient should immediately be told to lay supine looking straight. The air bubble will then move toward the center of the anterior chamber, and the peripheral iridectomy will become functional. The recovery is immediate.

A case of posterior chamber phakic lens can develop pupil block due to retained viscoelastic material, closure of iridotomy by the haptic, or by inflammatory exudates. There is ballooning of the peripheral iris. The treatment lies in making additional iridotomies or a surgical iridectomy. Hyperopic eyes are more prone to pupil block than myopic eyes. If malignant glaucoma occurs, as has been reported in a myopic case, the crystalline lens, the phakic refractive lens and the iris are forced forward, increasing the pupil block. This condition is an ocular emergency.[8]

Inflammatory Reaction

In every operated case there is a certain inflammatory reaction as manifested by aqueous flare and deposition of pigment cells on the implanted intraocular lens. These cells disappear in a few weeks.

Early severe reaction is manifested as synechia and exudates. It calls for intensive treatment. In some cases, explantation may be needed.

Size Mismatch

A small phakic lens may show decentration. It may also move and knock on ciliary processes causing pigment release and inflammation. A larger lens would push the iris anteriorly, as well as press the ciliary body. In both cases, the lens needs explantation or exchange.

Hyphema

Hyphema can occur if a manual iridectomy is done at the time of lens implantation. It may come from the iridectomy site or from a tear at the iris root. The latter is possible in iris-fixated lens, if iris is not properly held and passed through the claw.

Cataract

A localized cataract as a result of instrumental trauma is possible with every kind of lens implantation.

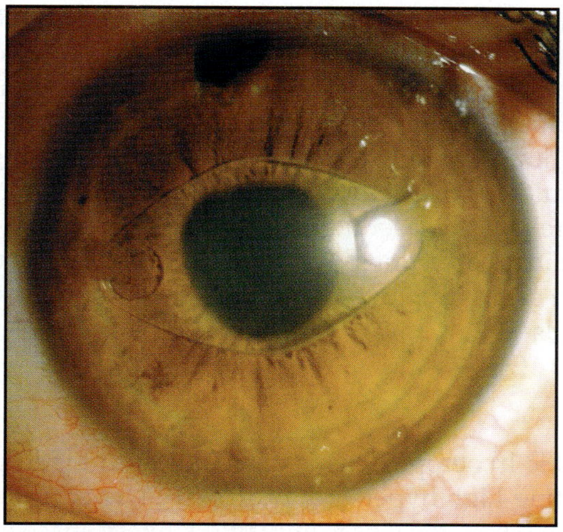

Figure 20-8. Acute uveitis 3 weeks after phakic iris fixated implant in a 25-year-old patient. There is a small hypopion in addition to exudates in the pupil and on the lens. The patient had been careless about the use of prescribed medicines.

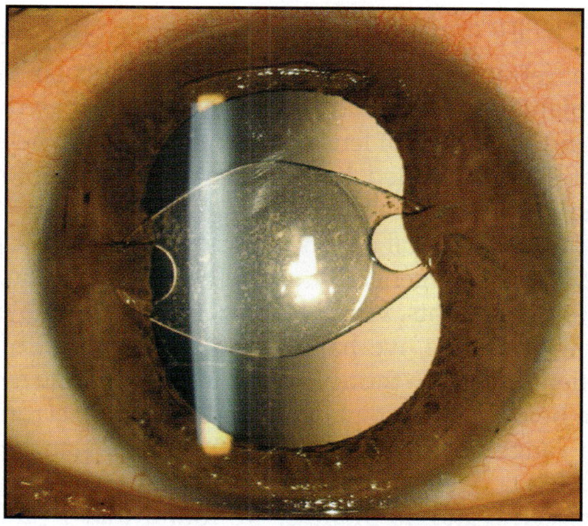

Figure 20-9. The same eye 4 days after the start of anti-inflammatory treatment.

Late

Ovalization of the Pupil

Ovalization occurs with angle-supported lens as a result of mechanical tucking of the iris by haptic pressure or by ischemic and fibrotic changes in the periphery of the iris caused by haptic pressure. Once it starts, the change is progressive. Explantation is advised.

Inflammatory Reaction

An inflammatory reaction of an acute or subacute nature can occur with any phakic lens because unlike an in-the-bag lens, every phakic lens has a contact with the uveal tissues. Ciliary congestion, deposits on the IOL including KPs, and synechia and exudates formation are some signs. The patients need to be followed and assessed regularly. In some cases explantation is in order to save further problems. The inflammation is easy to handle in a case of iris-fixated lens, because the lens is independent of the pupil and the crystalline lens (Figures 20-8 and 20-9).

Cataract Formation

An angle-supported or an iris-supported lens is not responsible for initiating or progressing a cataract, because the crystalline lens is far away and there is no interference with aqueous circulation. However, the same cannot be said about the phakic lenses in the posterior chamber. Cataract has been reported frequently with phakic posterior chamber lenses (Fechner et al, 17.8%, Fink, 75%, Menezo et al, 25% and 33.3%).[9-11] Depending upon the design and version, more or less phakic lens to crystalline lens contact is unavoidable. Adhesions might form. We cannot trivialize this complication.

Glaucoma

A closure of the peripheral iridotomy by the lens haptic, inflammatory or pigment cells, plus obstruction of the pupil by the lens optic can precipitate an attack of glaucoma. Iris bombe is quite evident. If done in time, Nd:YAG iridotomy or a manual iridectomy relieves the problem.

A potential long-term complication is the development of pigmentary glaucoma, as a result of pigment shedding from the ciliary processes and the posterior pigment epithelium of iris. There is no posterior chamber lens design that can avoid pigment shedding.

Erosion of the Iris

A mismatched phakic posterior chamber lens can erode the iris by friction and pressure. The problem is that it is not easy to judge if there is a mismatch. Excessive and uneven shallowing of the anterior chamber periphery, pigment deposits on the lens and the angle of the anterior chamber, micro-hyphema, and signs of inflammation should alert to the possibility of iris erosion. The presence of a transillumination defect will leave no doubt.

Endothelial Loss

Endothelial cell loss can occur due to surgical trauma, implant-endothelial touch, acute or chronic inflammation, and glaucoma. A strict vigil should be kept on the endothelial cell counts, whatever the design of lens used. Many earlier anterior chamber designs have shown moderately severe loss of cells.

Surgical Results

The refractive results in phakic intraocular lens implantation are good, because they are based on sound principles of lens power calculation. Excellent tables are provided by lens makers for their own designs.

In adults, visual results hold no surprises, because their vision is generally stable before operation. In younger patients, visual results are more variable.

In our clinic, we have operated on a total of 15 patients between the ages of 7 and 14 years, the mean age being 11. These patients had refractive errors in the range of +5.00 D to +11.00 D the mean being +7.00 D. After following up on the patients for between 6 and 48 months, we found that 1 patient lost 1 line and 1 had no change while the remaining 13 gained between 1 and 5 lines, the mean gain of all 15 being 2.2 lines. No secondary operations were done. One patient had moderate inflammatory reaction that resolved with treatment. The average endothelial cell loss was 3%.

Future Plans and Development

The ideal phakic IOL has not been developed. This ideal lens would include:

- Long track record
- Ease of implantation
- Availability for examination with or without pupil dilatation
- Minimum contact with the uveal tissues
- No interference with aqueous movement
- No danger of cataract formation
- No danger of decentration
- No danger to the corneal endothelium
- Ease of explantation

Laser refractive surgery scores over a phakic lens in that beyond a few months to a year, regular lifetime attention is not required. It also reduces or removes existing astigmatism, which a phakic lens normally does not. There shall never be an "implant and forget" design. Lifelong care shall be necessary for the young patients of today by the third, fourth, and even fifth generation of ophthalmologists, who shall have to be trained to deal with millions of today's and tomorrow's implanted lenses.

The most important issue in hyperopia is the presence or development of amblyopia, which usually develops at a young age. Some treatment modality shall have to be provided to very young children, be it a revolutionary form of contact lens, an intracorneal lens, an IOL, or an acceptable form of laser refractive surgery. This will surely happen, but will begin at a slow pace. The art of orthoptic and pleoptic treatment does not attract many followers, because of its lack of remunerative glamour. Gradually, it has degenerated to the level of mere patching. There is a need to recultivate this highly useful way of reducing the misery of amblyopia. There may be laser adjustable phakic lenses, so that the final corrections can be accurately made. Long-term safety in terms of decades shall be the watchwords.

Summary

Phakic hyperopic lens is an important modality for treating high hyperopia, provided there is sufficient space where the lens is implanted. Every space in the anterior segment is adversely affected by the growth in the volume of the crystalline lens. Therefore, not every patient is suitable for a hyperopia phakic lens.

What the eye needs is an optic with the smallest haptic. All the benefits are derived from the optic and all the problems are the handiwork of the haptics. Being an invasive procedure for an otherwise healthy eye, a phakic lens implantation is not to be taken lightly. It is not a single event as an act of insertion, but is the beginning of a lifelong intraocular process that requires regular monitoring for inflammation, synechia, pigment shedding, glaucoma, cataract formation, and endothelial status. Endothelial cells can be lost in every kind of phakic IOL, due to a variety of known (clinical and subclinical inflammation, glaucoma, and endothelial touch) and unknown reasons. Only a laser flare meter can monitor subclinical inflammation. Because most of the patients are relatively young, we have to keep a perspective of scores of years, in planning, selecting, and performing surgery.

Our visual results in younger group of patients after phakic lens implantation are highly encouraging. Further studies of this nature are needed to establish the advantages and the long-term safety.

References

1. Alio JL, Mulet E, Shalaby AMM. Artisan Phakic iris Claw Intraocular Lens for High Primary and Secondary Hyperopia. *J Refract Surg.* 2002;18:697-707.
2. Strampelli BS. Opportabilitadi lenti acrilliche in camera anteriore nella aphachia e nei vizi di refrazione. *Ann Ottamol Clin Oculist.* 1954;80:75-82.
3. Barraquer J. Anterior chamber plastic lenses: results and conclusions from 5 years experience. *Trans Ophthalmol Soc UK.* 1959;79:393.
4. Baikoff G, Joly P. Surgical correction of severe myopia using an anterior chamber implant in the phakic eye. Concept—results. *Bull Soc Belge Ophthalmol.* 1989;233:109-25.

5. Fyodorov SN, Zuyev VK, Aznabayev BM. Intraocular correction of high myopia with negative posterior chamber lens. *Ophthalmosurgery*. 1991;3:57-58.
6. Fechner PU, van der Heijde GL, Worst JGF. The correction of myopia by lens implantation into phakic eyes. *Am J Ophthalmol*. 1989;107:659-663.
7. Zaldivar R, Davidorf J, Oscherow S, et al. Combined posterior chamber phakic intraocular lens and laser in situ keratomileusis:bioptics for extreme myopia. *J Refract Surg*. 1999;14:294-305.
8. Kodjikian L, Gain P, Donate D, et al. Malignant glaucoma induced by a phakic posterior chamber intraocular lens for myopia. *J Cataract Refract Surg*. 2002;28:2217-2221.
9. Fechner PU, Haigis W, Wichmann W. Posterior chamber myopia lenses in phakic eyes. *J Cataract Refract Surg*. 1996;22:178-182.
10. Fink AM, Gore C, Rosen E. Cataract development after implantation of staar collamer posterior chamber phakic lens. *J Cataract Refract Surg*. 1999;25:278-282.
11. Menezo JL, Peris-Martinex C, Cisneros A, et al. Posterior chamber phakic intraocular lenses to correct high myopia, a comparative study of Staar and Adatomed models. *J Cataract Refract Surg*. 2001;17:32-42.

Suggested Reading

Pol, BAE van der, Worst JGF. Iris Claw intraocular lenses in children. *Documenta Ophthalmologica*. 1996;92:29-35.

Baikoff G, Arne JL, Bokobza Y, et al. Angle-fixated anterior chamber phakic intraocular lens for myopia of -7 to -19 diopters. *J Refract Surg*. 1998 May-Jun;14(3):282-93.

Fechner PU, Haigis W, Wichmann W. Posterior chamber myopia lenses in phakic eyes. *J Cataract Refract Surg*. 1996 Mar;22(2):178-82.

Fechner PU. Intraocular lenses for the correction of myopia in phakic eyes: short-term success and long-term caution. *Refract Corneal Surg*. 1990 Jul-Aug;6(4):242-4.

Fechner PU, Singh D, Wolff K. Iris claw lens in phakic eyes to correct hyperopia: preliminary study. *J Cataract Refract Surg*. 1998;24:48-56.

Fechner PU, Wichmann W. Correction of myopia by implantation of minus optic (Worst iris claw) lenses into the anterior chamber of phakic eyes. *Eur J Implant Surg*. 1993;5:55-59.

Fechner PU, van der Heijde GL, Worst JG. The correction of myopia by lens implantation into phakic eyes. *Am J Ophthalmol*. 1989 Jun 15;107(6):659-63.

Fechner PU. Cataract formation with a phakic IOL. *J Cataract Refract Surg*. 1999 Apr; 25(4):461-2.

Fyodorov SN, Zuew VK, Tumanyan NR, Suheil AJ. Clinical and functional follow-up of minus IOL implantation in high grade myopia. *Oftalmochirurgia*. 1993;2:12-17.

Kashani AA. Phakic posterior chamber intraocular lenses for the correction of high myopia. *J Refract Surg*. 1996 May-Jun;12(4):454-6.

Krumeich JH, Daniel J, Gast R. Closed-system technique for implantation of iris-supported negative-power intraocular lens. *J Refract Surg*. 1996 Mar-Apr;12(3):334-40].

Landesz M, Worst JG, Van Rij G, Houtman WA. Opaque iris claw lens in a phakic eye to correct acquired diplopia. *J Cataract Refract Surg*. 1997 Jan-Feb;23(1):137-8.

Menezo JL, Martinez MC, Cisneros AL. Iris-fixated Worst claw versus sulcus-fixated posterior chamber lenses in the absence of capsular support. *J Cataract Refract Surg*. 1996 Dec;22(10):1476-84.

Menezo JL, Cisneros A, Hueso JR, Harto M. Long-term results of surgical treatment of high myopia with Worst-Fechner intraocular lenses. *J Cataract Refract Surg*. 1995 Jan;21(1): 93-8.

Menezo JL, Avino JA, Cisneros A, et al. Iris claw phakic intraocular lens for high myopia. *J Refract Surg*. 1997 Sep-Oct;13(6):545-55.

Perez-Santonja JJ, Iradier MT, Benitez del Castillo JM, et al. Chronic subclinical inflammation in phakic eyes with intraocular lenses to correct myopia. *J Cataract Refract Surg*. 1996 Mar;22(2):183-7.

Perez-Santonja JJ, Bueno JL, Zato MA. Surgical correction of high myopia in phakic eyes with Worst-Fechner myopia intraocular lenses. *J Refract Surg*. 1997 May-Jun;13(3):268-81;discussion 281-4.

Perez-Santonja JJ, Iradier MT, Sanz-Iglesias L, et al. Endothelial changes in phakic eyes with anterior chamber intraocular lenses to correct high myopia. *J Cataract Refract Surg*. 1996 Oct;22(8):1017-22.

Perez-Santonja JJ, Hernandez JL, Benitez del Castillo JM, et al. Fluorophotometry in myopic phakic eyes with anterior chamber intraocular lenses to correct severe myopia. *Am J Ophthalmol*. 1994 Sep 15;118(3):316-21.

Perez-Torregrosa VT, Menezo JL, Harto MA, et al. Digital system measurement of decentration of Worst-Fechner iris claw myopia intraocular lens. *J Refract Surg*. 1995 Jan-Feb; 11(1):26-30.

Sanders DR, Brown DC, Martin RG, et al. Implantable contact lens for moderate to high myopia: phase 1 FDA clinical study with 6 month follow-up. *J Cataract Refract Surg*. 1998 May;24(5):607-11.

Singh, D, Correspondence. Iris claw lens usage in India. *Eur J Implant Ref Surg*. 1989;1:285-287.

Singh, D, Singh IR, Singh, R. Use of the worst-Singh lobster claw intraocular lens in children. *Ophthalmic Practice*. 1987;5:18-20.

Trindade F, Pereira F, Cronemberger S. Ultrasound biomicroscopic imaging of posterior chamber phakic intraocular lens. *J Refract Surg*. 1998 Sep-Oct;14(5):497-503.

Wiechens B, Winter M, Haigis W, et al. Bilateral cataract after phakic posterior chamber top hat-style silicone intraocular lens. *J Refract Surg*. 1997 Jul-Aug;13(4):392-7.

Zaldivar R, Davidorf JM, Oscherow S. Posterior chamber phakic intraocular lens for myopia of -8 to -19 diopters. *J Refract Surg*. 1998 May-Jun;14(3):294-305.

Zaldivar R, Davidorf JM, Oscherow S, et al. Combined posterior chamber phakic intraocular lens and laser in situ keratomileusis: bioptics for extreme myopia. *J Refract Surg*. 1999 May-Jun;15(3):299-308.

Chapter Twenty-One

Ultrasound Biomicroscopy of the Artisan Phakic Intraocular Lens in Hyperopic Eyes

Mihai Pop, MD; Yves Payette, MSc; and Magdi Mansour, MD, MSc

This chapter is condensed from material originally appearing in the Journal of Cataract and Refractive Surgery, *Volume 28, 1799-1803, October 2002 and is reprinted with the permission of Elsevier Science Inc.*

Introduction

In 1986, the first iris-claw intraocular lens (IOL) was implanted in a phakic eye by Worst and Fechner. Since then, several different models of this IOL have been developed. To date, versions for the treatment of myopia have been implanted in eyes worldwide without any published reports of abnormal pupil function or contact between the phakic IOL and the natural lens.[1,2] Still, some authors have expressed concern over the potential for this iris-claw IOL to damage the iris or the corneal endothelium.[3-5]

There is only a preliminary report in the literature about the Artisan iris-claw lens for hyperopia (model 203),[6] which in 2000 to 2001, was being investigated in clinical trials in the United States. The purpose of the present study was to describe the position of that phakic IOL relative to adjacent structures in the anterior segment. Examination of the anterior chamber was performed with ultrasound biomicroscopy (UBM). UBM is a simple technique that has been described previously for determining the postoperative fixation of other phakic IOLs, including the Artisan iris-claw lens for myopia, the collamer posterior chamber ICL (STAAR) for myopia and hyperopia, and the ZSAL-4 anterior chamber IOL for myopia.[2,7-9]

Patients and Methods

Patients

The Artisan iris-claw phakic IOL (model 203, Ophtec, Boca Raton, Fla) was implanted in 4 eyes of 3 patients. In Patient 1, a +4.00 D IOL was implanted in the left eye, which had a refraction of +3.00 – 1.25 x 108 D. Patient 2 underwent bilateral IOL implantation. Refraction in the right eye was +5.00 – 1.00 x 180 D and a +5.00 D IOL was implanted; the left eye refraction was +8.50 – 1.25 x 177 D and it received a +6.00 D implant. Patient 3 was implanted with a +4.00 D IOL in the left eye, which had a refraction of +3.75 – 0.75 x 70 D.

All patients received approval to undergo surgery from Health Canada on the Special Access Programme by the Therapeutic Product Medical Devices Bureau. The surgeries were approved by the ethics review board and all patients signed an informed consent form. A comprehensive ophthalmic screening examination, including gonioscopy and iris examination, was performed before surgery. Patients with any of the following findings were ineligible for the procedure: intraocular pressure (IOP) >21 mmHg, endothelial cell count <2000 cells/mm^2, or a history of glaucoma, uveitis, diabetic retinopathy, or iris atrophy.

The Iris-Claw Phakic Intraocular Lens for High Hyperopia

The intraocular iris-claw phakic Artisan lens (IOL) for hyperopia (model 203, Ophtec) is available in 1.00 D increments from +3.00 D to +12.00 D. It is constructed of polymethylmethacrylate, measures 8.5 mm in length by 5.0 mm in width, and the 5.0 mm optic has a convex-concave shape with a total height of 1.0 mm. Each of the IOL's two haptics is composed of 2 arms with merging claws at the ends that are used to fix the IOL to the mid-peripheral iris stroma. The opening created by the merging claws of the haptic measures 2.2 mm wide by 1.55 mm long.

The Artisan IOL is inserted with the pupil constricted and the anterior chamber filled with viscoelastic. After it is introduced into the anterior chamber, the lens is rotated with the haptics at 3- and 9 o'clock using a Sinskey-type IOL manipulating instrument. The optic is centered over the pupil. Iris entrapment is performed by holding a knuckle of iris with a specially designed, disposable enclavation needle (Ophtec OD-125) while gently pressing the center of one haptic over the knuckle, thus grasping iris tissue with both claws. The same procedure is repeated with the other haptic. Once the lens is fixated, manual peripheral iridectomy is performed.

Ultrasound Biomicroscope Examination

Pre- and postoperative examinations were performed using the Humphrey ultrasound biomicroscope, model 840 (Humphrey Instruments, Dublin, Calif). This system uses a 50-MHz transducer with a probe and has an axial and lateral resolution of 50 µm that provided sampling resolution on scans of 5 µm, as described by the manufacturer.

For the examination, the cornea was anesthetized with topical proparacaine 0.5%. Depending on the size of the eye aperture, a 20-, 22-, or 24-mm eye cup filled with sterile gonioscopic solution was inserted between the upper and lower eyelids. The patient was asked to fixate on a ceiling target with the fellow eye to maintain accommodation and fixation.

All eyes were scanned by a single operator. Cross-sectional images were taken through the cornea, iris, ciliary body and lens, starting from the nasal to the temporal side and from the superior to the inferior side, thus providing 360-degree coverage of the anterior chamber. Axial vertical and axial transverse sections were examined through the central cornea to the central lens. All measurements were made using the calipers provided by the UBM system software on the 2-dimensional image recorded by the UBM. The brightness of the echogram represented the intensity of the original echo.

Echograms were taken where needed in the anterior chamber to measure the preoperative anterior chamber depth (ACD) and the postoperative distance between the IOL and the corneal endothelium (endothelial-optic distance). The anterior chamber depth was measured from the corneal endothelium to the anterior surface of the lens capsule and the endothelial-optic distance was measured from the corneal endothelium to the anterior surface of the IOL. The distance between the IOL and the lens was also measured from the posterior surface of the IOL to the anterior surface of the lens capsule. In addition, the closest distance form the farthest point of the haptic to the angle of the anterior chamber was measured.

ACD and axial length were also determined by ultrasonography, using the Ocuscan (Alcon, Fort Worth, Tex) standard ultrasonograph. The ultrasonograph measured the ACD from the corneal epithelium to the anterior lens capsule; the axial length was evaluated from the corneal epithelium to the macula.

RESULTS

Preoperative gonioscopic examination was normal for all eyes, although it was observed that the natural iris arch seemed more pronounced than it is in myopic eyes. At 1 month after surgery, intraocular pressure ranged from 16 to 18 mmHg, and there were no signs of postoperative pupillary block or other postoperative complications.

The postoperative UBM examination was performed between 24 and 317 days after surgery. Preoperative and postoperative anterior segment measurement data are summarized in Table 21-1. UBM-determined anterior chamber depth ranged from 2.70 mm to 3.25 mm preoperatively. Postoperatively, the pseudo-anterior chamber depth (endothelial-optic distance) measured 2.03 mm to 2.54 mm. A space was maintained between the anterior lens capsule and the posterior surface of the IOL in all eyes (range, 0.35 mm to 0.79 mm). The distance from the end of the haptic to the angle of the anterior chamber ranged from 1.46 mm to 2.47 mm.

Figures 21-1 through 21-5 depict the position of the IOL's optic edge and haptics relative to the iris. In

Table 21-1

Preoperative and Postoperative Anterior Segment Measurements

			Preoperative		Postoperative			Days After Surgery
Eye #	*Patient #/Eye*	*Lens Power (D)*	*ACD[1] (mm)*	*ACD[2] (mm)*	*Pseudo ACD (mm)*	*IOL to Lens (mm)*	*Haptic to Angle of Anterior Chamber (mm)*	
1	1/OD	+4	3.56	3.25	2.22	0.79	1.75	317
2	2/OD	+5	3.10	2.95	2.16	0.59	2.47	66
3	3/OS	+4	2.76	3.05	2.54	0.57	1.46	24
4	2/OS	+6	3.22	2.70	2.03	0.35	1.47	66

[1] Performed with the standard ultrasonograph from the corneal epithelium to the anterior lens capsule
[2] Performed with the UBM from the corneal endothelium to the anterior lens capsule
ACD = anterior chamber depth

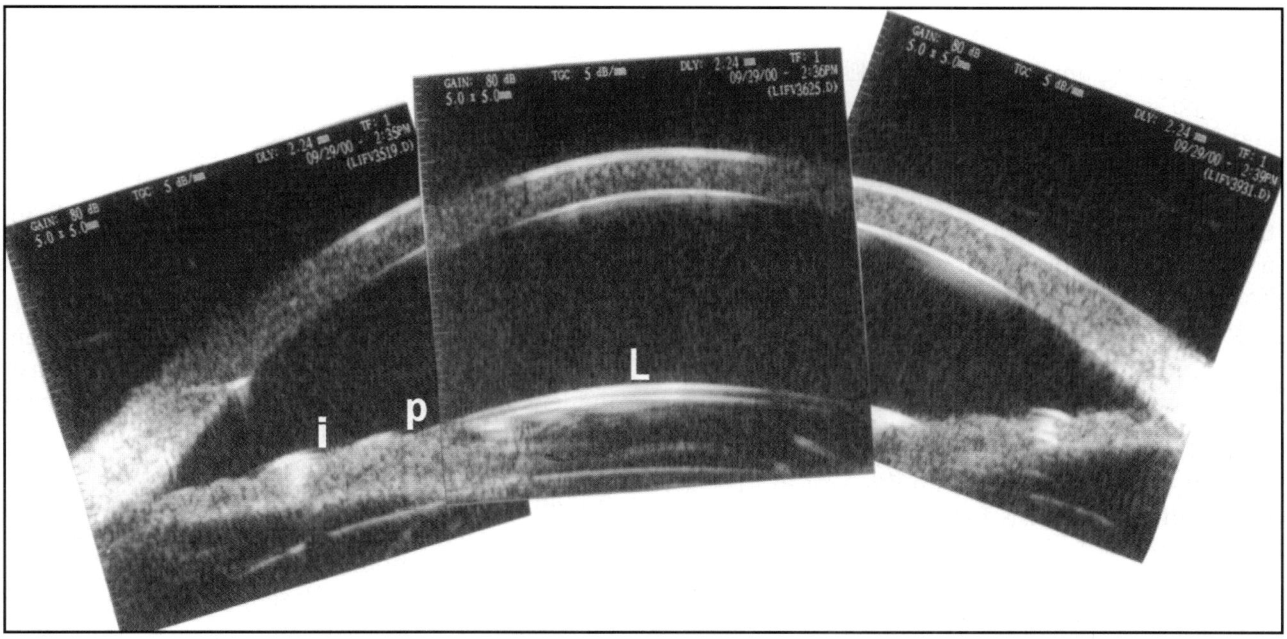

Figure 21-1. Postoperative composite picture of 3 longitudinal axial UBM echograms of the iris-claw phakic IOL for Patient 1. The IOL (L) indentation (p) into the iris (i) can be seen. Scale is 1:17.

Figure 21-1, where the postoperative longitudinal axial UBM picture of the IOL position through the central cornea was combined with 3 separate echograms, the optic edges are seen indenting the iris.

Figure 21-2 shows the marginal optical zone of the IOL and haptic at the edge of iris and indicates protrusion of the optic edge into the iris.

Figures 21-3 and 21-4 illustrate the postoperative lateral vertical UBM echograms of the IOL's haptic in two separate eyes. The portion shown is between the haptic and the optical zone. The optical zone of the IOL is anterior to the image seen. Both the pigment layer and the anterior stroma of the iris are visible, and the two arms of the haptic and the shadowing behind it through the iris and lens capsule can be seen as well.

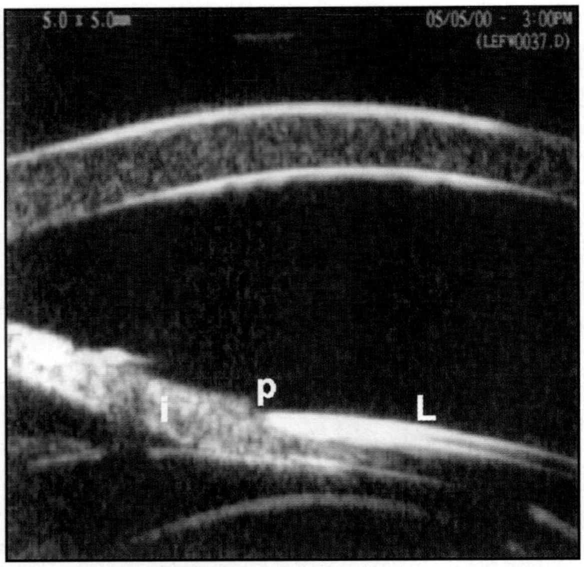

Figure 21-2. Postoperative longitudinal transverse echogram of the iris phakic IOL (L) for Patient 2 showing edge of lens optic protruding (p) into iris (i).

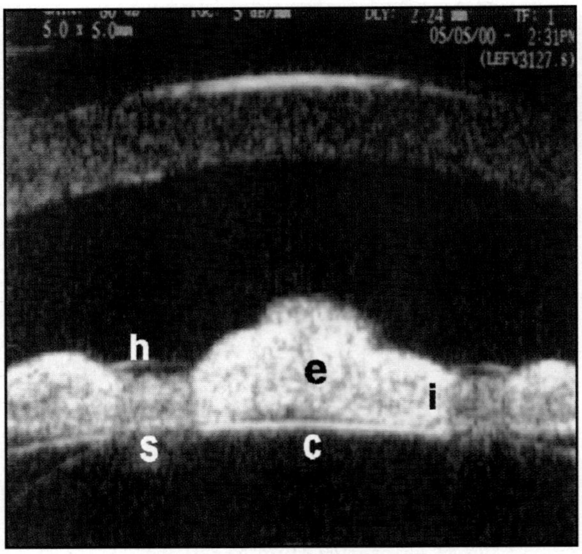

Figure 21-3. Postoperative lateral transverse UBM echogram of the iris-claw phakic intraocular lens for Patient 3 showing the two arms of the haptics (h) near to the site of entrapment and the shadowing (s) behind it through the iris (i), the iris entrapment (e) and the lens capsule (c). Haptics are beneath the iris tissue, showing indentation of the arms.

In the echograms of the study eyes, the optic edge could be seen protruding into the iris (Figures 21-1 and 21-2). Indentation of the iris by the haptic arms was observed as well (Figures 21-3 and 21-4). A comparison of Figures 21-3 and 21-4 indicates that the magnitude of the latter indentation is greater nearer to the site of iris entrapment. Figure 21-5 is a previously unpublished photo showing the optic impinging on the iris as well as the open iridectomy.

Discussion

Several observations were made in this early evaluation of 4 eyes implanted with the Artisan iris-claw phakic intraocular lens for treatment of hyperopia. The pseudo-anterior chamber created after IOL implantation measured approximately 30% less in depth than the natural anterior chamber. However, a distance of 2.03 to 2.54 mm was still maintained between the anterior surface of the IOL optic and the corneal endothelium. In no eye was the IOL touching the lens capsule, and the distance between the anterior surface of the lens capsule and the posterior surface of the IOL ranged from 0.35 to 0.79 mm. These measurements for the distance between the IOL and both the endothelium and the crystalline lens are similar to those we reported previously for myopic eyes implanted with the Artisan iris-claw phakic lens.[2]

Examination of the echograms, however, revealed both the optic edge of the hyperopic phakic IOL and its haptics seemed to indent iris tissue. Comparison of the echograms from 2 different eyes indicated the magnitude of the indentation increased closer to the site of iris entrapment (Figure 21-3 and 21-4). Such indentation was not observed in our study of myopic eyes.[2] As the preoperative gonioscopy indicated, these hyperopic eyes had a more pronounced natural iris arch than their myopic counterparts, one might postulate that the lens indentation into iris tissue was secondary to inadequate vaulting of the hyperopic phakic lens relative to the natural iris arch of the hyperopic eye. An alternative explanation might be that lens indentation into the iris was due to pupillary block. However, that hypothesis would be refuted by the fact that postoperative IOP remained normal in the implanted hyperopic eyes.

Although we observed the iris was indented by the optic edge and haptics, the iris pigment layer seemed to be undisturbed except within a small area of the iris entrapment. The UBM echograms also showed the pigment layer was slightly folded on itself within the iris entrapment, and that may present an area from which pigment dispersion could occur. So far, in this small group of eyes with limited follow-up, complications from pigment dispersion—ie, pigmentary dispersion glaucoma, have not occurred. Based on the echogram findings, however, we expect some eyes will develop pigment erosion secondary to phakic IOL indentation, and complications from this IOL-intraocular tissue

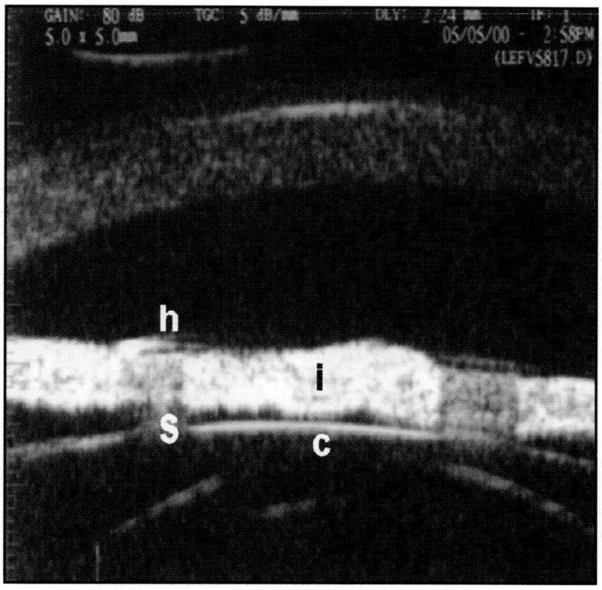

Figure 21-4. Postoperative lateral transverse UBM echogram of the iris-claw phakic intraocular lens for Patient 2 showing the two arms of the haptics (h) near to the IOL optic and the shadowing (s) behind it through the iris (i) and the lens capsule (c). Haptic at the left seems to be in close contact with the iris.

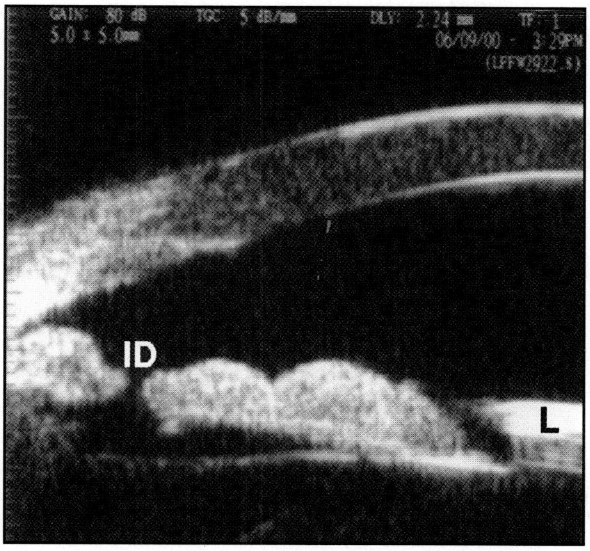

Figure 21-5. Postoperative longitudinal transverse echomgram of the Artison Phakic IOL. Iridotomy (ID) is clearly visible as is the IOL (L).

interaction remain to be studied in a larger group of eyes.

Based on this preliminary study, future pigment erosion seems probable in the phakic Artisan lens for hyperopia, but no conclusions can be stated about the potential long-term consequences of the IOL indentation into iris. As a precaution, we would recommend that gonioscopy and iris vaulting assessment be part of the preoperative evaluation of candidates for the hyperopic iris-claw phakic lens. In performing those examinations, surgeons should be aware that individuals with a natural highly vaulted iris might be particularly susceptible to experience indentation of lens into iris tissue. In the future, refinements in lens design, consisting of shortening of the haptics or increase in lens vaulting, might eliminate the potential for iris indentation.

Summary

This preliminary study of 4 eyes revealed adequate space is maintained between the Artisan hyperopic IOL and the corneal endothelium, the angle, and crystalline lens. Haptic indentation into the iris was observed that might lead eventually to pigment erosion. Preoperative gonioscopy and maintenance of normal IOP postoperatively suggest the indentation is secondary to inadequate lens vaulting relative to the high natural arch of the iris in hyperopic eyes. IOL design modification to shorten the haptics or increase lens vaulting may resolve this problem.

References

1. Budo C, Hessloehl JC, Izak M, et al. Multicenter study of the Artisan phakic intraocular lens. *J Cataract Refract Surg.* 2000;26:1163-1171.
2. Pop M, Mansour M, Payette Y. Ultrasound biomicroscopy of the iris-claw phakic intraocular lens of high myopia. *J Refract Surg.* 1999; 15:632-635.
3. Menozo JL, Cisneros AL, Rodriguez-Salvador V. Endothelial study of iris-claw phakic lens: four year follow-up. *J Cataract Refract Surg.* 1998;24:1039-1049.
4. Menezo JL, Martinez MC, Cisneros AL. Iris-fixated Worst claw versus sulcus-fixated posterior chamber lenses in the absence of capsular support. *J Cataract Refract Surg.* 1996; 22:1476-84.
5. Menezo JL, Avino JA, Cisneros A, et al. Iris claw intraocular lens for high myopia. *J Refract Surg.* 1997;13:545-55.
6. Fechner PU, Singh D, Wulff K. Iris-claw lens in phakic eyes to correct hyperopia: preliminary study. *J Cataract Refract Surg.* 1998;24:48-56.
7. Fink AM, Gore C, Rosen E. Cataract development after implantation of the STAAR Collamer posterior chamber phakic lens. *J Cataract Refract Surg.* 1999;25:278-282.
8. Rosen E, Gore C. STAAR Collamer posterior chamber phakic intraocular lens to correct myopia and hyperopia. *J Cataract Refract Surg.* 1998;24:596-606.
9. Jimenez-Alfaro I, Garcia-Feijoo J, Perez-Santonja JJ, Cuina R. Ultrasound biomicroscopy of ZSAL-4 anterior chamber phakic intraocular lens for high myopia. *J Cataract Refract Surg.* 2001; 27(10):1567-73.

Chapter Twenty-Two

Presbyopic Lens Exchange for Hyperopia and Presbyopia

Kevin L. Waltz, OD, MD and R. Bruce Wallace III, MD, FACS

Introduction and Background

Modern cataract surgery has become a refractive procedure. Patients have become accustomed to the removal of the cataract and insertion of the IOL without complications. Recently, patient expectations have become very specific—achieving independence of glasses. Currently, patients must be counseled that these expectations are probably unreasonable and may not be obtainable. The patient may be willing to live with reading glasses after cataract surgery, but surgeons who routinely leave patients with significant refractive error for distance vision will see a steady decline in surgical volume.

Often, laser vision correction (LVC) surgeons are faced with unhappy patients, even though uncorrected distance vision is 20/20 or better postoperatively.[1] Sometimes these patients are left with uncorrected or iatrogenic higher order aberrations after surgery. This is common in low myopes who develop symptomatic presbyopia as a result of LVC. These patients are warned of the necessity for reading glasses after corrective surgery; however, some are still surprised and very upset that the improvement in distance vision is at the expense of near vision.

An alternative with potentially less compromise than LVC is a pseudoaccommodative intraocular lens (IOL). A pseudoaccommodative IOL corrects the distance vision in a similar way to a monofocal IOL; however, it also contains a mechanism to allow for additional focal points in the near range. Such mechanisms include an IOL with a multifocal optical design such as the Array Multifocal IOL (Advanced Medical Optics, Santa Clara, Calif), or an IOL with a mechanical anterior-posterior translation such as the CrystaLens (C&C Vision, Aliso Viejo, Calif). Since the mid to late 1990's, most worldwide markets have had at least one lens option that simulates accommodation while correcting distance refractive error. The FDA approved the Array Multifocal IOL (Figure 22-1) in the fall of 1997 for use in cataract patients over the age of 60. It subsequently received the CE mark from the European Union for the indication of correcting presbyopia in November 2001. Other pseudoaccommodative IOLs pursuing approval for cataract indication in the US and European Union include the Restor multifocal lens and the MA60D3 acrylic lens (Figures 22-2A and B) both from Alcon (Ft. Worth, Texas). The CrystaLens (Figure 22-3) is pursuing approval as well. Pseudoaccommodative IOLs pursuing approval exclusively in the European Union include the 1CU lens (HumanOptics, Erlangen, Germany) and the AcriTech Pair (Berlin).

Determining which refractive modality is best for each individual patient can be challenging for the modern ophthalmic surgeon. Monovision is the most common method of maintaining near acuity. Monovision essentially undertreats one eye to minimize the negative effect of a successful treatment in

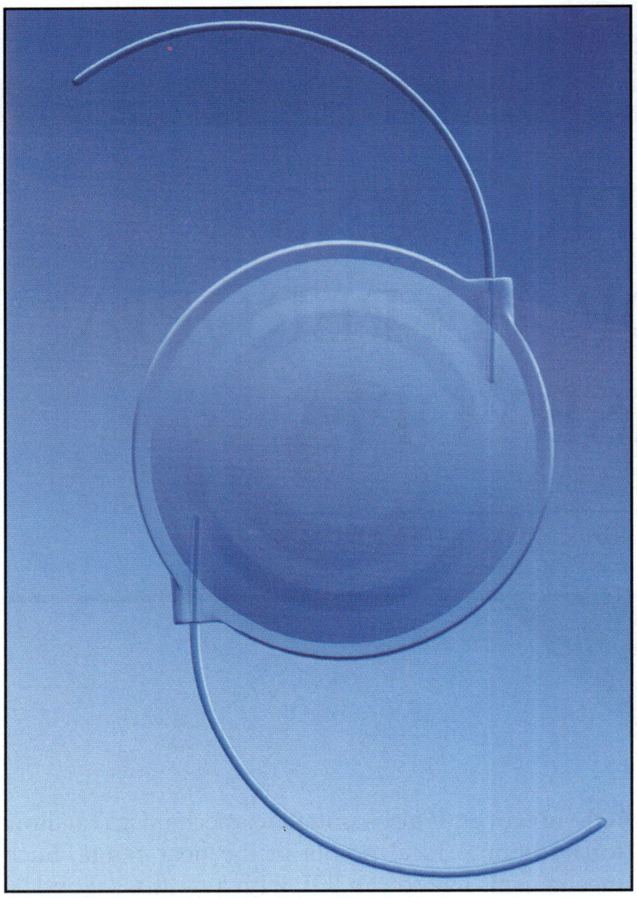

Figure 22-1. The AMO Array Multifocal IOL has a 13-mm overall diameter with a 6-mm silicone optic. It has PMMA haptics.

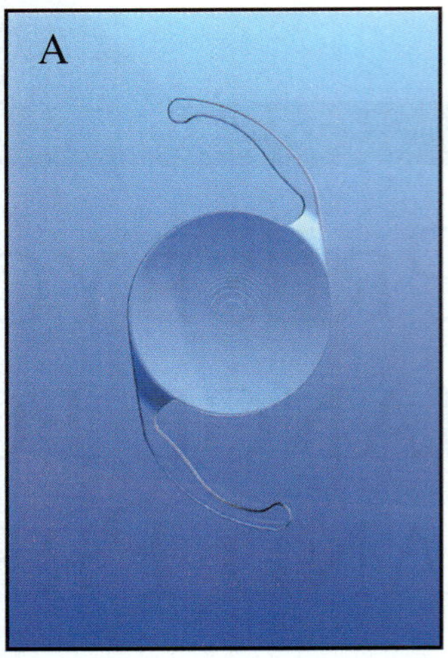

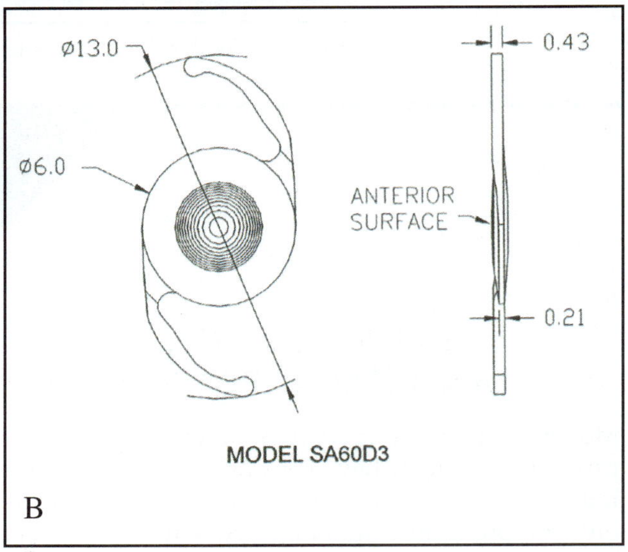

Figure 22-2A and B. The Alcon diffractive-refractive multifocal one-piece acrylic IOL.

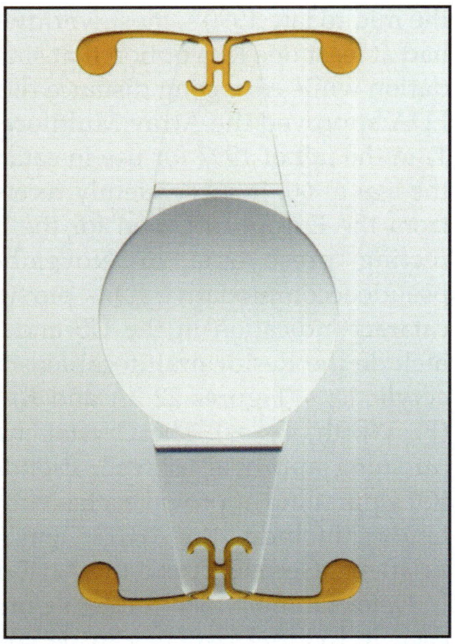

Figure 22-3. The C & C CrystaLens has a 4.5-mm silicone optic. It has a groove in each plate haptic to enhance the forward translational movement of the lens with accommodative effort.

both eyes for distance vision. Monovision works well in most patients, but will be unacceptable for a significant percentage of those who try it. Sometimes, additional surgery is required to reverse the process in those patients that cannot adapt. This is relatively easy to do with LVC, but can be more challenging with intraocular surgery. Another frequently overlooked aspect of monovision is the need to have the distance eye perfect. Because only one eye is focused for distance, the patient is very unforgiving of any blur. The near eye need not be perfect because the patient can effectively optimize near acuity by varying the working distance. As a result, the enhancement rate is much higher for the distance eye than for the near eye. Another negative of surgical monovision is the possible permanent reduction of stereoscopic vision.

Finding a safe, effective, and predictable treatment for presbyopia is the current Holy Grail of cataract and refractive surgery.[2] Contemporary options, including monovision and pseudoaccommodative IOLs, have significant risks and compromises that the surgeon and the patient must understand in order to be successful.[1-11] Monovision with LVC gives many patients good distance and near vision; however, monovision is not optimal with lens surgery due to the challenges faced when reversal is needed. The advantage of lens surgery is that most all lower order aberrations,[9-12] and some higher order aberrations, can be corrected in one procedure. Removal of the crystalline lens facilitates replacement of naturally occurring higher order aberrations with those of a manufactured lens. Another advantage of lens surgery is the prevention of possible cataracts and associated morbidity later in life.[13]

PRELEX stands for *PRE*sbyopic *L*ens *EX*change.[5] By definition, PRELEX is the surgical removal of the natural crystalline lens, and replacement with a pseudoaccommodative mechanism. The pseudoaccommodative mechanism is either a multifocal optic and/or an anterior/posterior translation of the optic simulating the natural process of accommodation. PRELEX is independent of the presence or absence of a cataract. Whether as a result of cataract surgery, or the natural aging process, PRELEX treats presbyopia. While the PRELEX procedure has been performed with several different types of intraocular lenses, most of the authors' experience is limited to the use of the Array Multifocal IOL. Therefore, unless otherwise indicated, the remainder of this discussion will be devoted to PRELEX with a multifocal IOL.

Patient Selection

Performing PRELEX on hyperopic patients not only improves the safety profile of the procedure, but also ultimately improves patient satisfaction. Hyperopic patients are usually better candidates for PRELEX than myopic or emmetropic patients. Because hyperopic patients typically have axial lengths of less than 24 mm, they are less at risk for retinal detachment than myopic patients.[14] Hyperopic patients frequently see halos preoperatively. Consequently, they are less bothered by halos postoperatively. The limitations of the natural hyperopic visual system are similar to those of distance dominant multifocal optical systems. Primarily, there are more challenges with near vision than with distance vision.[5]

PRELEX patients want to be less dependent on glasses after surgery. Most patients understand the need to wear glasses for some activities, perhaps most daily chores, but most are interested in becoming the least dependent on glasses and contacts as possible. Accordingly, the typical PRELEX patient is between 40 and 80 years old. Few patients younger than 40 favor lenticular surgery. Furthermore, few patients older than 80 feel the need to be less dependent on glasses. The typical age for a PRELEX patient having surgery exclusively for refractive reasons is 55 years old. The typical age for a PRELEX patient having surgery to correct cataracts is 62 years old.

When discussing treatment options with potential PRELEX patients, several points are emphasized. For one, the surgery is irreversible. While the IOL can be exchanged, the natural lens cannot be replaced. Risks of surgery include, but are not limited to, a potentially devastating intraocular infection, as well as retinal detachment. Patients with axial lengths greater than 24 mm are probably more at risk for retinal detachment. Selecting patients with axial lengths of 24 mm or less can minimize this risk. Another important discussion point is halos. The patient will see halos postoperatively. The halos never actually go away, but the patient's perception of them decreases with time. Multifocal implants create a new visual system, which requires some adaptation time. Most patients adapt within the first 3 months, but the adaptation process can take more or less time, depending upon the individual.[3,5]

Hyperopic patients are usually better candidates for PRELEX than myopic or emmetropic patients. The concept of refractive lensectomy for hyperopia has been with us for some time.[5,9-12] As mentioned before, eyes with axial lengths of less than 24 mm (typically hyperopes) are not associated with an increased risk of retinal detachment with intraocular surgery.[11] Visual aberrations created by multifocal optics are similar to what the hyperope naturally experiences. Halos tend to be less bothersome to the hyperopic patient postoperatively, because most experience them preoperatively. Hyperopes naturally have challenges with near vision. The myope typically can function quite well at near without correction. As a result, the hyperope functions better with a distant dominant multifocal optical system than the myope. This is not to say the myope cannot adapt, but it may be more challenging than for the hyperope.

PRELEX works best in hyperopes. Most ophthalmologists and optometrists believe there are many more myopes in the world than hyperopes. Therefore, many ophthalmic surgeons doubt that much of a market for hyperopic PRELEX exists. Contrary to many surgeons' perceptions, there are many more hyperopic patients than myopic patients. Approximately 50% of the adult population in developed countries is hyperopic, 20% emmetropic, and 30% myopic.[15,16] Although the typical 50-year-old myope is bothered by the need for glasses, most can function quite well at near without them. The typical 50-year-old hyperopic patient is very bothered by the need to wear glasses and usually cannot function

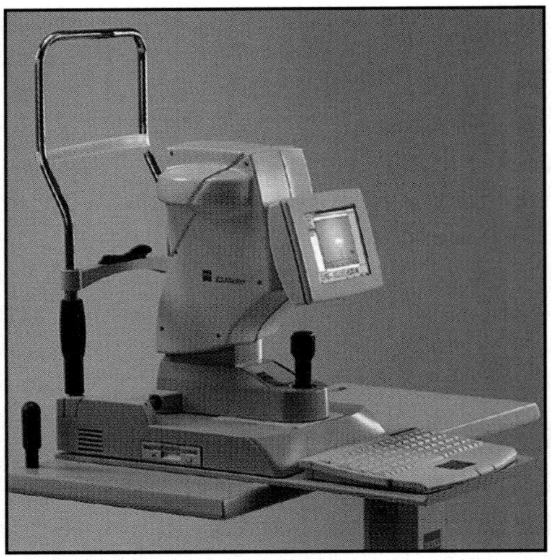

Figure 22-4. The IOL Master (Carl Zeiss Meditec, Dublin, Calif) optical coherence biometer.

without them for any visual task. Compounding the issue is the progressive deterioration of their situation with each passing year. Most presbyopic hyperopes consistently meet the primary criteria for PRELEX; the desperate desire to be less dependent on glasses.

Preoperative Testing for PRELEX

The most critical preoperative tests for PRELEX are those used to determine the correct IOL power. If the correct IOL power is selected initially, the remainder of the process is much easier for both the surgeon and the patient. Classic preoperative biometry includes tests for axial length and corneal curvature. These two measurements account for the majority of the preoperative variability. The most accurate way to determine axial length is by immersion A-scan biometry or optical coherence biometry (Figure 22-4). Routine applanation biometry is not consistently accurate enough to achieve the desired refractive results of both surgeon and patient. Corneal curvature can be determined by either manual keratometry or corneal topography; however, topography will be the most accurate when performing astigmatic correction at the time of lenticular surgery.[17,18]

Other preoperative measurements can be helpful in determining the best IOL power. For axial lengths less than 22 mm, predicting the size of the anterior chamber becomes important. The depth of the anterior chamber relative to the total axial length predicts the effective lens position. The effective lens position is the actual position of the lens relative to the overall length of the eye. The effective lens position assumed by many IOL calculation formulas tends to be less accurate in eyes shorter than 22 mm.

Using an IOL formula that does not calculate the effective lens position accurately can be a source of error. The Holladay II formula is one that can accurately account for the effective lens position, where most other formulas cannot. Incorrect IOL powers are most often seen with short eyes that have relatively normal anterior chamber depths. In these cases, a hyperopic surprise can occur if the anterior chamber depth is not taken into account. The magnitude of the error can be as much as several diopters in eyes with very short axial lengths and/or very deep anterior chambers.

Preoperative Counseling

The key to a successful outcome with PRELEX is preoperative counseling. A technically perfect, safe, uneventful procedure that securely places the IOL into the capsular bag does not guarantee success. Additionally, the patient must understand and accept what will happen postoperatively before deciding to have surgery. The patient must not only be motivated to improve their visual system with PRELEX, but also be prepared to deal with some expected and unexpected challenges that the procedure can create.[5,19-21]

Realistic expectations about potential visual outcomes after PRELEX are important. Assuming the refractive target has been achieved, the patient can expect to have excellent unaided distance vision during the day. In fact, PRELEX patients frequently report their unaided distance vision during daylight hours to be the best it has ever been throughout their life.

Distance vision is usually less satisfying at night than during the day. When the pupil dilates at night, it creates a significant increase in unwanted visual sensations in all human optical systems. This is especially true after refractive corneal procedures, including LASIK (Figures 22-5 through 22-7). These unwanted visual sensations can manifest as starbursts, halos, and/or glare. Most PRELEX patients will experience an increase in these sensations after surgery as well. Subsequently, preoperative patient education is critical. The patient needs to be allowed to weigh these potential side effects against the anticipated benefits of the surgery.[5,19-21]

Near vision after PRELEX with the Array Multifocal IOL is usually best in dim illumination. Bright lights usually make near vision more difficult, but not always. The Array IOL has two optimal pupil sizes for near vision, 1.9 mm and 3.4 mm. Understanding how pupil size affects near vision is

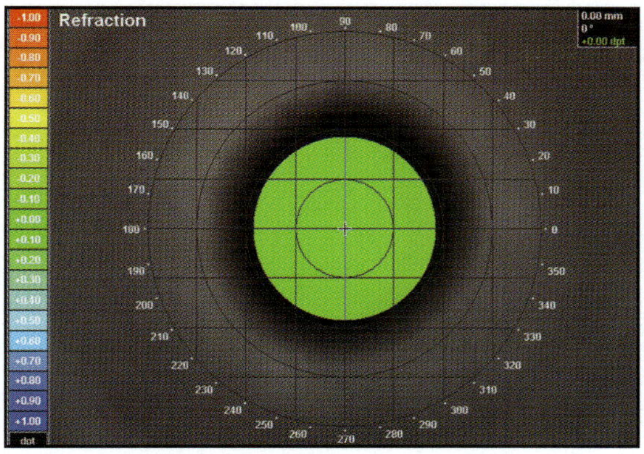

Figure 22-5. Wavefront analysis of a 27-year-old female patient after successful uneventful LASIK. The wavefront was measured using the Tracey Visual Function Analyzer. Above is a refractive map. The scale in diopters is to the left. Each box on the grid represents 1 mm^2. This represents an essentially perfect wavefront result with a 4 mm pupil.

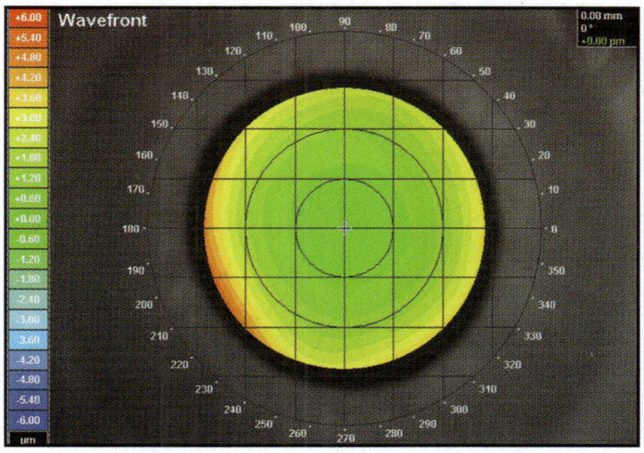

Figure 22-6. Same eye as in Figure 22-5. This measurement is taken through a 6 mm pupil. As seen here, the visual function of a successful LASIK patient is worse with a dilated pupil.

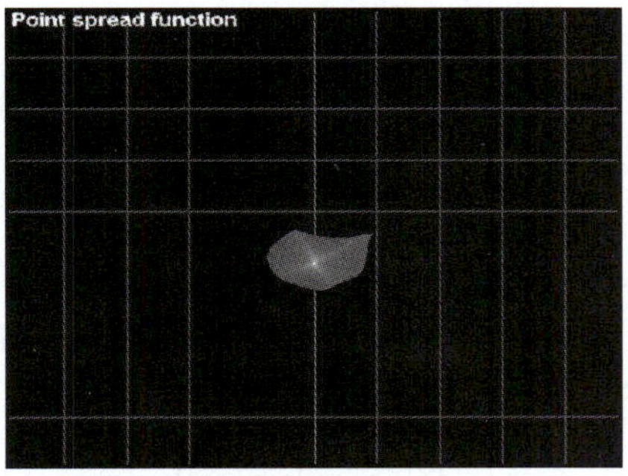

Figure 22-7. Point spread function of the eye imaged in Figures 22-5 and 22-6. This represents what the eye sees when viewing a single point source of light. Note that there is a halo around the point source and a starburst radiating from the halo. The patient is 20/15 uncorrected, but admits to seeing halos and starbursts at night. This is not a problem because appropriate preoperative counseling was given. The patient is happy and quite satisfied with the results of surgery.

important. Near vision is dependent upon the pinhole effect with the smaller pupil size. The larger pupil size relies upon the Array optical system for near vision.

When the pupil is 1.9 mm in diameter, the patient benefits from the pinhole effect. With the pinhole effect, there is a limited amount of diffraction related vision loss. The central distance dominant zone of the Array IOL is 2.1 mm in diameter. As the pupil size becomes smaller than 2.1 mm, the human optical system becomes diffraction limited. Diffraction progressively limits acuity as the pupil becomes smaller than 2 mm. When the pupil is approximately 2 mm, the effect of the Array near zone is excluded. Patients with small pupils read best in bright light.

The optical add of the Array IOL is best at a pupil size of 3.4 mm (Figures 22-8 through 22-10). At this pupil size, the relative light distribution of the Array favors the near vision in that almost 50% of the light is devoted to the near focal point. Patients with this size pupil tend to perform near visual tasks better in dimmer light. Some patients have pupils naturally larger than 3.4 mm. These patients may choose to increase the light intensity when reading to constrict their pupils to the optimal 3.4 mm size for Array optics.

Some PRELEX surgeons prefer to routinely surgically dilate the pupils of older patients at the time of surgery. This practice can create challenges for both the patient and the surgeon. One consequence of increasing pupillary diameter, in any patient, is a marked increase in higher order aberrations (see Figures 22-5 through 22-7). Few other things will quickly and consistently create unwanted higher order aberrations. This remains true when implanting the Array IOL. If a patient has very small pupils, less than 2 mm in the undilated state, implanting the

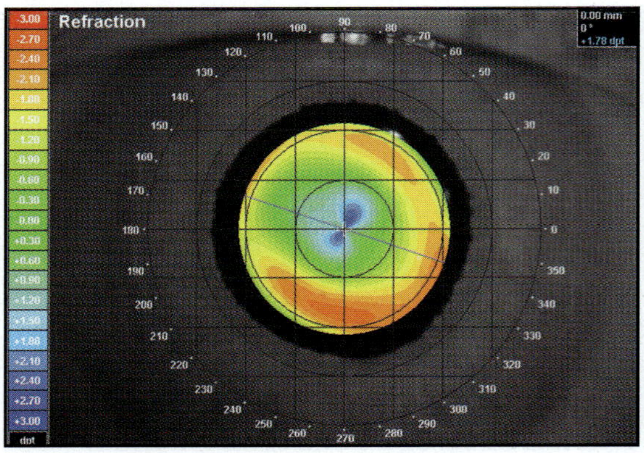

Figure 22-8. Refraction map of a PRELEX patient with an Array IOL. Note the central zone is relatively hyperopic. The myopic donut surrounding the central zone provides the add power.

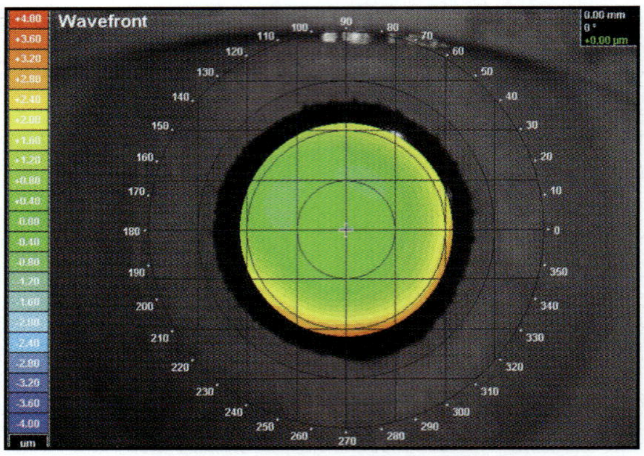

Figure 22-9. Wavefront map of eye in Figure 22-8. The central zone has zero wavefront error and the surrounding donut creates a predictable zone of too much convergence, or negative wavefront error in microns. This creates spherical aberration which, in turn, creates the add allowing the patient to see well at near. Wavefront maps with multifocal IOLs are variable and depend on pupil size, as seen here.

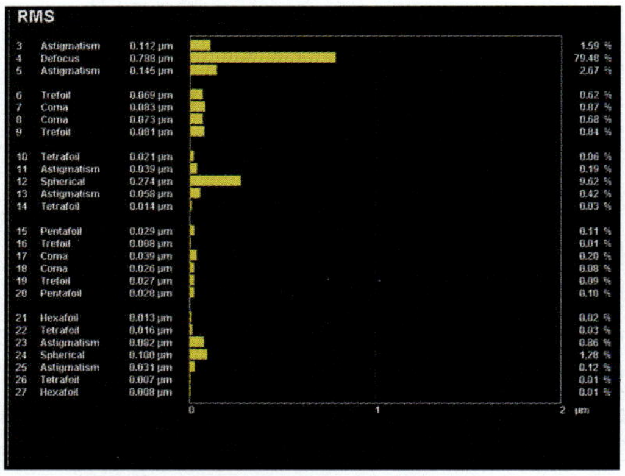

Figure 22-10. RMS wavefront plot of the eye in Figures 22-8 and 22-9. Spherical aberration is noted in line 12. One of the anomalies of multifocal IOL wavefront analysis is demonstrated here. The wavefront analyzer averages the power of the IOL over the entire measured area. Because the analysis includes the add of the multifocal IOL, the multifocal optic will always be measured as too myopic.

Array without surgically dilating the pupil may be the best choice. After the procedure, the patient's distance and near vision should be evaluated. Most likely the patient will have excellent near vision from the pinhole effect, and will not need further intervention. If no surgical treatment for small pupils is desired, often a myopic endpoint, approximately -0.50 D, is beneficial. This does not materially hurt distance vision, but helps significantly with near vision.

The normal physiological responses of potential PRELEX patients can be beneficial in predicting the best candidates. For instance, myopes and hyperopes react very differently, and predictably, to loss of accommodation. As a result, the reaction to PRELEX can be anticipated based upon this information. To illustrate this, two hypothetical scenarios will be examined—one a hyperope wearing +2.00-D spheres, and the other a myope wearing -2.00-D spheres.

Every hyperopic patient's visual system is stressed by the constant need to accommodate. Not only must the hyperopic patient use accommodation to see objects clearly at distance, but even more so for objects at near. Glasses typically correct the manifest hyperopia, but not the latent hyperopia. For the hyperope wearing +2.00-D spectacles, the total hyperopic correction, including manifest and latent components, is probably closer to +3.00 D.

This patient allows the actual accommodative effort to lag behind the accommodative demand (under-accommodation) in an effort to decrease stress on the visual system. As a result, the hyperope has a constant blur that becomes progressively worse as the accommodative demand increases. The onset of cataracts only exacerbates the problem. Additionally, hyperopic spectacles create base-out prism. Base-out prism makes convergence more difficult, which further stresses the hyperopic visual system.

Hyperopic patients benefit the most from PRELEX. Both uncorrected distance and near vision are better postoperatively than preoperatively. Reducing dependency on spectacles eliminates the need to overcome base-out prism. (This can be demonstrated quite easily with a trial frame.) The hyperope's typical unwanted visual sensation is a halo. Halos are familiar to hyperopes. As a result, seeing halos after PRELEX is not that troublesome.

Unlike the hyperope, the myope likes to over-accommodate at distance. The patient wearing -2.00 D in spectacles most likely only has -1.50 D of myopia. The myopic patient tends not to over-accommodate at near. The typical myope very closely matches the accommodative demand with the accommodative effort at near. This gives the myope excellent corrected and uncorrected near vision. Also of benefit is base-in prism, created by myopic spectacles. Base-in prism makes convergence easier, which decreases stress on the myopic visual system.

Myopic patients benefit the least from PRELEX. Distance vision is similar preoperatively and postoperatively. However, uncorrected near vision is often not as good postoperatively as preoperatively with the natural lens. Most myopes notice this loss. Reducing dependency on spectacles also eliminates the benefit of base-in prism. Consequently, the patient must exert more effort in convergence. In contrast to the hyperope, the myope's typical unwanted visual sensation is a starburst. Halos are unfamiliar to myopes. As a result, seeing halos after PRELEX can be more troublesome for the myope.[5]

Both myopes and hyperopes have certain challenges with PRELEX. All patients experience an adaptation period that involves learning to use the new visual system created by the Array. Shortly after surgery, distance vision is good with the Array, but near vision is more challenging to learn. Myopes and hyperopes perceive these challenges differently. Consequently, adaption differs due to their inherently dissimilar experiences preoperatively.

The PRELEX Procedure

PRELEX is lenticular surgery. PRELEX cases performed for purely refractive reasons are similar to the removal of a very soft cataract. PRELEX is an unforgiving surgery. Only very experienced lenticular surgeons should attempt this type of surgery. Because most readers will already be experts at lenticular surgery, this discussion will concentrate on the particular points of surgery that may vary from routine lenticular surgery. The primary difference between a PRELEX procedure and a routine lenticular surgery is an intense effort to correct the pre-existing corneal cylinder. For optimal vision, the PRELEX patient needs to have less than 0.75 D of cylinder postoperatively.

Generally, the preferred treatment for pre-existing cylinder is corneal relaxing incisions at the time of surgery. Corneal relaxing incisions are predictable, safe, and effective to about 2.00 D. Corneal relaxing incisions become less predictable with amounts of cylinder greater than 2.00 D, but are still safe and effective. The surgeon may consider staging the PRELEX procedure with LVC to treat cylinder greater than 2.00 D. Details regarding corneal relaxing incisions and LVC to correct cylinder can be found in the references.[22,23]

Cylinder can be treated with LVC either before or after the lenticular portion of the procedure. In certain cases, creating the corneal flap prior to lenticular surgery can be advantageous. Doing so enables the surgeon to lift the flap at any time after the lenticular procedure and apply the required laser treatment When treating cylinder with LVC prior to lenticular surgery, pre-LVC topography and post-LVC topography are very helpful. With this information, corneal curvature measurements can be adjusted for the Array IOL calculation. The adjustment is slightly technique dependent and needs to be customized, similar to an A-constant for an IOL. The change in corneal curvature from the pre- to post-LVC topography should be multiplied by 0.72 to correct for the new corneal curvature. For example, if LVC flattens the corneal curvature by 2.00 D, multiply 2.0 X 0.72 to arrive at 1.44 D. This is the amount that needs to be added to the originally calculated IOL power to arrive at the new IOL power.

Surgical preparation for PRELEX differs slightly from routine lenticular surgery. One variation is in the way dilation is achieved. Instead of drops, pieces of sterile sponges soaked in a cocktail of anesthetic, antibiotic, and dilating drops are placed in the inferior cul-de-sac preoperatively. This minimizes the deleterious effects the preservatives have on the corneal surface and keeps the patient more comfortable during and after surgery. Also, a better dilation is achieved through this method versus drops. Sometimes the pupil will be dilated asymmetrically toward the prior position of the sponge in the inferior cul-de-sac. This is a minimal annoyance.

Minimizing the endothelial impact of surgery is important. There are many viscoelastics available to protect the cornea from the minimal ultrasound energy expended during a typical PRELEX procedure. A capsulorrhexis slightly smaller than the lens optic is created and centered on the apex of the cornea. The anterior capsular opening should be between 4.5 mm and 5.5 mm. By covering the edge of the optic with the capsule, the predictability of the refractive outcome can be enhanced and posterior capsule opacification discouraged.

Maintaining a centered multifocal IOL is critical to the success of the PRELEX procedure. It is necessary to meticulously clean the posterior capsule, but not the anterior capsule. Once the capsular bag has been

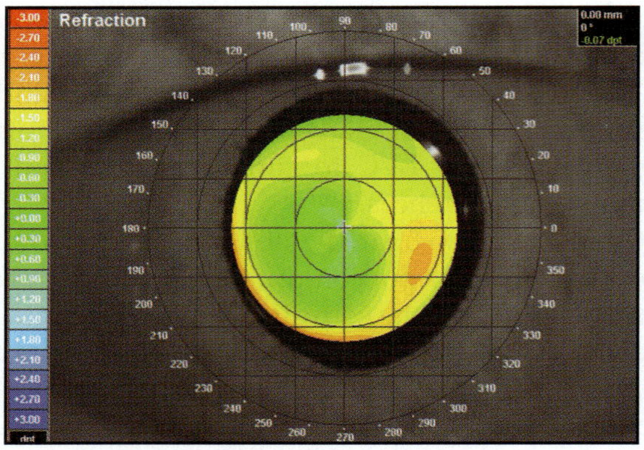

Figure 22-11. Refractive map of a PRELEX eye with Array lens approximately 10 minutes prior to YAG capsulotomy. It appears the lens is decentered, however, by exam, the IOL is perfectly centered. Distance vision is 20/20 uncorrected, but the patient complains of recently decreased near vision. The capsule is clear, but is actually bending the IOL and moving its optical center. Capsular bending also decreases the effective add power of the IOL.

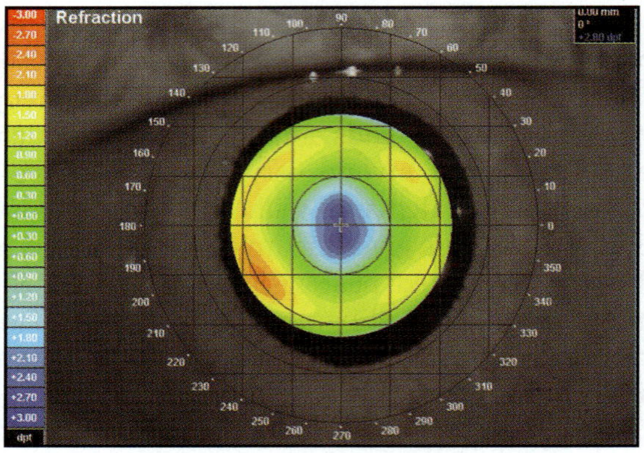

Figure 22-12. Refractive map of the eye in Figure 22-11 approximately 20 minutes after YAG capsulotomy. The bending forces of the capsule have now been released and the add portion of the IOL has reappeared. The patient reported immediate improvement in near vision.

adequately cleaned and inflated with viscoelastic, the IOL is implanted. After IOL implantation, the viscoelastic is removed. The IOL is then rotated in the capsular bag two full rotations. Rotating the IOL helps the surgeon clean the fornices of the capsular bag of any residual viscoelastic. Also, lenticular remnants are more easily identified in the capsular bag with this method.

Some PRELEX surgeons have reported occasional late decentration of the Array IOL. This is most likely related to retained viscoelastic within the capsular bag. If the viscoelastic is not completely removed, it prevents equal circumferential adhesion of the capsule and allows late dislocation of the IOL as the capsule contracts. This can be virtually eliminated by the addition of two full IOL rotations after the lens has been placed in the bag.

PRELEX patients are very sensitive to the Maddox rod effect of a wrinkled posterior capsule. Rotating the lens haptics into a position to create a vertical fold in the posterior capsule is helpful. The vertical fold serves several purposes. For one, the Maddox rod effect of a vertical capsular fold is horizontal. This is much less symptomatic than the Maddox rod effect of a horizontal or oblique fold in the capsule. The vertical fold also confirms that both haptics are in the bag, and the bag is intact. Additionally, the fold ensures that the haptics are in the best position to allow the optic to stay centered in case of slight nasal decentration of the capsule.

PRELEX and YAG Capsulotomy

Most surgeons report a higher YAG capsulotomy rate in patients with multifocal IOLs than in patients with monofocal IOLs. Patients with early posterior capsule opacification report their near vision being affected long before distance vision. Many patients request YAG capsulotomies with unaided vision of 20/20 at distance and J2 or J3 at near. This is a puzzling and troubling phenomenon for both surgeons and patients alike.

Wavefront analysis clearly explains this increase in capsulotomies in patients with multifocal IOLs. Capsular contraction causes bending of the multifocal IOL. This causes apparent shifting of the optical center and loss of the effective add power. YAG capsulotomies relieve the capsular contraction and distortion caused by capsular bending (Figures 22-11 and 22-12).

PRELEX Enhancements

Postoperative dry eye can affect visual quality after PRELEX. Tear supplements and punctal occlusion are helpful to overcome glare, fluctuating vision, and difficulty reading due to poor tear function.

As mentioned previously, halos are expected during the immediate postoperative period. Many patients can lessen the annoyance of halos with the use of Alphagan-P (brimonidine tartrate 0.15%, Allergan, Irvine, Calif), which helps to reduce pupil dilation in scotopic conditions. Typically, patients notice an improvement in symptoms with the use of

Alphagan-P; however, many report the improvement is not worth the hassle of drops, even once a day.

Unwanted postoperative hyperopia can be addressed with LVC, conductive keratoplasty, or rarely IOL exchange. For low levels of hyperopia (~1.00 D), moving the IOL out of the capsular bag into the ciliary sulcus can be of benefit. Recent access to low power IOLs (AQ5010V, STAAR) can help to remedy postoperative hyperopia or myopia. In addition to LVC and IOL exchange, certain levels of myopia can be treated with a mini-RK.

Postoperative cylinder interfering with acceptable visual function is usually addressed with corneal relaxing incisions (CRIs). Prior to performing these procedures, corneal stability should be documented with sequential corneal topography.

Infrequently, pupillary miosis prevents PRELEX patients from achieving useful uncorrected near vision. If this persists, argon laser pupilloplasty to one or both eyes can restore visual function at near.

After surgery, patients need to be reminded that PRELEX presents the brain with a whole new visual system. Patients can expect to experience a learning curve toward less dependence on glasses and less bother with unwanted visual imagery.

Summary

PRELEX is the best surgical option for most hyperopic presbyopes. Refractive lens exchange with a multifocal IOL can provide excellent stereoscopic unaided distance and near vision without disturbing central corneal integrity. With proper patient selection, patient counseling, and precise surgery, PRELEX provides a significant and measurable improvement in the quality of life for hyperopic presbyopes.

References

1. Holladay JT, Dudeja DR, Chang J. Functional vision and corneal changes after laser in situ keratomileusis determined by contrast sensitivity, glare testing, and corneal topography. *J Cataract Refract Surg.* 1999;25;663-69.
2. McLeod SD. The challenge of presbyopia. *Ophthalmology.* 2002;109:1572-1574.
3. Fine IH, Hoffman RS, Packer M. Clear-lens extraction with multifocal lens implantation. *Int Ophthalmol Clin.* 2001;41:113-121.
4. Kuchle M, Hguyen NX, Langenbucher A, et al. Implantation of a new accommodative posterior chamber intraocular lens. *J Refract Surg.* 2002;18:208-216.
5. Waltz KL, Wallace RB. PRELEX: surgery to implant multifocal intraocular lenses. *Ophthalmic Practice.* 2001:19(8): 343-346.
6. Dick HB, Krummenauer F, Schwenn O, et al. Objective and subjective evaluation of photic phenomena after monofocal and multifocal intraocular lens implantation. *Ophthalmology.* 1999;106:1878-1886.
7. Pieh S, Weghaupt H, Skorpik C. Contrast sensitivity and glare disability with diffractive and refractive multifocal intraocular lenses. *J Cataract Refract Surg.* 1998;24:659-662.
8. Haring G, Gronemeyer A, Hedderich J, de Decker W. Stereoacuity and anisekonia after unilateral and bilateral implantation of the Array refractive multifocal intraocular lens. *J Cataract Refract Surg.* 1999;25:1151-56.
9. Siganos DS, Pallikaris IG. Clear lensectomy and intraocular lens implantation for hyperopia from +7 to +14 diopters. *J Refract Surg.* 1998;14:105-113.
10. Kolahdouz-Isfahani AH, Rostamiam K, Wallace D, Salz JJ. Clear lens extraction with intraocular lens implantation for hyperopia. *J Refract Surg.* 1999;15:316-323.
11. Fink AM, Gore C, Rosen ES. Refractive lensectomy for hyperopia. *Ophthalmol.* 2000;107:1540-1548.
12. Osher RH. Controversies in cataract surgery. *Audiovis J Cat Implant Surg.* 1989;5:3.
13. Klein BE, Klein R, Kristine L. Incidence of age-related cataract over a 10-year interval: The Beaver Dam Eye study. *Ophthalmology.* 2002;109:2052-2067.
14. Verzella F. Refractive surgery of the lens in high myopes. *Refract Corneal Surg.* 1990;6:273-275.
15. Katz J, Tielsch JM, Sommer A. Prevalence and risk factors for refractive errors in an adult inner city population. *Invest Ophthalmol Vis Sci.* 1997;38:334-340.
16. Sorsby A, Leary GA, Richards MJ. Correlation ametropia and component ametropia. *Vision Res.* 1962;2:309-318.
17. Zaldivar R, Shultz MC, Davidorf JM, Holladay JT. Intraocular lens power calculations in patients with extreme myopia. *J Cataract Refract Surg.* 2000;26;668-74.
18. Holladay JT. How to prevent refractive surprise. *Review of Ophthalmology.* 1999;April:97-101.
19. Featherstone KA, Bloomfield JR, Lang AJ, et al. Driving simulation study: bilateral array multifocal versus bilateral AMO monofocal intraocular lenses. *J Cataract Refract Surg.* 1999;25:1254-1262.
20. Steinert RF, Post CT, Brint SF, et al. A progressive, randomized, double-masked comparison of a zonal-progressive multifocal intraocular lens and a monofocal intraocular lens. *Ophthalmology.* 1992;99:853-861.
21. Steinert RF, Aker BL, Trentacost DJ, et al. A prospective study of the AMO Array zonal-progressive multifocal silicone intraocular lens and a monofocal intraocular lens. *Ophthalmology.* 1999;106:1243-1255.
22. Gills JP, Gayton JL. Reducing pre-existing astigmatism. In: Gills JP, Fenzl R, Martin RG, eds. *Cataract Surgery: The State of the Art.* Thorofare, NJ: SLACK Incorporated; 1998; 53-66.
23. Nichamin LD, Wallace RB. Reducing astigmatism. In: Wallace RB, ed. *Refractive Cataract Surgery and Multifocal IOLs.* Thorofare, NJ: SLACK Incorporated; 2001:167-172.

Chapter Twenty-Three

Accommodating Intraocular Lenses

J. Stuart Cumming, MD, FACS, FRCOphth

Conventional monofocal intraocular lenses (IOLs), which provide a single focal distance, offer excellent visual rehabilitation. However, the majority of patients receiving these IOLs require reading glasses or bifocals for either distance vision or near vision. Multifocal IOLs that provide multiple focal distances for both near and distance vision offer an alternative to cataract patients seeking vision at distance and near without spectacles.[1,2] The multifocal intraocular lenses, however, are associated with a reduction of visual quality, because more than one image is projected on the retina simultaneously.[1] This loss of image quality can affect visual performance and has led to an interest in developing alternative modalities for correction of near and intermediate vision in pseudophakic patients.

Observations Leading to the Development of the Accommodating Lens

It is known that a certain number of patients implanted with standard monofocal intraocular lenses appear to have functional near vision following lens implantation. This effect can be attributed to one or a combination of factors that include myopia, small pupil size resulting in increased depth of focus, and minus cylinder,[3-7] and/or forward movement of the intraocular lens possibly induced by the accommodative effort of the ciliary muscle.[8-10]

Lens design may play a role in the phenomenon of accommodation in pseudophakia. In 1989 it was noted that a few elderly patients implanted with single-piece silicone plate haptic lenses had excellent near vision when it was measured through the distance correction in a dimly lit room, behind the phoropter.[11] This method of examination effectively reduces the effect of small pupil size, myopia and minus cylinder—ie, the factors that account for pseudoaccommodation. This suggested that movement of the optic by ciliary muscle action was responsible for the ability of these patients to see at near. In ten of these carefully-selected patients implanted with silicone plate haptic lenses, A-scans were done, first following cycloplegia and then compared to A-scans following pilocarpine administration. The average vitreous cavity length was approximately 0.7 mm longer following pilocarpine administration, suggesting that the ciliary muscle was responsible for forward movement of the silicone plate haptic lens.[11] Other published reports have shown that the ciliary muscle not only maintains its strength through the aging process, but experiences an increase in force.[12-15]

Anterior movement of the optic has been reported by Hardman Lea et al[16] and by Niessen and colleagues.[17] In these two similar studies, anterior chamber depth was decreased following pilocarpine administration, indicating forward movement of standard looped IOLs. However, while there was a significant difference in anterior chamber depths with pilocarpine as compared to cyclopentolate, the magnitude of this difference was reported to be approximately 0.2 to 0.25 mm, considerably smaller than the 0.7 mm change described above.

It was noted in 1990[11] that the plate haptic silicone lenses of STAAR (Monrovia, Calif) (AA4203) and Chiron (Emeryville, Calif) (C10) had the same optic size (6.0 mm) and refractive index (1.41) as the Allergan (Irvine, Calif) SI18 silicone lens, but their A constants were significantly different. The uniplanar plate lens A constant was found to be 119.0 and the posterior-vaulted loop lens 117.2. This difference in the A constants could amount to a difference of 1.50 D more power for a plate lens compared to a loop lens for implantation into the same eye. The difference in A constants is a reflection of the average location of the optics of each lens design along the axis of the eye, the optic of the uniplanar plate lens locating more posteriorly than that of the posterior-vaulted loop lens.

There are forces acting during the process of fibrosis that tend to move a plate lens posteriorly and a loop lens anteriorly. By slit lamp observation, the capsular bag can be seen to shrink-wrap the plate lens. The ectodermal cells under the anterior capsule cause contraction of the bag which in turn exerts end-to-end pressure on the plates. The plates are flexible but will not buckle. The plates therefore flex; however, because the anterior capsule is fibrosed and inelastic, the plates are forced posteriorly with anterior capsule contraction. This is in contrast to the effects of fibrosis on a loop lens. As the bag contracts, the flexible loops (which in most lens designs are 12.5 mm or more in diameter) are indirectly in contact with the ciliary muscle through the ovalized and distorted capsular bag and are moved centrally. As the pseudophake changes focus from distance to near during the period of fibrosis, and assuming that the ciliary muscle contracts, this could induce an increase in vitreous cavity pressure, which would tend to move the optic of a loop lens anteriorly—ie, "myopic shift," and because the loops are indirectly in contact with the ciliary muscle they would tend to be moved centrally. Further evidence that constriction of the ciliary muscle increases vitreous pressure is the observation that the vitreous face of aphakic patients can be seen to bulge forward upon ciliary muscle contraction.[11]

Based upon these observations, pre- and postoperative biometry measurements were made of the length of the vitreous cavity in patients implanted with silicone plate and silicone loop lenses.[19] A method of calculating the postoperative vitreous cavity length to compare it to the preoperative length was devised by Alan Ritter, MScEE, a biometric engineer. A comparison was made of the change in vitreous cavity lengths from preop to postop between the two lens designs. In the silicone plate haptic group, the spread of the optic along the axis of the eye was 1.45 mm and 50% of the time the vitreous cavity was shortened, the greatest increase in vitreous cavity length being only 0.77 mm. The plate lenses, therefore, locate up against the vitreous face in the posterior part of the capsular bag space, which is approximately 5.0 mm deep in a 70-year-old. In the eyes implanted with silicone prolene loop lenses (Allergan SI 18), the optic had a spread of 3.15 mm in its location along the axis of the eye, and in 80% of the patients, the vitreous cavity was lengthened by as much as 2.17 mm.

A comparison was made of the uncorrected visual acuities (UCVAs) at 5 to 6 weeks postoperatively comparing 253 loop lens model Allergan SI18 implanted eyes to 503 plate lens models STAAR AA4203 and Chiron C10 implanted eyes (surgery done by the same surgeon).[20] Of those patients with good potential acuity, 93% of patients with plate lenses and 84% of patients with loop lenses had UCVAs of 20/40 or better, representing a statistically significant difference of uncorrected vision in favor of the plate lens.

From these observations, it would appear that plate lenses, which consistently locate in the posterior part of the capsular bag space up against the vitreous, have the greatest potential for forward movement upon ciliary muscle constriction and have proven superior uncorrected visions when compared to loop lenses.

Literature Relating to the Ciliary Muscle Action and Vitreous Pressure

The literature reveals several papers supporting the possible role of ciliary muscle contraction in causing an increase in vitreous pressure.

Busacca,[21] an Italian ophthalmologist practicing in São Paulo, Brazil, published an article in the French literature in 1955 describing his examination of a young aniridic patient. The patient was examined by gonioscopy after first instilling a parasympath-

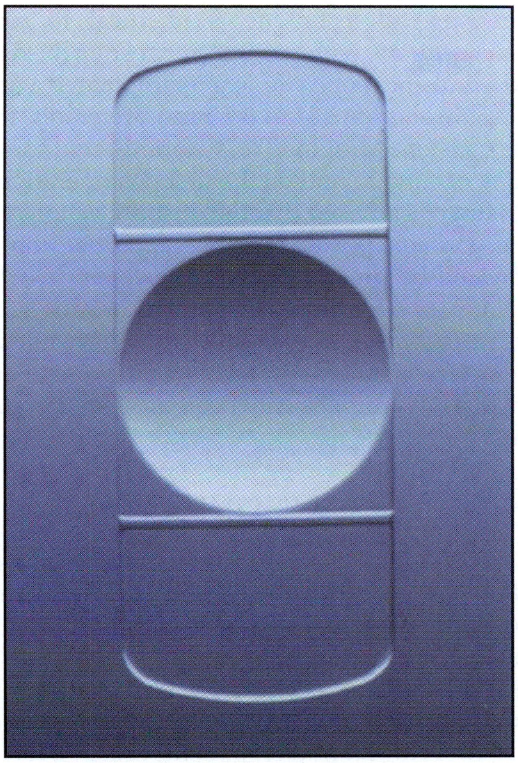

Figure 23-1. The first accommodating IOL (was implanted in England in 1991 in an 85-year-old lady).

omimetic, eserine, and later a parasympatholytic, atropine. Meticulous drawings were made of the change of shape of the ciliary body, the lens, and the location of the lens relative to the cornea and vitreous cavity. These changes were then transposed to graphic form. Upon studying the changes it became apparent that the ciliary muscle, like all muscles, redistributes its mass upon constriction and does so in such a manner that with contraction it encroaches on the vitreous cavity space and the lens equator is moved forward. Forward movement of the lens equator has also been reported in other publications.[21-23]

In 1986, Dr. D. Jackson Coleman[24] cannulized the anterior chamber and vitreous cavities in 10 primates and directly stimulated the ciliary muscle. He demonstrated a simultaneous decrease and increase in pressure in the anterior chamber and vitreous cavity respectively. Also in 1986, Dr. Spencer Thornton[24] demonstrated anterior movement in more than 20% of eyes from 200 patients implanted with PMMA loop lenses. The patients with accommodation had an accommodative range of up to 1.50 D.

The literature relating to the ciliary muscle redistributing its mass with constriction such that it encroaches on the vitreous cavity, together with the literature demonstrating an increase in vitreous cavity pressure with constriction, could explain the anterior movement of the optic in some patients.

Accommodating Lens Design

The first accommodating IOL, designed by the author, attempted to take advantage of a presumed increase in vitreous pressure upon constriction of the ciliary muscle. To increase the mechanical advantage of the ability of the optic of a plate lens to move forward, the length of the plates was increased and the overall length of the lens maintained at 10.5 mm (the same length as the standard plate lenses). Lengthening the plates required a smaller optic. The optical zones (the distance between the stakes) in 6 designs of 3-piece foldable lenses were measured and found to be less than 5.0 mm in all cases.[25] An optic of 4.5 mm, unencumbered by loop stakes, was therefore accepted for the accommodating lens and grooves or hinges were placed across the plates adjacent to the optic to decrease the resistance of the optic to forward movement.

Because the pseudophake constantly changes his or her focus during the postoperative period of fibrosis, an increase of vitreous pressure could cause anterior dislocation of the lens or cause the optic to fixate in a forward position. To prevent this and to ensure a maximal posterior location of the optic, it was postulated that the ciliary muscle should be paralyzed during the period of fibrosis.

The first accommodating lens (Figure 23-1) was implanted in England on March 12, 1991 in an 85-year-old woman. The surgery was done with capsulorrhexis and phacoemulsification through a 3.5 mm scleral tunnel incision. Atropine 1% was used postoperatively to prevent ciliary muscle contraction. The patient was examined on July 25, 1991 and by fogging from a maximum plus refraction to maximum minus while maintaining the best corrected distance vision, a 4.0-D accommodative amplitude was recorded. Biometry was performed with the eye fixing in the distance and then after the administration of pilocarpine. Three measurements were made for both the distance and near position of the optic. The average anterior chamber depth was 7.9 mm in the distance gaze pre-pilocarpine and 5.36 mm after pilocarpine. The average vitreous cavity length was 16.11 mm in distance gaze and 18.53 mm after pilocarpine. There was therefore an average decrease in the anterior chamber depth of 2.54 mm and increase

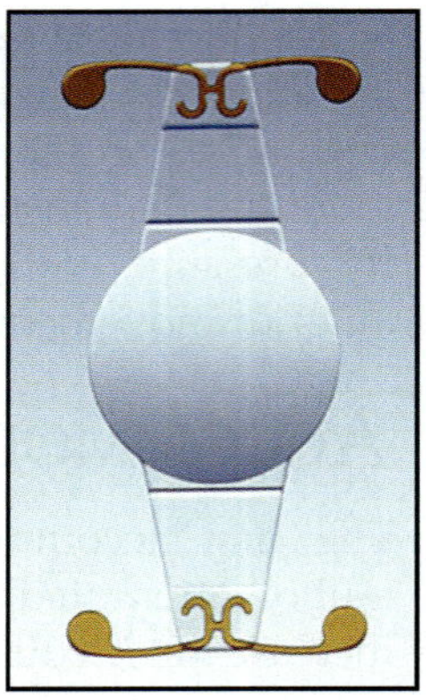

Figure 23-2. The final design was first implanted in 1998. There have been 4000 subsequent implantations over more than a 4-year period.

in vitreous cavity length of 2.42 mm following contraction of the ciliary muscle. This first implantation proved that with an appropriate intraocular lens design, the ciliary muscle could be utilized to provide movement of an optic along the axis of the eye and thereby provide accommodation in a pseudophake.

This first lens design was then implanted in 20 eyes by Prof. Jochen Kammann in Dortmund, Germany. Accommodation was demonstrated in all patients; however, several lenses had some degree of decentration and 5 dislocated anteriorly into the sulcus 2 to 3 months postoperatively.

Several lens designs were then implanted over the next 9 years by Prof. Kammann. When a lens design was deemed to be unacceptable due to postoperative complications, a new design and mould had to be made and lenses of several powers manufactured, sterilized and packaged. After implantation of the newly-designed lens, the patients had to be followed for several months to evaluate their visual performance and complication rate. The process of developing and evaluating a new accommodating lens design took at least 12 months.

The first 6 lens designs demonstrated limited accommodation and/or had complications of either decentration, anterior dislocation into the sulcus, or anterior vaulting. However, they all demonstrated some degree of accommodation. The final design (Figure 23-2), was first implanted in September 1998 and after 4000 implantations over more than a 4-year period, has given excellent visual results with excellent centration, and no dislocations have occurred. The major complication has been anterior vaulting caused by either a capsulorrhexis that is too large or by a clear corneal single-plane incision leading to wound leak with a resulting sudden drop in pressure in the anterior chamber.

The surgical technique is identical to routine cataract surgery with a 5.0 mm capsulorrhexis and phacoemulsification. The lens is implanted without folding through a 3.5- to 3.7-mm, preferably multiplane incision. Atropine 1% is administered topically the day of surgery and on the first postoperative day. The patient is advised that the distance vision will be stable 1 week postoperatively and that the near vision will be present 2 weeks postoperatively and will improve over time. The patients are advised not to wear reading glasses, because the ciliary muscle in these cataract patients (who have an average age of more than 70 years) has not been used for 25 years or more.

Results

The initial safety clinical trials for the final accommodating lens design, the AT-45 (C&C Vision, Aliso Viejo, Calif), were conducted in Germany and Mexico. The patients were not preselected for their ability to achieve good uncorrected results. These initial trials were essentially without complications.

The first clinical trial on patients selected for bilateral implantation was conducted by Dr. Arturo Chayet in Tijuana, Mexico. These patients had to have the potential for good vision, a corneal cylinder of 1.00 D or less, and a cataract in both eyes. The first lens was implanted in January 1999. Fourteen patients were implanted bilaterally, and the last 2 implantations were done February 7, 2000. The uncorrected bilateral visions 4 years postoperatively of 6 of these patients are as follows: 5 of the patients could see equal to or better than 20/30 and J3 (79%) and 100% saw 20/40 and J3 or better. With the distance-corrected vision and no add, 5 of the 6 patients could see 20/25 and J3 or better (83%) and 1 patient reported with PCO and had acuities of 20/30 and J3. Centration and postoperative inflammation has been minimal. Of the 11 eyes examined at 4 years, there have been 3 YAG capsulotomies.

The FDA clinical trial began in March, 2000 and the last lens was implanted in November, 2002. A total of 497 eyes were implanted in the study with the goal of reporting on 300 at a follow-up interval of 1 year. The postoperative uncorrected distance, uncorrected near, distance-corrected near, best-corrected near, and distance-corrected intermediate visions are tabulated on Tables 23-1 through 23-6, which show the results of visual acuity values reported at the end of 1 year.

Studies have been conducted on several lens designs to demonstrate either anterior movement of the optic or a change in refractive power in eyes

Table 23-1

Uncorrected Distance Visual Acuity

n=371

	N	%
20/20 or better	184	49.6
20/25 or better	269	72.5
20/32 or better	211	83.8
20/40 or better	339	91.4
20/41-20/100	28	7.5
Worse than 20/100	4	1.1

Table 23-2

Best-Corrected Distance Visual Acuity

n=370

	N	%
20/20 or better	313	84.6
20/25 or better	359	97.0
20/32 or better	366	98.9
20/40 or better	368	99.5
20/41-20/100	2	0.5
Worse than 20/100	0	0.0

Table 23-3

Uncorrected Near Visual Acuity

n=368

	N	%
J1 or better	161	43.8
J2 or better	256	69.6
J3 or better	328	89.1
J4-J10	37	10.1
Worse than J10	3	0.8

Table 23-4

Near Visual Acuity Through the Distance Correction

n=369

	N	%
J1 or better	98	26.6
J2 or better	208	56.4
J3 or better	337	91.3
J4-J10	32	8.7
Worse than J10	0	0.0

Table 23-5

Best Corrected Near Visual Acuity

n=369

	N	%
J1 or better	258	69.9
J2 or better	356	96.5
J3 or better	365	98.9
J4-J10	369	100
Worse than J10	0	0.0

Table 23-6

Intermediate Visual Acuity Through the Distance Correction

n=368

	N	%
J1 or better	351	95.4
J2 or better	365	99.2
J3 or better	366	99.5
J4-J10	2	0.5
Worse than J10	0	0.0

implanted with an accommodating lens. Twenty of the Type II accommodating lenses were implanted in 1992. Biometry was done on 13 of these eyes in 1994, first with a mydriatic and later with pilocarpine. Eleven eyes showed an average forward movement of the optic of 1.0 mm, and in 2 eyes the optics moved posteriorly by 0.3 mm and 0.1mm.

In March 1995, a similar study was conducted on the Type III lens, which demonstrated an average anterior movement of 0.83 mm in 5 eyes.

Anterior movement of the optic has also been demonstrated by dynamic retinoscopy. In 6 eyes in patients with a mean age of 71 years, the power changes ranged from 1.00 to 5.00D, with an average

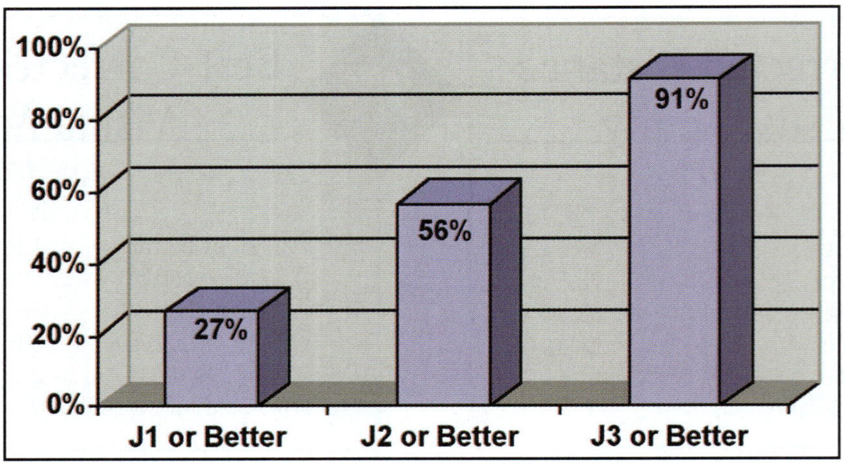

Figure 23-3. Monocular near vision through the distance correction 1 year postoperative (369 eyes).

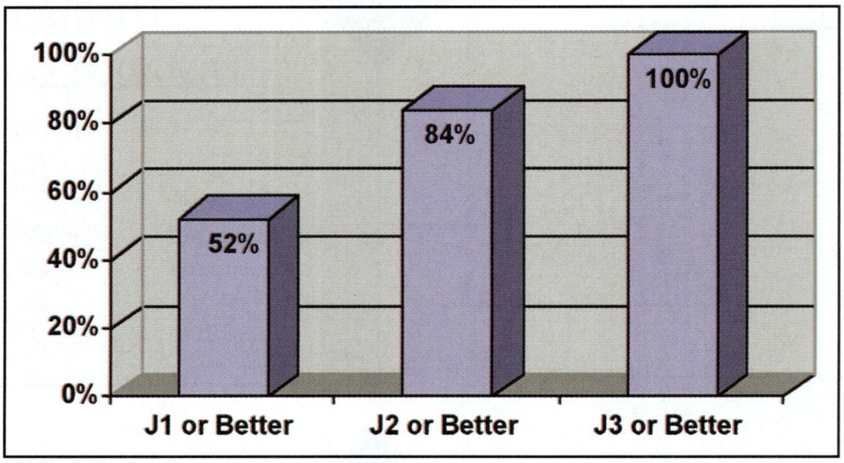

Figure 23-4. Binocular near vision though the distance correction 1 year postoperative (124 eyes).

of 3.33 D.[26] This was consistent with their near points of accommodation.

The final phase of the FDA clinical trial, after 1-year follow-up, was completed in January, 2003 after implanting 497 eyes and following 300 patients for at least 1 year. The FDA required that the A constant (119.0) and formula (SRK-T) be consistent for all the eyes implanted with the Model AT-45 lens, the CrystaLens. The examinations were all conducted under standardized lighting conditions, and the University of Minnesota reading card was used for intermediate (80 cm) and near (40 cm) vision measured with a marked cord.

The FDA also required that a contrast sensitivity test, with and without glare, be conducted. This was done using the Stereo Optical Optec (Chicago, Ill) 1600 Vision Tester.

The results of the various examinations are demonstrated by the bar graphs in Figures 23-3 through 23-11.

Summary

The evidence is encouraging that a safe and effective IOL design that can accommodate to change the refractive power of the eye has been developed. The FDA clinical trial has been completed. More than 90% of 124 bilaterally-implanted patients can see J2 or better at intermediate and near, and 20/30 or better at distance without correction twelve months postoperatively after implantation with the C&C Vision accommodating lens Model AT-45, the CrystaLens. The majority of these patients do not use glasses or have a reduced dependency on glasses.

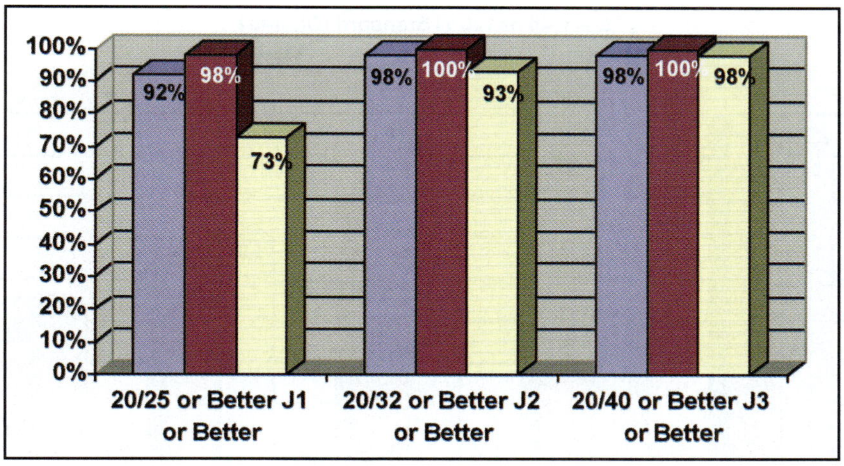

Figure 23-5. Binocular uncorrected distance, intermediate, and near visual acuity 1 year postoperative (124 eyes).

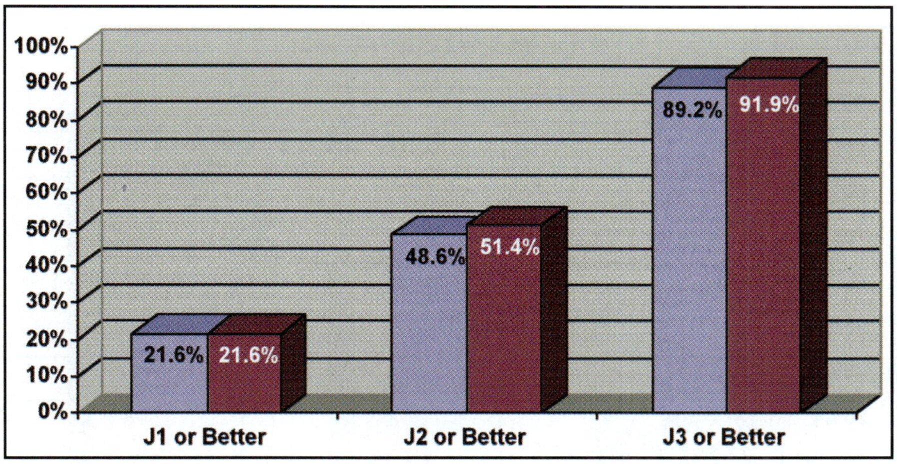

Figure 23-6. Monocular near visual acuity through the distance correction short and long axial lengths 1 year postoperative.

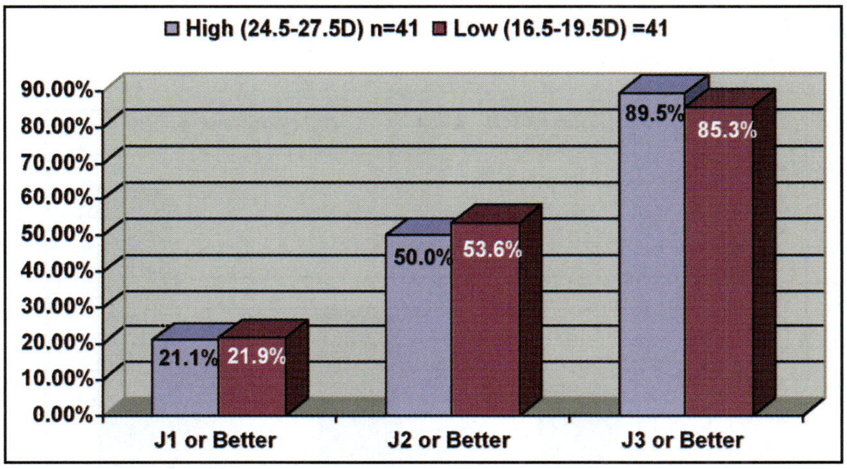

Figure 23-7. Monocular near visual acuity through the distance correction highest and lowest powered lenses 1 year postoperative.

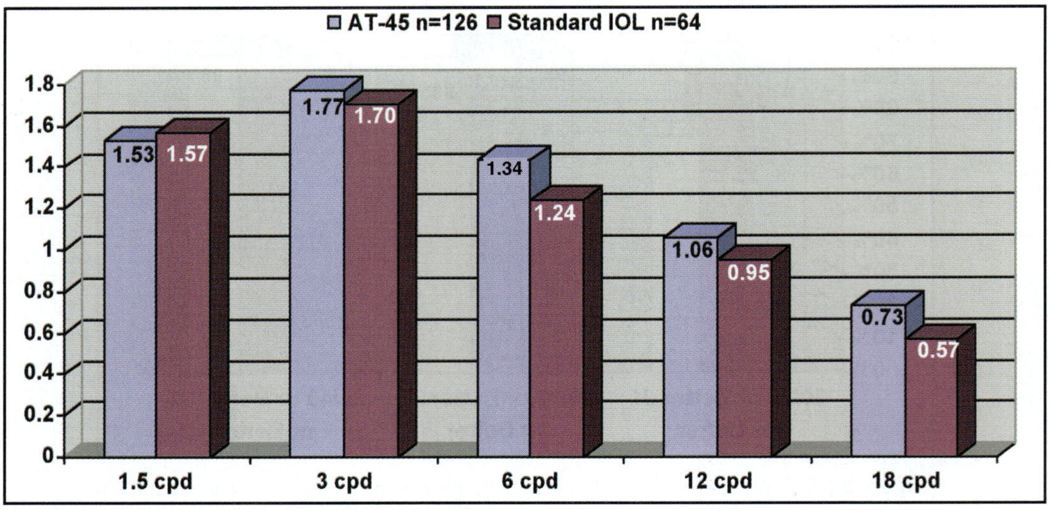

Figure 23-8. Log contrast sensitivity through the distance correction with glare AT-45 versus standard IOL. The luminance was 3cd/m2 3 lux glare, 6 months or more postoperatively.

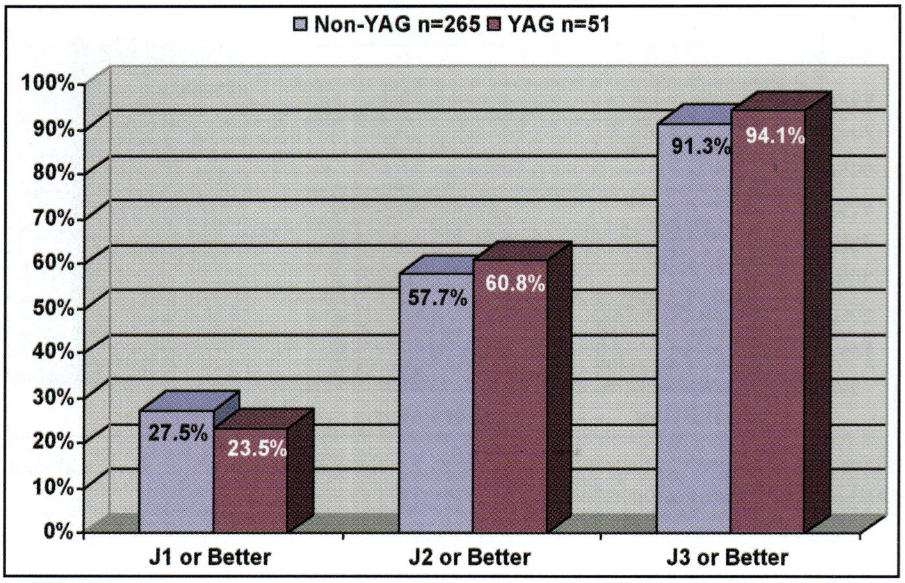

Figure 23-9. Near vision though the distance correction. YAG group versus non-YAG group, 1 year postoperative.

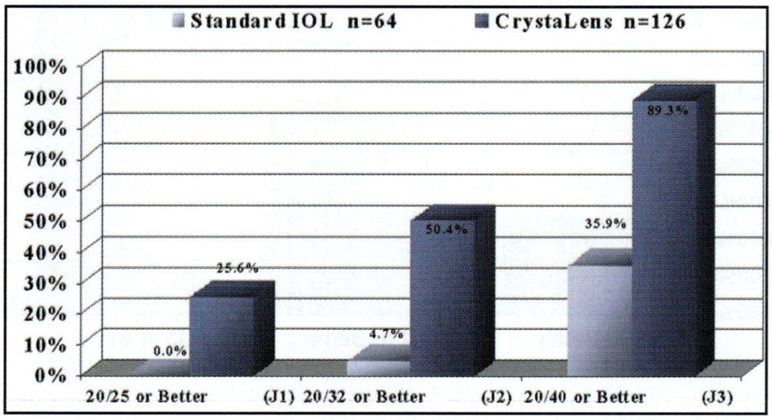

Figure 23-10. Near visual acuity through the distance correction, CrystalLens vs standard IOL.

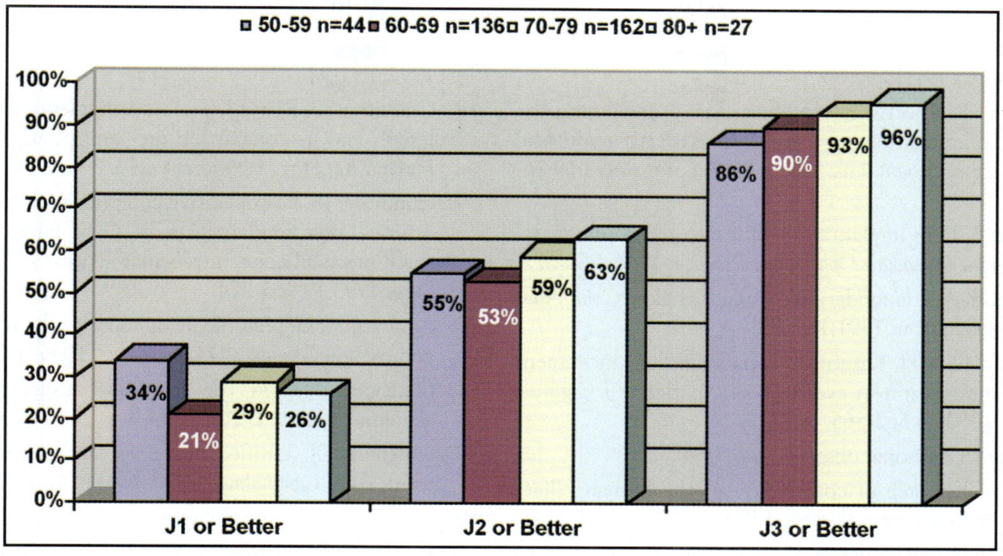

Figure 23-11. Monocular near vision through the distance correction by age decade, 1 year postoperative.

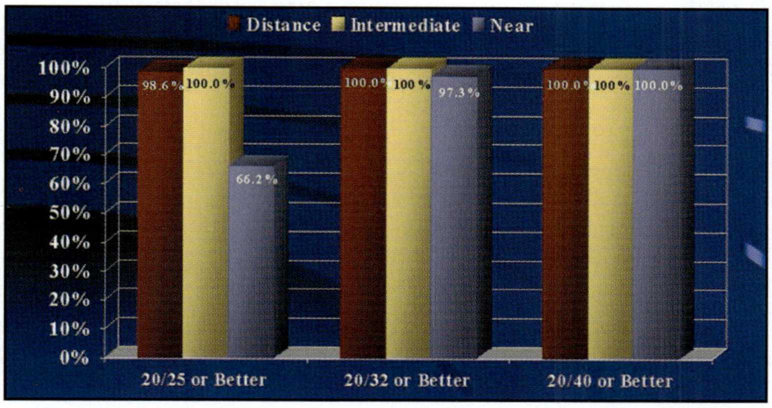

Figure 23-12. Summary of uncorrected visual acuity near, intermediate, and distance for patients within ±0.50 D of Plano in each eye (n=74).

Accurate biometry and keratometry are essential to eliminate or reduce dependence on spectacles. Careful monitoring of the preoperative measurements revealed the best uncorrected visions were obtained using either immersion biometry or the IOL Master with the third generation software for the axial length measurements and manual keratometry.

Figure 23-12 demonstrates the results that can be obtained if the preoperative measurements are carefully taken and the correct A constant of 119.00 and the SRK-T formula are used. The 74 patients implanted bilaterally and with a postoperative refraction of ± 0.50 D all had excellent vision at distance, intermediate and near.

The author wishes to thank the clinical investigators, consultants, and the staff of C&C Vision for their hard work and expertise that have made the clinical trial so successful.

References

1. Steinert R. A prospective comparative study of the AMO array zonal-progressive multifocalsilicone intraocular lens and a monofocal intraocular lens. *Ophthalmology*. 1999; 106:7;1243-1255.
2. Lindstrom, RL. Food and Drug Administration study update. One-year results from 671 patients with the 3M multifocal intraocular lens. *Ophthalmology*. 1993;100:91-97.
3. Huber C. Planned myopic astigmatism as a substitute for accommodation in pseudophakia. *Am Intraocular Implant Soc J*. 1981;7:244-249.
4. Huber C. Myopic astigmatism: a substitute for accommodation in pseudophakia. *Doc Ophthalmol*. 1981;52:123-178.
5. Nakazawa N, Ohtsuki K. Apparent accommodation in pseudophakic eyes after implantation of posterior chamber intraocular lenses. *Am J Ophthalmol*. 1983;96:435-438.

6. Trindade F, Oliveira A, Frasson M. Benefit of against-the-rule astigmatism to uncorrected near acuity. *J Cataract Refract Surg.* 1997;23:82-85.
7. Percival S. Prospectively randomized trial comparing the pseudoaccommodation of the AMO ARRAY multifocal lens and a monofocal lens. *J Cataract Ref Surg.* 1993;19:26-31.
8. Thornton S. Lens implantation with restored accommodation. *Current Canadian Ophthalmic Practice.* 1986;4:60-62.
9. Thornton S. Accommodation in pseudophakia. *Color Atlas of Lens Implantation.* 1991;159-162.
10. Lesiewaska-Junk H, Katuzny J. Intraocular lens movement and accommodation in eyes of young patients. *J Cataract Ref Surg.* 2000;26:562-565.
11. Cumming JS. Personal observations. 1990.
12. Fisher R. The force of contraction of the human ciliary muscle during accommodation. *J Physiol.* 1977;270:51-74.
13. Fisher R. The mechanics of accommodation in relation to presbyopia. In: Stark L, Obrecht G, eds. *Recent Research and Reviews from the Third International Symposium.* New York: Professional Press; 1987;42-4.
14. Fisher R. The mechanics of accommodation in relation to presbyopia. *Eye.* 1988;2:646-649.
15. Fisher R. The ciliary body in accommodation. *Trans Ophthalmol Soc UK.* 1986;105:208-219.
16. Hardman Lea S, Rubinstein M, Snead M, Haworth S. Pseudophakic accommodation? A study of the stability of capsular bag supported, one piece, rigid tripod, or soft flexible implants. *Br J Ophthalmol.* 1990;74:22-25.
17. Niessen A, De Jong L, Van der Heijde G. Pseudo-accommodation in pseudophakia. *Eur J Implant Ref Surg.* 1992;4:91-94.
18. Cumming JS, Ritter J. The measurement of vitreous cavity length and its comparison pre- and postoperatively. *Eur J Implant Ref Surg.* 1994;6:261-272.
19. Cumming JS. Postoperative complications and uncorrected acuities after implantation of plate haptic silicone and three-piece silicone intraocular lenses. *J Cataract Refract Surg.* 1993;19:263-274.
20. Busacca, A. La physiologie du muscle ciliaire etudiee par la gonioscopie. *Annales D'Oculistique.* 1955; 1-21.
21. Coleman DJ. On the hydraulic suspension theory of accommodation. *Tr Am Ophth Soc.* 1986:LXXXIV;846-868.
22. Coleman DJ. Unified model for accommodative mechanism. *Am J Ophthalmol.* 1970; 69(19):1063-1079.
23. Thornton S. Lens implantation with restored accommodation. *Current Canadian Ophthalmic Practice.* 1986;4:60-62.
24. Kamman J. Vitreous-stabilizing, single-piece, mini-loop, plate-haptic silicone intraocular lens. *J Cataract Refract Surg.* 1998;24:98-106.
25. Twa M. Personal communication. Twa M. Shiley Eye Center. University of California, San Diego; 2001.

Section Six

Marketing Considerations

Chapter Twenty-Four

Marketing Hyperopic Refractive Surgery

Shareef Mahdavi, BA

Similar to the growing need to incorporate evidence-based approaches to clinical judgment and decision-making in refractive surgery, there is an equally significant need to do the same in the marketing of refractive surgery to patients. To begin, let us define marketing and its role for the refractive surgeon.

Marketing encompasses all the non-clinical activities directed toward attracting and communicating with interested refractive surgery candidates in the time period from when they first become aware of the procedure until after they have chosen to have it done.

This chapter will explore some of what has already occurred in the marketplace, the challenges that surgeons face, and recommendations for change for future marketing efforts. Although most of the issues apply to refractive surgery in general, a section at the end of the chapter will address special considerations for the hyperopic patient.

Marketing and Medicine

Very few surgeons have received any formal training in marketing. Unlike the state licensing required to become a physician, there is no such equivalent regarding the business aspects of medical practice. For a moment, imagine what "business of medicine" curriculum might look like spread out over several years: Didactic, laboratory, rounds, internships, and possibly even fellowships would be required. This curriculum would build skills in decision making that would serve any clinician faced with starting their own practice. The major courses would include finance, operations (ie, patient flow), information technology, human resources, sales/promotion, and customer service. And while marketing is deserving of its own course title and subject matter, companies have increasingly recognized that their ability to successfully market goods and services is impacted by each and every one of the main functional areas and vice-versa. To date, the author's experience has been that refractive surgeons over-emphasize the sales/promotion components and under-emphasize customer service. Ideally, these would be more evenly balanced and the effort and energy spent toward serving customers would match or exceed that spent attracting them. To understand why this is significant, it will be helpful to distinguish the marketing of products versus the marketing of services.

Marketing involves the commerce of both *products* and *services*. And while it is relatively easy for consumers to compare different products (commonly referred to as comparison shopping), it is rather difficult to compare services without actually having the service preformed. While there are many products that are components of refractive surgery, for this discussion we will view refractive surgery as primarily a service business. Why? Because there is no physical product that the prospective patient can hold, see, feel, touch or otherwise experience prior to purchase. Instead, the patient (the author will interchangeably refer to patients as consumers) must make a purchase decision based solely on the promise of future performance. At its core, the decision to have the procedure is a contract between a patient and a provider (the surgeon) to deliver on an expectation of improvement in unaided vision. Undergoing the procedure is an experience in and of itself (and one the author highly recommends all surgeons have). And afterward, while the buyer still does not take home a physical product, the service they have just purchased is one that offers even greater potential benefit than virtually any other product or service they will purchase during their lifetime.[1]

That last statement bears repeating: The emotional and functional impact of refractive surgery creates underlying benefits for the consumer that potentially exceed any other purchase they will make over their lifetime, regardless of the price paid for those other products and services. This statement is supported by the refrain heard from virtually every refractive patient: "That was the best money I've ever spent and I wish I had done it sooner." On a larger scale, it is also supported by surveys that indicate customer satisfaction levels ranging between 90% to 100%.[2]

In summary, refractive surgery enjoys some unique characteristics in the marketplace. It is a service (rather than a product) that offers tremendous emotional benefits and satisfaction. It is also a medical procedure that is paid for directly by the patient rather than via a third-party provider (in most cases). And because refractive surgery requires providers to conduct marketing to attract patients, I use the hybrid term *medical-retail* to describe the larger consumer category that covers refractive surgery and other procedures and services that are offered directly to and paid directly by consumers.

Market Research

Any medical procedure performed today has typically undergone a process that began with basic scientific research. Soon after the point of discovery, research is conducted to better understand and validate the procedure and determine its effect on the human body. Marketing's version of this process is simply known as market research. There is a science to the process of understand consumer motivation for making purchase decisions. Research conducted by VISX (Santa Clara, Calif), Alcon (Fort Worth, Tex), TLC (St. Louis, Mo) and other major manufacturers and providers in refractive surgery has yielded several key findings over the years:[1]

- Refractive surgery is a highly *considered* purchase, taking months and even years for the decision process to be completed.
- There are several significant barriers to the adoption of refractive surgery, including fear, price, and a belief that the offering will continue to improve and evolve (which defers interest).
- Refractive surgery offers tremendous emotional benefits that are often unique to each individual but have in common an ability to impact the lifestyle and enjoyment for all individuals.

Based on periodic reviews of the literature, it appears that these findings have remained fairly consistent over the past 10 years. The decision to have refractive surgery, unlike many "impulse" purchases, is usually made only after a fair amount of research has been done by the consumer. This research takes the form of reading news stories, conducting internet searches, interviewing surgeons and staff, speaking with other consumers who have already had the procedure, and consulting close family members or friends. As with most consumer purchases, the consumer goes through a series of stages when considering refractive surgery, as shown in Table 24-1. Lin MacMaster, a principal with the marketing research firm Strategic Partners Group in McLean, Va, summarized refractive surgery as follows:

> *Laser vision correction is likely the most highly considered purchase decision in the history of consumer marketing. Compared with similar research conducted to understand why and how decisions are made to purchase expensive automobiles or new homes, the amount of emotional and mental effort expended by the refractive surgery patient greatly exceeds that put forth in these other consumer purchases.*[1]

And while both the rational and emotional reasons for choosing refractive surgery are becoming better understood, there is still relatively little known about the timing of the decision. While follow-up interviews with patients after the procedure indicate that they have long considered having it done, it has been difficult to pinpoint specific triggers that answer the question "why did you have it done now?" In all likelihood, the answer is also highly patient specific and would fall under one of several main "triggers" that ultimately get "pulled" in the

Table 24-1

Decision Process

Awareness →	*Interest* →	*Consideration* →	*Action*
News stories Advertising Public relations Activities	Recommendation from a friend, "trigger" event	Seminar Consultation View surgery	MD/OD recommendation, support of family or friend

Consumers go through a decision process when considering refractive surgery. Listed at each of the four steps there are some of the key "milestones" that occur in order for a consumer to move from one step to the next.

patient's decision-making process. These triggers include increasing frustration over the inability to perform a certain activity that would be enabled by improved vision, a missed opportunity that resulted from the inability to find one's corrective lenses, and a threshold reached in desire to gain perceived freedom and independence in daily activities that had previously been hampered by the use of glasses. MacMaster concluded from their qualitative research that:

> *The process of being fitted with one's first pair of glasses is often very painful emotionally. It is an admission to self of being flawed and now being separated from the world surrounding them. Contact lenses helped mask or cover the flaw; laser vision correction is powerful because it heals and removes the flaw, enabling the patient to return to a sense of being whole, of being one with the world.*[1]

Specific Challenges

This next section of the chapter will deal with four essential questions that are faced by those attempting to market refractive surgery:

- What messages should be used to attract potential candidates?
- What (or who) is the competition?
- What are the best ways to attract patients?
- How should unhappy patients be handed?

Messages

The marketing efforts to date have largely focused on two main messages—technology and price—that attempt to generate interest in having the procedure. These messages come in the form of communication with patients in advertising, patient brochures, and quotes in media coverage. They also come in the form of seminars, consultations, and Q & A that occurs between staff and prospective candidates. It is increasingly common to see an advertisement, for example, that touts either the "latest technology" or the "lowest price" or even both.

The problem with these approaches is that they work against the interests of both surgeon and patient. Many surgeons truly believe that acquiring new technology will somehow create an advantage in the local marketplace that will be appreciated and actualized by prospective patients. These acquisitions require significant investment in equipment and training followed by significant education of both staff and patients. They are often justified and rationalized by using a heuristic approach to risk-reward analysis: If the provider is the first to acquire and promote the new technology, patients will respond through growth in procedural volume. Thus, investment is justified by having perceived advantage of offering something new and unique to the marketplace. While these precepts do work in traditional marketing, they have not had a similar effect in creating sustainable growth in refractive surgery demand among consumers. Again, the reason(s) for this failure can be found by understanding the market research findings. Patient communications that lead with a message about technology generally serve to confuse patients. Typically, a patient has overcome significant fear just to get to the point of serious inquiry and consideration of refractive surgery (Figure 24-1). Because refractive surgery is a medical service, there is an implicit belief that the tools and techniques being used by the provider (ie, the surgeon) are valid and legitimate. In other words, the type of technology being used by the surgeon does not weigh heavily in the decision process. When technology is suddenly thrust into the mix of patient communication, the consumer is forced to think about this in addition to their innate fear. Contrary to the assumptions of most providers, the message confuses the patient, and the decision is delayed. When you consider how many different

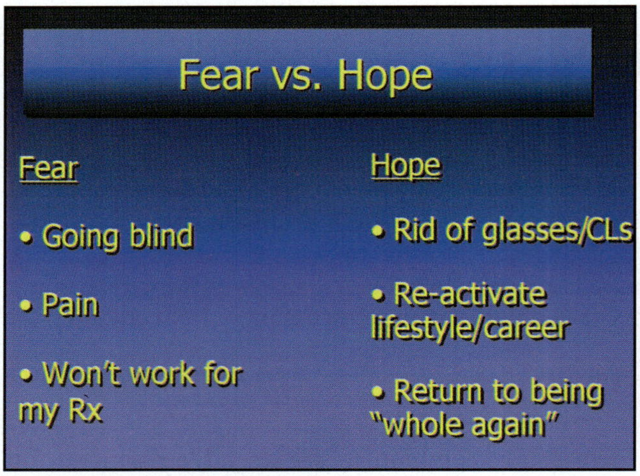

Figure 24-1. The consumer decision process involves resolving the conflict between hope and fear.

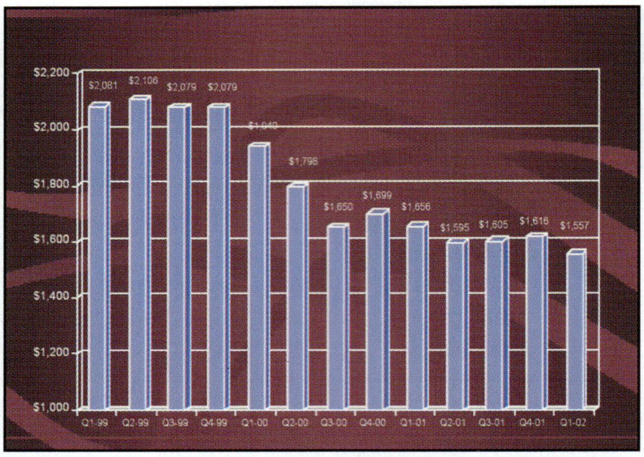

Figure 24-2. Average prices charged for LASIK have dropped approximately 20% in the past several years. (Chart courtesy of MarketScope.)

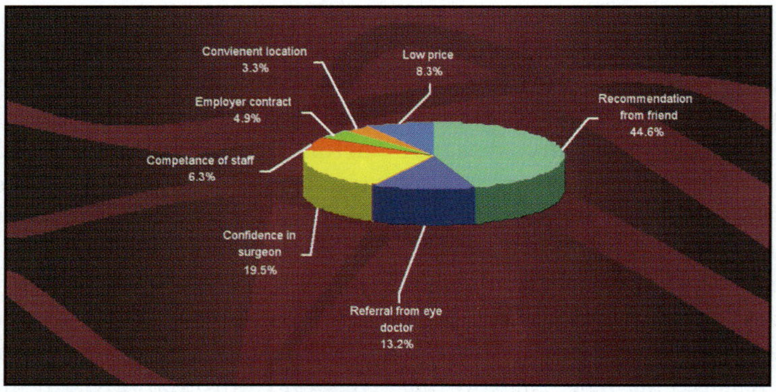

Figure 24-3. Reasons for selecting refractive surgeon. (Chart courtesy of MarketScope.)

technology messages have been promoted in just the first 10 years of refractive surgery (many of which have failed in the marketplace), it becomes easy to understand why consumers are confused. These messages have compounded to the point where consumers have been trained to believe that they should wait simply because something new and possibly better awaits just around the corner.

Messages that promote price and especially low price (eg, discount LASIK) have been equally harmful to the development and growth of the category. As seen in Figure 24-2, average prices being charged by doctors across the United States began declining in the year 2000 after being steady or increasing over the previous 3 years. The reasons for these price decreases seemed to revolve around notions of "increased competition" and a belief that consumers would respond in even greater numbers if the price were lowered. Corporate-owned laser centers emerged, offering prices 50% to 75% lower than what had previously been seen in the market. Individual surgeons began to either lower prices or create tiered-pricing that charged different fees depending on the level of refractive error, experience of the surgeon (versus an associate), or complexity of the treatment. As the figure shows, none of these pricing strategies have led to increased acceptance (as measured in overall procedures performed on a quarterly basis). In fact, the opposite has happened. As prices declined, so have procedure volumes. And while it may be impossible to precisely account for all the reasons why volumes have declined, it is safe to conclude that lower prices have not led to increased demand on an aggregate basis. This is also supported by survey data. See Figure 24-3, which continues to place price as a low influencer in a patient's decision to have refractive surgery in the first place.

As with the messages on technology, the emphasis on pricing and price promotion (often referred to

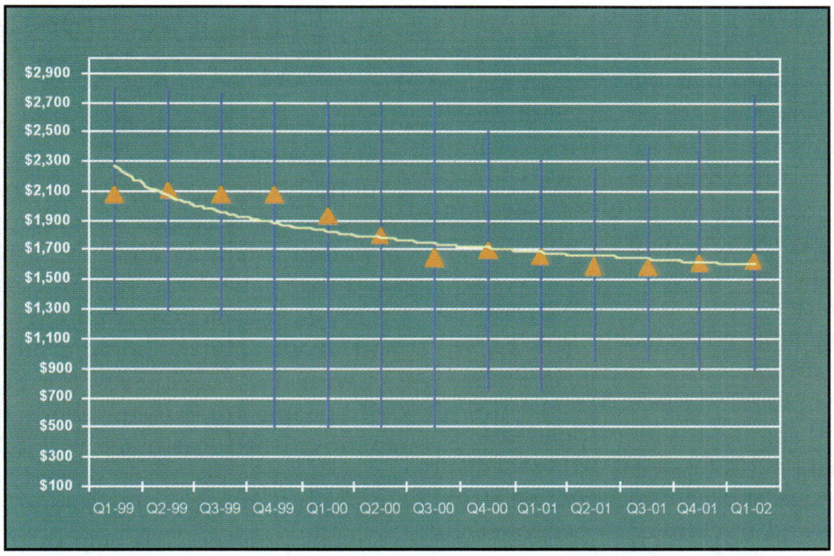

Figure 24-4. LASIK price trends. The range of prices offered by providers is indicated by the vertical bars at each quarterly time point. The increasing spread in the range served to confuse consumers as little effort was taken to differentiate service levels at the different price points. (Chart courtesy of MarketScope.)

as the "value-pricing" business model) has likewise confused patients and consumers. It has been very difficult for consumers to make decisions comparing what appear to be similar service offerings at very different price points. The wide range of pricing (Figure 24-4) available in a market serves to invoke fears about quality of the providers and credibility of the offering. As with common retail practices, price-focused messages have also trained interest patients to wait until the next "sale" or "special" so that they can make the purchase at the best possible price. While this works in more established product categories, it often fails miserably in service categories (accounting, legal, building contractors) and has not helped fuel market growth in the refractive surgery category.

As an alternative, this author recommends that surgeons begin focusing their messages across all mediums on personal attention, quality of care, safety, access to information on benefits/risks, outcomes, satisfaction rates, and qualifications. Within these categories, there are multiple ways to create differentiation and uniqueness in each service offering that will increasingly attract patients and begin to reduce the chaos and confusion that currently surrounds refractive surgery and interested candidates.

Competition

The way that providers define competition in refractive surgery is a root cause of the problems regarding the messages given to consumers. Surgeons have tended to view refractive surgery as a limited pool of candidates that they are battling to win over from other surgeons in their market area. They are, in essence, fighting for their fair share of the pie. In the author's view, this unnecessarily constrains marketing efforts by focusing on share of the market when the focus should be on growing the size of the market. And this is unfortunate, because the pool of available refractive surgery candidates (based on age, income and refractive error) is actually growing and is expected to grow over the next decade at a rate that exceeds current penetration rates of refractive surgery within that pool of candidates. Hence, there is little need to "compete" for patients but a great need to conduct marketing that serves to better "attract" patients and their disposable income. In reality, the refractive surgeon is competing for those discretionary dollars against other potential purchases that are in the same or even higher price range. This competitive landscape includes vacations, jewelry, home improvement, home theaters, spas... the list goes on and on. Because these other products and services can all be financed via monthly payments, the refractive surgeon would help level the field by ensuring that patient financing is an integral part of the offering.

Attracting New Patients

Although direct promotional techniques have emerged as a primary means of generating both awareness and interest in refractive surgery, special consideration needs to be given due to the length of time required for most candidates to make a decision. Recent data indicate that the average patient takes 8 months to come to a decision, with nearly one-third of patients taking more than a year to decide.[3] Additionally, advertising has proven prohibitively expensive for the majority of surgeons because it requires a commitment to significant sums of money in order achieve a "breakthrough" in the ability to reach target candidates. Likewise, the provider must sustain advertising levels with enough frequency to generate sufficient inquiry to justify the expense in the first place. Many surgeons who attempt advertising fail to either spend enough money, fail to create a professional advertisement with a strong message and call-to-action, or fail to adequately capture and track interest generated by the advertising. Those who have failed may come to the conclusion that "advertising doesn't work," when in fact it might well have been their phone answering system that was unable to process the calls that were generated.

Regardless of the amount of money available for advertising, the refractive surgeon would do well to focus efforts on sourcing patients who are "closer to home" in terms of their knowledge of the practice. Staying in contact with patients already treated will help increase the referrals from those patients. These "alumni" from the practice, given the high rate of satisfaction and strong emotional benefits from LASIK, serve as the single best source of new patient generation available to the practice. The practice, then, should be highly motivated to make it easy and convenient for current and past patients to refer potential new ones. In addition, sending communications in the form of newsletters and announcements to current patients as well as the patients of doctors who refer to you (eg, optometrists) is a good way of seeding the ground for future refractive patients.

One issue that serves as an obstacle to new business is the surgeon's belief in laser vision correction for him- or herself: If the surgeon is a candidate yet has not chosen to have the procedure, what kind of message does that send to patients? Most likely it's the wrong one. The same goes for staff and employees who come into contact with prospective refractive patients. Having gone through the procedure makes one automatically better able to identify and empathize with the needs and concerns of prospective patients. Not having done so (when one is a candidate) becomes a barrier to acceptance that will, without question, shine through to the prospective patient.

Handling Dissatisfied Patients Post-Surgery

While nearly all patients are happy with their outcomes, some are not. This may be due to uneven wound healing, postoperative complication, or simply unmet expectations. Regardless, the key is to pay attention promptly and have a protocol in place to help that patient move from dissatisfaction to neutrality to satisfaction. It may require multiple visits and significant hand holding, but the stakes are high: As with most businesses, a satisfied customer will tell 3 people immediately about their experience, but an unsatisfied customer will tell 10! The goal of every refractive surgeon should be to build a system that strives to prevent unhappy customers and also contains provisions to help the occasional unhappy customer achieve greater levels of satisfaction. Historically, the main reason as to why patients leave a practice has to do with how they were treated by the surgeon and staff,[7] which often has little or nothing to do with the clinical aspects of their care.

Farsighted Patients—Special Considerations

In many respects, the process for handling hyperopic patients is no different from handling myopic patients. The considerations around patient communication and customer service are identical. Differences do emerge, however, when one considers that the results to date for hyperopia have been inferior to those achieved for myopic patients of similar levels of refractive error. This gap in outcomes is being lessened through the use of eye trackers to assist with the longer procedure time in hyperopic treatment as well as improved software to help combat regression of effect. However, the results are simply not to the level achieved in myopia, and this impacts the expectations that are given to prospective hyperopic LASIK patients.

On one hand, presbyopic hyperopes are (or should be) grateful for anything that can help them see without glasses. The loss of accommodation serves to make near, mid-range, and distance vision virtually impossible without the help of corrective lenses. Their myopic counterparts typically enjoy at least decent near vision when they remove their corrective lenses. Thus, refractive surgery should be highly valued by the hyperope. On the other hand, the level of penetration of refractive surgery with hyperopic patients is much lower than that for myopic patients. Hyperopes represent at least one-third of the candidates but less than 10% of procedures being done. This level is similar to that experienced by most contact lens dispensers, where only 10% to 15% of the lenses sold are to hyperopic patients.[4]

While attempting to separate cause from effect in understanding why the penetration rate is lower among hyperopes, the need arises to develop a better understanding of the functional vision needs for this group. More survey and research data need to occur to understand when the hyperopic patient's vision begins to "go bad" (from the patient's perspective, often not until the early 40's). And then deeper understanding needs to go into how it affects everyday tasks. Some hyperopes seem to get along quite well with a blur for distance and help for their near vision only. Others are debilitated for all tasks, even requiring correction in order to apply makeup in a mirror less than 1 meter away.

For the time being, patient counseling should include a thorough discussion of daily functional tasks and which ones are most affected. Reasonable expectations should be given that are different from those applied to myopic patients.

Summary

Ten recommendations for more effective refractive marketing:

1. Be willing to commit the time and energy to build and maintain a refractive component to your practice.
2. Hire and train the best telephone-skilled communicator you can find to field calls from inquiring patients.
3. Generate patients and referrals from current patients and those of your referring doctors before ever attempting to pay for outside advertising.
4. Surgeon and staff should all have the procedure if they are candidates.
5. Set a price and be willing to provide value that exceeds your price.
6. Do not discount.
7. Make refractive surgery part of every discussion with every patient and not just reserved for those who show interest.
8. Offer patient financing to all interested patients, not just those who ask.
9. Consistently recognize and thank patients and others who refer new patients.
10. Be patient and have a long-term approach to the business.

References

1. MacMaster, Linda. *Consumer Research Findings Among Candidates Considering Laser Vision Correction.* Presentation at VISX University Boston, April 1997.
2. http://www.lasikprk.com/VisionPlaceIII/bb/safety_data.htm
3. David Harmon. Trends in Refractive Surgery. ASCRS Philadelphia, June 2002
4. Field experience of the author.

INDEX